theclinics.com

CLINICS IN PODIATRIC MEDICINE AND SURGERY

Advances in the Treatment of the Diabetic Foot

GUEST EDITOR
Thomas Zgonis, DPM

CONSULTING EDITOR
Vincent J. Mandracchia, DPM, MSHCA

July 2007 • Volume 24 • Number 3

SAUNDERS

An Imprint of Elsevier, Inc.
PHILADELPHIA LONDON TORONTO MONTREAL SYDNEY TOKYO

W.B. SAUNDERS COMPANY
A Division of Elsevier Inc.

1600 John F. Kennedy Blvd., Suite 1800, Philadelphia, PA 19103-2899

http://www.theclinics.com

CLINICS IN PODIATRIC MEDICINE AND SURGERY
July 2007
Editor: Patrick Manley

Volume 24, Number 3
ISSN 0891-8422
ISBN-13: 978-1-4160-5054-4
ISBN-10: 1-4160-5054-X

Reprints. For copies of 100 or more of articles in this publication, please contact the Commercial Reprints Department, Elsevier Inc., 360 Park Avenue South, New York, New York 10010-1710 Tel.: (212) 633-3813, Fax: (212) 462-1935, e-mail: reprints@elsevier.com

Clinics in Podiatric Medicine and Surgery (ISSN 0891-8422) is published quarterly by Elsevier Inc., 360 Park Avenue South, New York, NY 10010-1710. Months of publication are January, April, July, and October. Business and Editorial Offices: 1600 John F. Kennedy Blvd., Suite 1800, Philadelphia, PA 191023-2899. Customer Service Office: 6277 Sea Harbor Drive, Orlando, FL 32887-4800. Periodicals postage paid at New York, NY, and additional mailing offices. Subscription prices are $189.00 per year for US individuals, $297.00 per year for US institutions, $97.00 per year for US students and residents, $227.00 per year for Canadian individuals, $360.00 for Canadian institutions, $254.00 for international individuals, $360.00 per year for international institutions and $130.00 per year for Canadian and foreign students/residents. To receive student/resident rate, orders must be accompanied by name of affiliated institution, date of term, and the *signature* of program/residency coordinator on institution letterhead. Orders will be billed at individual rate until proof of status is received. Foreign air speed delivery is included in all *Clinics* subscription prices. All prices are subject to change without notice. POSTMASTER: Send address changes to *Clinics in Podiatric Medicine and Surgery*, Elsevier Periodicals Customer Service, 6277 Sea Harbor Drive, Orlando, FL 32887-4800. **Customer Service: 1-800-654-2452 (US). From outside of the US, call 1-407-345-1000.**

Clinics in Podiatric Medicine and Surgery is covered in *Index Medicus and EMBASE/Excerpta Medica.*

Printed in the United States of America.

CONSULTING EDITOR

VINCENT J. MANDRACCHIA, DPM, MSHCA, Chief Medical Officer; Staff Podiatrist, Section of Podiatric Surgery, Department of Surgery, Broadlawns Medical Center; Clinical Professor, Department of Podiatric Medicine and Surgery, College of Podiatric Medicine and Surgery, Des Moines University–Osteopathic Medicine Center, Des Moines, Iowa

GUEST EDITOR

THOMAS ZGONIS, DPM, FACFAS, Assistant Professor; Director, Externship and Reconstructive Foot and Ankle Fellowship Training Programs, Department of Orthopaedics/Podiatry Division, University of Texas Health Science Center at San Antonio, San Antonio, Texas

CONTRIBUTORS

ERNST CHANTELAU, MD, PhD, Professor of Medicine, Diabetes Foot Clinic; Department of Endocrinology, Diabetes and Rheumatology, Heinrich-Heine-University Düsseldorf, Düsseldorf, Germany

SAMIR CHHAYA, MD, Assistant Professor of Radiology, Department of Radiology, University of Texas Health Science Center, San Antonio, Texas

A. LEE DELLON, MD, PhD, Professor of Plastic Surgery and Neurosurgery, Johns Hopkins University; Director, Dellon Institutes for Peripheral Nerve Surgery, Baltimore, Maryland; Professor of Plastic Surgery, Neurosurgery, and Anatomy, University of Arizona, Tucson, Arizona

RAIMUND FIEDLER, MD, Department of Technical Orthopaedics, Münster University Hospital, Münster, Germany

ROBERT G. FRYKBERG, DPM, MPH, Adjunct Professor, Midwestern University, Glendale, Arizona; Chief, Podiatry Department, Carl T. Hayden Veterans Affairs Medical Center, Phoenix, Arizona

GLENN GARCIA, MD, Assistant Professor of Radiology and Associate Director of Radiology Residency Program, Department of Radiology, University of Texas Health Science Center, San Antonio, Texas

GIOVANNI GHIRLANDA, MD, Professor of Medicine, Università Cattolica del Sacro Cuore, Roma, Italy; and Director, Diabetes Clinic, Policlinico A. Gemelli, Roma, Italy

RYAN T. HAGINO, MD, FACS, Associate Professor of Surgery, Division of Vascular and Endovascular Surgery, University of Texas Health Science Center at San Antonio, San Antonio, Texas

MATT HEILALA, DPM, Foot and Ankle Institute, Austin, Texas; Private Practice, Anchorage, Alaska

WARREN S. JOSEPH, DPM, FIDSA, Attending Podiatrist, Veterans Affairs Medical Center, Coatesville, Pennsylvania

PAUL J. KIM, DPM, Foot and Ankle Institute, Austin, Texas; Assistant Professor, Arizona Podiatric Medicine Program, Midwestern University Division of Dentistry and Medicine, Glendale, Arizona

RENATE KIMMERLE, MD, PhD, Board Qualified Specialist in Endocrinology and Diabetology, Practice of Endocrinology and Diabetes, Düsseldorf, Germany

ARMIN KOLLER, Dr med, MD, Department of Technical Orthopaedics, Münster University Hospital, Münster, Germany

MARK A. KOSINSKI, DPM, Professor, Department of Medicine, New York College of Podiatric Medicine, New York; Instructor, Department of Surgery, New York Medical College, Valhalla, New York

BRADLEY M. LAMM, DPM, AACFAS, Head of the Podiatry Section, Director of Podiatric Residency Program, Rubin Institute for Advanced Orthopedics, International Center for Limb Lengthening, Sinai Hospital of Baltimore, Baltimore, Maryland

RAYMOND LIMET, MD, PhD, Professor, Department of Cardiovascular Surgery, University Hospital Liège, Liège, Belgium

REBECCA A. LOREDO, MD, Associate Professor of Radiology and Chief of Musculoskeletal Division, Department of Radiology, University of Texas Health Science Center, San Antonio, Texas

LORENA MANCINI, MD, Diabetologist, Diabetic Foot Clinic, Policlinico A. Gemelli, Roma, Italy

STEFAN A. MEISSNER, MD, Department of Orthopaedics, Münster University Hospital, Münster, Germany

ALI OZNUR, MD, Department of Orthopaedics and Traumatology, Guven Hospital, Ankara, Turkey

MAIKE PODELLA, MD, Department of Technical Orthopaedics, Münster University Hospital, Münster, Germany

LUDGER W. POLL, MD, PhD, Board Certified Diagnostic Radiologist, Practice of Radiology and Nuclear Medicine, Duisburg, Germany

THOMAS S. ROUKIS, DPM, FACFAS, Chief, Limb Preservation Service; Director, Complex Lower Extremity Surgery; and Research Fellowship, Vascular/Endovascular Surgery Service, Department of Surgery, Madigan Army Medical Center, Tacoma, Washington

JOHN J. STAPLETON, DPM, AACFAS, Clinical Instructor and Fellow, Reconstructive Foot and Ankle Surgery, Department of Orthopaedics/Podiatry Division, University of Texas Health Science Center at San Antonio, San Antonio, Texas

JOHN S. STEINBERG, DPM, Foot and Ankle Institute, Austin, Texas; Assistant Professor, Department of Plastic Surgery, Georgetown University School of Medicine, Center for Wound Healing, Washington, District of Columbia

HENDRIK VAN DAMME, MD, PhD, Department of Cardiovascular Surgery, University Hospital Liège, Liège, Belgium

GLENN M. WEINRAUB, DPM, FACFAS, Foot and Ankle Institute, Austin, Texas; The Permanente Medical Group, Kaiser Permanente, Department of Orthopaedic Surgery, Union City, Hayward, California

BRIAN WITTMAYER, DPM, Surgical Resident, Carl T. Hayden Veterans Affairs Medical Center, Phoenix, Arizona

THOMAS ZGONIS, DPM, FACFAS, Assistant Professor; Director, Externship and Reconstructive Foot and Ankle Fellowship Training Programs, Department of Orthopaedics/Podiatry Division, University of Texas Health Science Center at San Antonio, San Antonio, Texas

CONTENTS

FORTHCOMING ISSUES

October 2007

Adult Acquired Flatfoot
Adam M. Budny, DPM and Jordan P. Grossman, DPM, *Guest Editors*

January 2008

Lower Extremity Radiology
Denise Mandi, DPM, *Guest Editor*

April 2008

The Charcot Foot
Lee C. Rogers, DPM, *Guest Editor*

RECENT ISSUES

April 2007

Medical Management of the Podiatric Patient
Jonathan M. Labovitz, DPM, *Guest Editor*

January 2007

Residency Training
George F. Wallace, DPM, MBA, *Guest Editor*

October 2006

Implants in Foot and Ankle Surgery
Jesse B. Burks, DPM, MS, *Guest Editor*

July 2006

Diagnosis and Treatment of Peripheral Nerve Entrapments and Neuropathy
Babak Baravarian, DPM, *Guest Editor*

ELSEVIER
SAUNDERS

Clin Podiatr Med Surg
24 (2007) xiii–xiv

CLINICS IN PODIATRIC MEDICINE AND SURGERY

Foreword

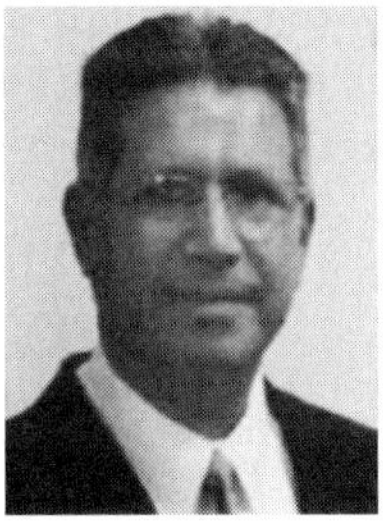

Vincent J. Mandracchia, DPM, MSHCA
Consulting Editor

> To dream too much of the person you would like to be is to waste the person you are.
>
> —Anonymous

Here comes the hardest part: clearly recognizing our positives and negatives, our individual strengths and weaknesses. Looking internally without those annoying "rose-colored glasses" is never easy, and it's awfully convenient to just forget about it and hope that we won't ever have to look at ourselves from a critical point of view. But there comes a time—whether it is thrust upon us as a component of the aging process or as an opportunity to make a significant career move or adjustment—when we understand the need to perform a self-evaluation.

Notice, I said "self-evaluation"—not how we perceive ourselves to be by our peers' standards, but by our own standards. This is not an easy thing to do, especially if we consider ourselves to be what we do for a living and not who we are. Some may argue that they are one in the same; I do not agree. Who we are makes up what we have become. A career is part of our makeup, not the entirety of it. How many times have we seen those individuals who have made their career their whole existence? What is our usual response? "That person needs to get a life." How ironic.

This is a great challenge for each of us from a professional and personal point of view. Marcus Aurelius, emperor of the Roman Empire, said, "We are troubled not by the things of the world but, rather, by our perception of

doi:10.1016/j.cpm.2007.05.001

those things." I am reminded of how we think of ourselves professionally, how we present ourselves to our patients, our peers, and other health professionals. Is the quality of care rendered the most important aspect of our professional lives or whether or not we have umpteen certifications, some of which make no sense? Does being a good test-taker constitute a certifiable knowledge of one's craft? For that matter, is the opposite true? Are we foot and ankle surgeons, podiatrists, foot specialists, biomechanical foot and ankle specialists, and so forth, or does it really matter? And if it does, to whom does it matter most: us (the individual), our colleagues, or our patients? Is it shameful to be a podiatrist, or is it noble to be the best podiatrist possible?

We need to give due diligence to examining our lives from all aspects. Socrates stated that "the unexamined life is not worth living," and William James suggested that the most important discovery in psychology is that by "changing the interior states of our minds, we can change the exterior dimensions of our lives." Our profession is made up of many individuals who bring much enrichment to the practice of podiatry. Yet so many voices and opinions are never heard because of lack of confidence and perceived weakness that is nothing more than peer-labeling and the unfortunate belief that this labeling is accurate. It is essential to remember that beliefs lead to emotions that eventually translate into behaviors, whether or not the beliefs are substantiated. Perception is indeed often interpreted as reality.

I would challenge each and every one of us to look internally and decide what positive contributions can be offered to make things better. Pick a cause that you believe will improve the stagnant systems that some group decided must be in place and that you must abide by, both in your professional and personal life. You are likely to become stronger, more confident, and more self-reliant. Interestingly, not everyone will welcome those traits in you... what a great realization! It takes courage to change yourself and the things around you—but as Ambrose Redmoon said: "Courage is not the absence of fear, but rather the judgment that something else is more important than fear." What is more important to you?

Vincent J. Mandracchia, DPM, MSHCA
Chief Medical Officer
Department of Surgery
Broadlawns Medical Center
1801 Hickman Road
Des Moines, IA 50314, USA

E-mail address: vmandracchia@broadlawns.org

ELSEVIER
SAUNDERS

Clin Podiatr Med Surg
24 (2007) xv–xvi

CLINICS IN
PODIATRIC
MEDICINE AND
SURGERY

Preface

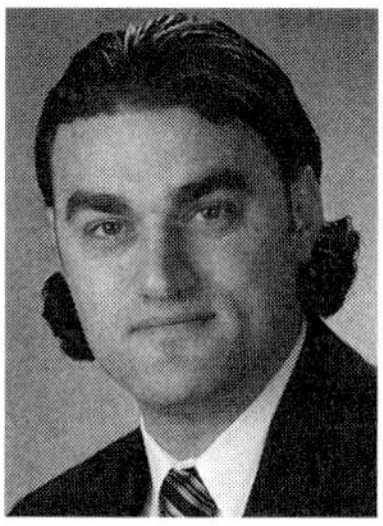

Thomas Zgonis, DPM, FACFAS
Guest Editor

It has been a great pleasure and honor to act as a Guest Editor in this exciting issue of *Clinics in Podiatric Medicine and Surgery* focusing on advances in the treatment of the diabetic foot. Diabetes has become an epidemic within the United States and around the world. One of the most common reasons for hospitalization in patients with diabetes is related to a foot condition. The multidisciplinary team approach for the prevention and treatment of diabetes-related pathologies is a well-accepted concept around the world.

In this issue, I have selected a world-renowned faculty to share their opinions and expertise on the medical and surgical treatment of the diabetic foot. Internists, endocrinologists, infectious disease specialists, cardiovascular surgeons, vascular surgeons, neurosurgeons, and foot and ankle surgeons from Europe and United States are just few of the invited authors contributing to this issue on the management of the diabetic foot.

I would like to thank the consulting editor, Dr Vincent J Mandracchia, for allowing me to moderate this great international issue, as well as my wife, Kristen, and our new addition to the family, Labrini Sophia, for their understanding and support throughout this intensive work and personal commitment.

0891-8422/07/$ - see front matter
doi:10.1016/j.cpm.2007.04.002

I hope you find this issue exciting and enjoy the different opinions, theories and surgical approaches to the treatment of the diabetic foot. I certainly appreciate and am thankful to the invited authors for their generous contributions.

Thomas Zgonis, DPM, FACFAS
Department of Orthopaedics/Podiatry Division
The University of Texas Health Science Center at San Antonio
7703 Floyd Curl Drive, MSC 7776
San Antonio, TX 78229, USA

E-mail address: zgonis@uthscsa.edu

ELSEVIER
SAUNDERS

Clin Podiatr Med Surg
24 (2007) 365–382

CLINICS IN
PODIATRIC
MEDICINE AND
SURGERY

Current Perioperative Treatment of Patients with Type 1 and Type 2 Diabetes

Giovanni Ghirlanda, MD[a,b,*], Lorena Mancini, MD[c]

[a] *Università Cattolica del Sacro Cuore, Roma, Italy*
[b] *Diabetes Clinic, Policlinico A. Gemelli, Roma, Italy*
[c] *Diabetic Foot Clinic, Policlinico A. Gemelli, Roma Italy*

Diabetes mellitus is the most common metabolic disease, and its incidence is rapidly increasing in epidemic proportions all over the world owing to the aging of the general population, reduced physical activity, and an excess of caloric intake [1,2]. Diabetes mellitus predisposes to clinical conditions that require surgery (Table 1) on the other hand diabetic patients share the same surgical risk as the general population, as a result they have an increased risk of surgical interventions [3–5]. Diabetes-related hospital stays are longer and are associated with a greater mortality and morbidity rate, with a huge burden on health care costs [6–9]. A team approach is highly desirable in the evaluation of the diabetic patient undergoing surgical intervention because of the complexity and severity of this disease. A perioperative management plan should be agreed on by the diabetologist, the surgeon, and the anesthesiologist and should take into account parameters such as the type of diabetes, the quality of previous and current metabolic control, the current pharmacologic treatment, the type of intervention, and the postoperative course foreseen. Perioperative management protocols have been developed and implemented, leading to a better outcome without any cost increase [10–17]. This article reviews the following issues: the classification of diabetes, the pathophysiology of glucose metabolism during surgical stress, the evaluation of operative risk, and the perioperative management of blood glucose and metabolic control.

Drs. Ghirlanda and Mancini have no disclosures to declare.

* Corresponding author. Servizio di Diabetologia, Largo A. Gemelli 8, 00168 Roma, Italy.

E-mail address: gghirlanda@rm.unicatt.it (G. Ghirlanda).

doi:10.1016/j.cpm.2007.03.005

Table 1
Diabetes complications and related surgery

Complication	Intervention
Cataract	Cataract surgery
Diabetic retinopathy	
Hemorrhage	Vitrectomy
Retinal detachment	Scleral buckling
Macroangiopathy	
Neuropathic foot ulcer	Debridement
Ischemic gangrene	Amputation Revascularization
Brain ischemia	Carotid artery surgery
Nephropathy	
End-stage renal disease	Peritoneal dialysis Arteriovenous fistula Kidney graft
Autonomic neuropathy	
Gastroparesis	Gastrostomy
Erectile dysfunction	Penile implant
Ischemic heart disease	
Angina, myocardial infarction	Cardiac bypass graft surgery Balloon angioplasty
Infectious disease susceptibility	
Gangrenous cholecystitis	Cholecystectomy
Peritonitis	Laparotomy
Foot osteomyelitis	Amputation
Necrotizing soft tissue infection	Fasciectomy

Diabetes classification and pathophysiology

Most diabetic patients are classified into two main categories [18–21]: (1) those with type 1 diabetes, which is caused by an absolute lack of insulin secretion [22], and (2) those with type 2 diabetes, which is characterized by the presence of insulin resistance and inadequate insulin secretion [23]. Type 1 diabetes is caused by autoimmune destruction of insulin-secreting pancreatic β cells and requires intensive insulin treatment, usually administered through a multiple-injection regimen or, in selected patients, delivered by an insulin pump. Blood glucose must be strictly monitored in type 1 diabetic patients because they tend to be metabolically unstable and to have broad glycemic fluctuations that can easily lead to a catabolic state with enhanced lipolysis and proteolysis resulting in ketoacidosis [22]. Insulin resistance, which is a feature of type 2 diabetes [24,25], often characterizes other clinical conditions of enhanced cardiovascular risk. Many type 2 diabetic patients also have intra-abdominal (visceral) obesity, hypertension, atherogenic dyslipidemia (high triglycerides and low levels of high-density lipoprotein cholesterol), and elevated PAI-1 levels [26–30]. The clustering of these abnormalities, which is referred to as the "metabolic syndrome," explains why patients with type 2 diabetes are at increased risk for macrovascular complications such as myocardial infarction, peripheral arterial disease, and stroke [31,32]. In many patients, diabetes remains undiagnosed for a long period of time; therefore, they show significant target organ damage when the disease is recognized [33]. Different regimens may be used in the treatment of type 2 diabetes combining diet, several classes of oral hypoglycemic agents, and insulin [23].

The metabolic response to surgical stress and anesthesia

Surgery is a compendium of diabetogenic stimuli [34]. Anxiety over the forthcoming intervention, a fasting state, anesthesia, surgical maneuvers, and any other stress elicit a complex neuroendocrine response leading to inhibition of insulin action and secretion [35–38] and to stimulation of counterregulatory hormones such as glucagon [39,40], catecholamines [41,42], cortisol [43–45], and growth hormone [46,47]. Although this hormonal imbalance is overcome in normal subjects by increased insulin secretion, in diabetic patients it results in enhanced insulin resistance that induces a reduction in peripheral glucose uptake, an increase in hepatic glucose production, and fat and protein breakdown. As a consequence, there is a risk for diabetic ketoacidosis in type 1 diabetes and for hyperglycemic hyperosmolar states in type 2 diabetes. These complications are also promoted by surgery-induced fluid losses, dehydration, fluid underreplacement, prolonged bed rest, and hypothermia that are common in the perioperative period [48–51]. It is easy to argue that insulin therapy is required in the majority of diabetic patients undergoing surgery.

Spinal, epidural, and other regional anesthesia techniques block most stress-induced metabolic and hormonal responses [51–59]. High doses of opioids may also inhibit this response, and a clear-cut advantage among these techniques is not yet evident. Patients treated with neural blockade resume oral feeding earlier than after general anesthesia and have a lesser disruption of their usual life; conversely, the risk of local infections and vascular damage is more likely with regional techniques. General anesthesia is associated with more hemodynamic stability in patients with autonomic neuropathy and prepares them better for possible complications [60,61]. The choice of the type of anesthesia depends more on a careful evaluation of the clinical status of the patient than on the superiority of one technique in comparison with another.

Preoperative evaluation

The mainstay of preoperative assessment is a thorough medical history and physical examination [15–17]. It is necessary to ascertain the type of diabetes, the details of the pharmacologic regimen, the timing of meals and medications, and the ability of the patient to deal with the disease and to manage potential problems such as hypoglycemia. A specific assessment of the symptoms related to chronic microvascular, macrovascular, and neurologic complications must be performed. All chronic complications correlate with the duration of the disease; therefore, evidence of one complication must prompt the physician to search for the others. Patients with an ischemic or a neuropathic foot often have cardiac or cerebrovascular atherosclerosis as well as visceral neuropathy (ie, lung, stomach, urinary bladder). All of these findings have important implications for anesthesia. The aim of these inquiries is the formulation of a thorough intraoperative and postoperative management plan [62]. Some aspects are so peculiar, frequent, and severe that they are treated separately.

Cardiovascular system

The excess mortality of diabetic patients is almost entirely due to cardiovascular diseases [63]. Global cardiovascular risk in diabetic men is four times greater than in their non-diabetic counterparts, and in diabetic women the difference is even more pronounced [64–67]. Diabetic patients without a history of coronary heart disease have the same cardiovascular mortality as non-diabetic patients who sustain a cardiac attack; therefore, diabetes is considered an equivalent of coronary heart disease [68–70].

Coronary atherosclerosis is more precocious, more extensive, and more severe in diabetic patients, although typical symptoms may be absent, particularly in women [71,72]. Silent ischemia is common in diabetes and is related to autonomic neuropathy and sympathetic and vagal cardiac denervation [73–75]. These patients often have tachycardia at rest, orthostatic hypotension, and a decrease of R-R variations during the Valsalva maneuver and must be regarded to be at high risk for silent ischemia and cardiorespiratory complications during anesthesia [76–78]. The threshold for suspicion of coronary heart disease must be lower in patients aged more than 60 years, in those with a duration of diabetes longer than 15 years, and in those with a diabetic foot, macroalbuminuria or impaired renal function, or peripheral or autonomic neuropathy [79,80]. In these patients, an exercise electrocardiographic test should be performed. Pharmacologic stress testing with imaging techniques (echocardiography, radionuclide study) should be performed in patients who are unable to exercise, as is common in patients with a diabetic foot [81–87]. A specific cardiomyopathy may occur in diabetic patients without evidence of coronary artery disease. This condition is probably multifactorial. Chronic metabolic imbalance, enhanced apoptosis by oxidative stress, the abnormal presence of glycated structural proteins, and calcium overload of cardiomyocytes are the possible underlying causes [88,89]. The main alteration is an impairment in diastolic filling rather than a decreased left ventricular systolic performance, and the clinical presentation is a congestive heart failure that may be silent and unmasked by any perioperative stress [90,91].

Kidney and urinary tract

In Western countries, diabetes is the leading cause of end-stage renal disease, and type 1 diabetic patients are one of the major cohorts of candidates for kidney transplantation. Diabetic nephropathy is common after 10 years of type 1 disease and may be present at diagnosis in type 2 diabetes [92–97]. Microalbuminuria is an early marker of nephropathy in type 1 patients, whereas in type 2 patients it is a predictive factor of cardiovascular mortality [98–101]. Urinary tract infections are also common in diabetes owing to the well-known susceptibility to infections and the impairment in bladder emptying in the presence of autonomic neuropathy [102,103]. Renal failure is the most frequent major complication in diabetic patients undergoing general and cardiac surgery, affects about 7% of patients, and causes longer hospital stays with increased morbidity and mortality [104]. Proteinuria, an increased serum creatinine level, advanced age, anemia, and a positive cardiovascular history are risk factors for perioperative renal dysfunction. A complete urinalysis to rule out infections and to assess proteinuria, serum creatinine, and electrolyte levels is mandatory before surgery. Renal hypoperfusion must be avoided through appropriate volume replacement, always watching for latent heart failure. Problems seen after contrast-based radiologic procedures that are common in patients with an ischemic foot are now less frequent with the use of isotonic non-ionic dyes. With careful hydration and the prophylactic use of *N*-acetyl cysteine, this complication is now rare [105–108].

Respiratory system

Lung function is impaired in diabetes, and clinical infections are more frequent in diabetic patients, although a direct correlation with metabolic control is not clearly demonstrated [109–111]. In type 1 diabetes, respiratory function tests may show a progressive impairment that correlates with autonomic neuropathy, but the clinical relevance of this finding needs to be ascertained [112,113]. Obesity that often is associated with diabetes also impairs lung function; therefore, an early mobilization and the use of mucolytic aerosol are useful to minimize the infectious risk.

Diabetic joint stiffness

Diabetes mellitus is associated with abnormalities in the skin and periarticular tissues, resulting in affections that limit joint movement. Typical diabetes-associated conditions include palmar flexor tenosynovitis, Dupuytren disease, carpal tunnel syndrome, Charcot arthropathy, and shoulder-hand reflex dystrophy [114–117]. In all of these conditions, advanced glycation end products are thought to form from nonenzymatic glycation of collagen proteins, resulting in the presence of pathologic connective tissue that, together neuropathy and microangiopathy, leads to the limitation of joint mobility [118]. When the atlanto-occipital joint is involved and the extension of the occiput on the cervical spine is impaired, endotracheal intubation may be difficult or even impossible. A positive prayer sign (the patient's inability to press the hands together to achieve a complete overlapping of palms and fingers) is highly correlated to the cervical spine involvement and may be a marker of difficult intubation. This condition is underdiagnosed and usually is not ruled out in the routine evaluation of diabetic patients before anesthesia; however, its prevalence is as high as 20% to 30%, especially in type 1 diabetes, and difficulties in performing laryngoscopy and intubation are reported to be tenfold more common in diabetic patients when compared with non-diabetic patients [119–121].

In patients with diabetic neuroarthropathy such as Charcot's foot, stiffness of joints is frequent, and the patient during surgery must be carefully positioned in the operatory bed to avoid musculoskeletal or neurovascular injuries.

Gastrointestinal system

Visceral neuropathy leads to vagal denervation with delayed gastric emptING, reduced peristalsis, and antroduodenal incoordination up to gastric paresis, and esophageal reflux with an increased risk of vomiting and aspiration of gastric contents [122,123]. Considerations in such patients should include a prolonged presurgery fasting time, the use of an aspiration tube, and the inhibition of acid secretion. Optimal fluid and electrolyte balance is mandatory to favor the gastrointestinal motility. Prokinetic drugs are widely used, but their efficacy is not yet fully ascertained [124,125].

Infectious risk

Diabetes increases the risk of morbidity and mortality from infectious diseases, and infections account for most diabetes-related hospital admissions [126–128]. Hyperglycemia impairs polymorphonuclear and macrophage functions such as chemotaxis, phagocytosis, and bactericidal activity [129–133]. The presence of micro- and macroangiopathy and the delayed wound healing further promote infections in diabetic patients. Wound pressure develops quickly, and during bed stays bone prominence must be carefully protected. During hospital admission, patients with an ischemic foot may quickly experience calcaneal wound pressure that may lead to infection and worsen the outcome [134]. Ancillary surgical procedures must be performed with strict aseptic techniques, and antibiotic therapy must be performed using a full dosage regimen with bactericidal agents.

Perioperative treatment of diabetes mellitus

Diabetic patients scheduled for elective surgery should be prepared in an outpatient setting through a strict collaboration among the physicians concerned, that is, the diabetologist, surgeon, and anesthesiologist [7,14,135]. The preparatory plan must consider the type and duration of diabetes, the potential complications, the actual treatment, the surgical procedure scheduled, the type of anesthesia chosen, and the time necessary before the patient can resume his or her habitual diabetes regimen. It is also important to ascertain the degree of compliance of the patient, his or her ability to face diabetes-related problems, and the presence of hypoglycemia unawareness. Patients must be hospitalized in good metabolic control and with their nutritional status optimized. Hyperglycemia is detrimental for diabetic and non-diabetic patients, whereas tight glycemic control improves clinical outcomes [8,136–146].

Continuous intravenous insulin infusion is considered the best way to control blood glucose during surgery because it ensures an effective tissue delivery of the hormone and a simple and rapid titration owing to the short half-life of the intravenous insulin. Although many protocols have been advocated for the management of diabetic patients during surgery and in critical care units, there is no consensus on the best way to achieve optimal results in terms of glycemic control without important side effects [147–152]. Each hospital must choose its own strategy to train a multidisciplinary team devoted to the improvement of treatment of diabetic patients.

Recently, data about a protocol that has been implemented with good results at multiple institutions have been published [153]. Although there is no general agreement about the glycemic goals during surgery, the American Association of Clinical Endocrinologists and the American Diabetes Association have recently recommended in a hospital setting a range between 80 and 110 mg/dL for patients admitted in intensive care units and a random blood glucose level less than 180 mg/dL with a mean glycemia around 110 mg/dL in non–critically ill patients [154]. Some concerns have been raised about these recommendations. They are not evidence based because the data are derived mainly from the study of patients in a single intensive care unit and not from controlled protocols [155]. Moreover, a recent article has been published that questions such tight control [156]. Very tight blood glucose control is associated with an increased risk of hypoglycemia, the symptoms of which are often masked in patients hospitalized for different illnesses or even anesthetized [157]. Although surgical patients are not prone to hypoglycemia due to increased insulin resistance during a hospital stay, the harmful effects of hypoglycemia, especially in cardiac patients, cannot be underestimated [158,159]. It is difficult to overcome all of the problems connected to the achievement of an optimal glycemic target without increasing the risk of hypoglycemia. Currently, a mean blood glucose level of 130 mg/dL with daily fluctuations in the range of 100 to 160 mg/dL is a good target for all hospitalized patients. In patients undergoing cardiac surgery, a more strict control of glycemia is strongly advised.

Patients scheduled for elective surgery must be operated on in the best possible conditions so that interventions can be postponed if the patient's metabolic control is not optimal [160–162]. Patients with non-optimal metabolic control should be admitted almost the day before surgery and treated with insulin to normalize blood glucose. In general, surgery must be scheduled early in the morning to avoid a protracted fasting and to allow a longer surveillance period.

A surgical intervention is defined as minor if the patient can resume oral food intake about 6 hours after operation. Surgery is defined as a major intervention when oral food intake cannot be resumed until 6 hours after operation or when protracted general anesthesia (ie, longer than 1 hour) is required.

Minor surgery

Type 2 diabetic patients treated with diet or oral hypoglycemic agents

Metformin should be discontinued 48 hours before surgery and resumed after the assessment of renal function [163–167]. Oral hypoglycemic agents should not be administered on the morning of intervention, and blood glucose should be checked before intervention and then every 1 to 2 hours until the patient resumes oral food intake and their usual drug regimen; as a rule, no additional treatment is necessary. If unexpected hyperglycemia occurs, single doses of regular insulin or a short-acting analogue should be administered.

Type 2 diabetic patients treated with insulin or type 1 diabetic patients

Long-acting insulin should be discontinued. On the evening before intervention, intermediate insulin can be administered although in reduced doses because the patient is in a semifasting state in view of the forthcoming operation. The experience with the new peakless insulin glargine as basal insulin is favorable; the day before the intervention, it can be injected at usual doses in patients undergoing minor surgery. Blood glucose should be checked at the beginning and then every hour throughout the intervention. Usual treatment should be restarted when oral food intake is resumed. Marked glycemic fluctuations should be avoided in these patients. If they occur, the following measures can be taken: either single doses of regular insulin or a short-acting analogue injected subcutaneously, or a short-lasting intravenous insulin infusion.

Major surgery

Patients undergoing major surgery must be treated with an intensive regimen of intravenous infusion of insulin, glucose, and potassium. Many protocols of insulin infusion have been published in recent years. These protocols use infusion algorithms that can be tailored to individual patients considering their clinical state and response to insulin infusion [14,15,142,148,151–153]. A simple protocol is the GIK regimen (insulin, glucose, potassium), in which insulin may be infused in the same bag with glucose and potassium or given separately by an infusion pump. The GIK regimen starts with an intravenous infusion of 500 mL of 5% glucose added with 8 units of regular insulin and 20 mEq of KCl at a rate of about 100 mL/h. If a reduction in the total amount of administered fluids is desirable, 10% glucose solutions with 16 units of insulin can be used. Adjustments of insulin concentration are made according to the values of blood glucose obtained hourly by portable devices. If the blood glucose is higher than desired, 5 units of insulin are added; if hypoglycemia occurs, it is enough to stop the infusion (Table 2). A bolus of 5 units of regular insulin may be injected at the beginning of infusion if the blood glucose is more than 200 mg/dL. This regimen is safe, simple, and effective, but it is necessary to change the whole infusion set if the patient experiences hyperglycemia and needs higher dosages of insulin. This change be prevented by administering glucose and potassium separately through one intravenous line and insulin, preferably with a pump, through another.

An infusion rate of 1 U/h is appropriate for the great majority of patients. The starting solution is prepared by adding regular insulin to normal saline (eg, 25 units of regular insulin in 250 mL of normal saline) at an infusion rate of 10 mL/h; glucose infusion is kept constant at 5 to 10 g/h. If blood glucose levels rise, the rate of insulin infusion can be increased by 0.5 U/h. A close watch on the two infusion lines is recommended so that they will not clog and their flow will not be altered by other infusion lines. The infusion of glucose and insulin must be continued to prevent an excessive catabolism until normal food intake is resumed. The mean amount of glucose required is about 120 g/day at a rate of 5 to 10 g/h. This amount is best achieved giving a 10% dextrose solution at 100 mL/h. This dosage of insulin applies to patients with normal insulin sensitivity, which varies considerably from one patient to another.

Table 2
Protocol for combined glucose, insulin, potassium infusion

Blood glucose (mg/dL)	Glucose, insulin, potassium infusion	
120–180	500 mL of 5% dextrose, 8 U insulin, 20 mEq KCl. Infusion rate 100 mL/h	500 mL 10% dextrose, 16 U insulin, 20 mEq KCl. Infusion rate 50 mL/h
181–280	Add insulin, 4 U	Add insulin, 8 U
>281	Add insulin, 8 U	Add insulin, 16 U

Higher dosages are necessary in conditions such as infections, hepatic disorders, obesity, neoplasms, and systemic illnesses.

Preoperative insulin requirements can be indicative of the amount of insulin needed during intraoperative infusion. Insulin requirements are ten times higher during extracorporeal circulation because of hypothermia and the aspecific binding of insulin to the surface and tubing of the apparatus used for extracorporeal circulation. Neurosurgery also markedly increases insulin requirements.

Emergency surgery

Usually, patients requiring emergency surgery are in bad metabolic control, and a careful balance between the urgency of the operation and the necessity to improve their metabolic status must be performed [167,168]. In these patients, a thorough medical history and physical examination must be performed to exclude possible diagnostic pitfalls, mainly if abdominal surgery is scheduled. Patients with diabetic ketoacidosis may have abdominal symptoms and even leukocytosis to stimulate a true surgical emergency [169,170]. Diabetic autonomic neuropathy of the gastrointestinal tract may cause gastroparesis, abdominal pain, intractable vomiting, and paralytic ileus that prompt the surgeon to operate. Patients with a diabetic foot infection, ulceration, or osteomyelitis may have emergency surgery for lower limb amputation or for the debridement of extensive infectious cellulitis or necrotizing fasciitis. Infection is always present in these cases and must be intensively treated [171–173]. When necessary, appropriate surgery must not be unduly postponed. A rapid correction of hydration and of electrolyte unbalance is mandatory, possibly through a central vein access. Continuous insulin infusion must be started immediately together glucose and electrolytes, with glucose monitored every hour and potassium every 2 to 4 hours and also postoperatively because late life-threatening hypokalemia is possible.

Back to home

Hospital admission should be reverted into a positive experience giving the opportunity to review with the patient all aspects of the treatment of his or her diabetes. A contact with a diabetes clinic must be guaranteed, especially if the drug regimen has been changed during the hospitalization. The importance of diet, a proactive self-management of the diabetes, and the implementation of physical activity must be presented as the cornerstones of the patient's future lifestyle.

References

[1] Wild S, Roglic G, Green A, et al. Global prevalence of diabetes: estimates for the year 2000 and projections for 2030. Diabetes Care 2004;27(5):1047–53.

[2] Yach D, Stuckler D, Brownell KD. Epidemiologic and economic consequences of the global epidemics of obesity and diabetes. Nat Med 2006;12(1):62–6.
[3] Goldman DR. Surgery in patients with endocrine dysfunction. Med Clin North Am 1987; 71:499–509.
[4] Rossini AA, Hare JW. How to control the blood glucose level in the surgical diabetic patient. Arch Surg 1976;111:945–50.
[5] Alberti KGMM, Thomas DJB. The management of diabetes during surgery. Br J Anaesth 1979;51:693–710.
[6] Risum O, Abdelnoor M, Svennevig JL, et al. Risk factors of recurrent angina pectoris and of non-fatal myocardial infarction after coronary artery bypass surgery. Eur J Cardiothorac Surg 1996;10(3):173–8.
[7] Jacober SJ, Sowers JR. An update on perioperative management of diabetes. Arch Intern Med 1999;159(20):2405–11.
[8] Umpierrez GE, Isaacs SD, Bazargan N, et al. Hyperglycemia: an independent marker of in-hospital mortality in patients with undiagnosed diabetes. J Clin Endocrinol Metab 2002;87(3):978–82.
[9] Rehman HU, Mohammed K. Perioperative management of diabetic patients. Curr Surg 2003;60(6):607–11.
[10] Levetan CS, Salas JR, Wilets IF, et al. Impact of endocrine and diabetes team consultation on hospital length of stay for patients with diabetes. Am J Med 1995;99(1): 22–8.
[11] Courtney L, Gordon M, Romer L. A clinical path for adult diabetes. Diabetes Educ 1997; 23(6):664–71.
[12] Larme AC, Pugh JA. Evidence-based guidelines meet the real world: the case of diabetes care. Diabetes Care 2001;24(10):1728–33.
[13] Markovitz LJ, Wiechmann RJ, Harris N, et al. Description and evaluation of a glycemic management protocol for patients with diabetes undergoing heart surgery. Endocr Pract 2002;8(1):10–8.
[14] Vora AC, Saleem TM, Polomano RC, et al. Improved perioperative glycemic control by continuous insulin infusion under supervision of an endocrinologist does not increase costs in patients with diabetes. Endocr Pract 2004;10(2):112–8.
[15] Smiley DD, Umpierrez GE. Perioperative glucose control in the diabetic or nondiabetic patient. South Med J 2006;99(6):580–9.
[16] Coursin DB, Connery LE, Ketzler JT. Perioperative diabetic and hyperglycemic management issues. Crit Care Med 2004;32(4 Suppl):S116–25.
[17] Scherpereel PA, Tavernier B. Perioperative care of diabetic patients. Eur J Anaesthesiol 2001;18(5):277–94.
[18] The Expert Committee on the Diagnosis and Classification of Diabetes Mellitus. Report of the Expert Committee on the Diagnosis and Classification of Diabetes Mellitus. Diabetes Care 1997;20:1183–97.
[19] The Expert Committee on the Diagnosis and Classification of Diabetes Mellitus. Follow-up report on the diagnosis of diabetes mellitus. Diabetes Care 2003;26:3160–7.
[20] American Diabetes Association position statement. Diagnosis and classification of diabetes mellitus. Diabetes Care 2007;30:S42–7.
[21] Wolfsdorf J, Glaser N, Sperling MA. American Diabetes Association. Diabetic ketoacidosis in infants, children, and adolescents: a consensus statement from the American Diabetes Association. Diabetes Care 2006;29(5):1150–9.
[22] Haller MJ, Atkinson MA, Schatz D. Type 1 diabetes mellitus: etiology, presentation, and management. Pediatr Clin North Am 2005;52(6):1553–78.
[23] Stumvoll M, Goldstein BJ, van Haeften TW. Type 2 diabetes: principles of pathogenesis and therapy. Lancet 2005;365(9467):1333–46.
[24] Lowell BB, Shulman GI. Mitochondrial dysfunction and type 2 diabetes. Science 2005; 307(5708):384–7.

[25] Bonora E, Formentini G, Calcaterra F, et al. HOMA-estimated insulin resistance is an independent predictor of cardiovascular disease in type 2 diabetic subjects: prospective data from the Verona Diabetes Complications Study. Diabetes Care 2002;25(7):1135–41.
[26] Kahn BB, Flier JS. Obesity and insulin resistance. J Clin Invest 2000;106(4):473–81.
[27] Mokdad AH, Ford ES, Bowman BA, et al. Prevalence of obesity, diabetes, and obesity-related health risk factors, 2001. JAMA 2003;289(1):76–9.
[28] Koh-Banerjee P, Wang Y, Hu FB, et al. Changes in body weight and body fat distribution as risk factors for clinical diabetes in US men. Am J Epidemiol 2004;159(12):1150–9.
[29] Sowers JR. Obesity as a cardiovascular risk factor. Am J Med 2003;115(Suppl 8A):37S–41S.
[30] McTigue KM, Garrett JM, Popkin BM. The natural history of the development of obesity in a cohort of young US adults between 1981 and 1998. Ann Intern Med 2002;136(12): 857–64.
[31] Cameron AJ, Shaw JE, Zimmet PZ. The metabolic syndrome: prevalence in worldwide populations. Endocrinol Metab Clin North Am 2004;33(2):351–75.
[32] Giles TD, Sander GE. Pathophysiologic, diagnostic, and therapeutic aspects of the metabolic syndrome. J Clin Hypertens (Greenwich) 2005;7(11):669–78.
[33] Unwin N, Shaw J, Zimmet P, et al. Impaired glucose tolerance and impaired fasting glycaemia: the current status on definition and intervention. Diabet Med 2002;19(9):708–23.
[34] Dagogo-Jack S, Alberti KG. Management of diabetes mellitus in surgical patients. Diabetes Spectrum 2002;15:44–8.
[35] Surwit RS, Schneider MS, Feinglos MN. Stress and diabetes mellitus. Diabetes Care 1992; 15(10):1413–22.
[36] Vranic M, Miles P, Rastogi K, et al. Effect of stress on glucoregulation in physiology and diabetes. Adv Exp Med Biol 1991;291:161–83.
[37] Mizock BA. Alterations in carbohydrate metabolism during stress: a review of the literature. Am J Med 1995;98(1):75–84.
[38] Gibson SC, Hartman DA, Schenck JM. The endocrine response to critical illness: update and implications for emergency medicine. Emerg Med Clin North Am 2005;23(3): 909–29.
[39] Chan TM. The permissive effects of glucocorticoid on hepatic gluconeogenesis: glucagon stimulation of glucose-suppressed gluconeogenesis and inhibition of 6-phosphofructo-1-kinase in hepatocytes from fasted rats. J Biol Chem 1984;259(12):7426–32.
[40] Fanelli CG, Porcellati F, Rossetti P, et al. Glucagon: the effects of its excess and deficiency on insulin action. Nutr Metab Cardiovasc Dis 2006;16(Suppl 1):S28–34.
[41] Halter JB, Beard JC, Porte D Jr. Islet function and stress hyperglycemia: plasma glucose and epinephrine interaction. Am J Physiol 1984;247:E47–52.
[42] Najmaii S, Redford D, Larson DF. Hyperglycemia as an effect of cardiopulmonary bypass: intraoperative glucose management. J Extra Corpor Technol 2006;38(2):168–73.
[43] Madsen SN, Engguist A, Badawi I, et al. Cyclic AMP, glucose and cortisol in plasma during surgery. Horm Metab Res 1976;8(6):483–5.
[44] McMahon M, Gerich J, Rizza R. Effects of glucocorticoids on carbohydrate metabolism. Diabetes Metab Rev 1988;4(1):17–30.
[45] Clarke RS, Bali IM, Issac M, et al. Plasma cortisol and blood sugar following minor surgery under intravenous anaesthetics. Anaesthesia 1974;29(5):545–50.
[46] Press M. Growth hormone and metabolism. Diabetes Metab Rev 1988;4(4):391–414.
[47] Dunger D, Yuen K, Salgin B. Growth hormone effects on glucose metabolism. Horm Res 2007;67(Suppl 1):37–42.
[48] Shangraw RE, Stuart CA, Prince MJ, et al. Insulin responsiveness of protein metabolism in vivo following bedrest in humans. Am J Physiol 1988;255:E548–58.
[49] Stuart CA, Shangraw RE, Prince MJ, et al. Bed rest–induced insulin resistance occurs primarily in muscle. Metabolism 1988;37(8):802–6.
[50] Nygren J, Thorell A, Efendic S, et al. Site of insulin resistance after surgery: the contribution of hypocaloric nutrition and bed rest. Clin Sci (Lond) 1997;93(2):137–46.

[51] Engquist A, Brandt MR, Fernandes A, et al. The blocking effect of epidural analgesia on the adrenocortical and hyperglycemic responses to surgery. Acta Anaesthesiol Scand 1977;21(4):330–5.

[52] Kehlet H, Brandt MR, Hansen AP, et al. Effect of epidural analgesia on metabolic profiles during and after surgery. Br J Surg 1979;66(8):543–6.

[53] Halter JB, Pflug AE. Effect of sympathetic blockade by spinal anesthesia on pancreatic islet function in man. Am J Physiol 1980;239(2):E150–5.

[54] Pflug AE, Halter JB. Effect of spinal anesthesia on adrenergic tone and the neuroendocrine responses to surgical stress in humans. Anesthesiology 1981;55(2):120–6.

[55] Kehlet H. The endocrine responses to regional anesthesia. Int Anesthesiol Clin 1988;26(3): 182–6.

[56] Kehlet H. The modifying effect of anesthetic technique on the metabolic and endocrine responses to anesthesia and surgery. Acta Anaesthesiol Belg 1988;39(3):143–6.

[57] Lattermann R, Schricker T, Wachter U, et al. Understanding the mechanisms by which isoflurane modifies the hyperglycemic response to surgery. Anesth Analg 2001;93(1): 121–7.

[58] Schricker T, Lattermann R, Fiset P, et al. Integrated analysis of protein and glucose metabolism during surgery: effects of anesthesia. J Appl Physiol 2001;91(6):2523–30.

[59] Karci A, Tasdogen A, Erkin Y, et al. The analgesic effect of morphine on postoperative pain in diabetic patients. Acta Anaesthesiol Scand 2004;48(5):619–24.

[60] Latson TW, Ashmore TH, Reinhart DJ, et al. Autonomic reflex dysfunction in patients presenting for elective surgery is associated with hypotension after anesthesia induction. Anesthesiology 1994;80(2):326–37.

[61] Keyl C, Lemberger P, Palitzsch KD, et al. Cardiovascular autonomic dysfunction and hemodynamic response to anesthetic induction in patients with coronary artery disease and diabetes mellitus. Anesth Analg 1999;88(5):985–91.

[62] Connery LE, Coursin DB. Assessment and therapy of selected endocrine disorders. Anesthesiol Clin North Am 2004;22(1):93–123.

[63] Garcia MJ, McNamara PM, Gordon T, et al. Morbidity and mortality in diabetics in the Framingham population: sixteen year follow-up study. Diabetes 1974;23(2):105–11.

[64] Stamler J, Vaccaro O, Neaton JD, et al. Diabetes, other risk factors, and 12-yr cardiovascular mortality for men screened in the Multiple Risk Factor Intervention Trial. Diabetes Care 1993;16(2):434–44.

[65] Abbott RD, Donahue RP, Kannel WB, et al. The impact of diabetes on survival following myocardial infarction in men vs women: the Framingham Study. JAMA 1988;260(23): 3456–60.

[66] Donahue RP, Goldberg RJ, Chen Z, et al. The influence of sex and diabetes mellitus on survival following acute myocardial infarction: a community-wide perspective. J Clin Epidemiol 1993;46(3):245–52.

[67] Yusuf S, Hawken S, Ounpuu S, et al. INTERHEART Study Investigators. Effect of potentially modifiable risk factors associated with myocardial infarction in 52 countries (the INTERHEART study): case-control study. Lancet 2004;364(9438):937–52.

[68] Haffner SM, Lehto S, Ronnemaa T, et al. Mortality from coronary heart disease in subjects with type 2 diabetes and in nondiabetic subjects with and without prior myocardial infarction. N Engl J Med 1998;339(4):229–34.

[69] Miettinen H, Lehto S, Salomaa V, et al. Impact of diabetes on mortality after the first myocardial infarction: the FINMONICA Myocardial Infarction Register Study Group. Diabetes Care 1998;21(1):69–75.

[70] Juutilainen A, Lehto S, Ronnemaa T, et al. Type 2 diabetes as a "coronary heart disease equivalent": an 18-year prospective population-based study in Finnish subjects. Diabetes Care 2005;28(12):2901–7.

[71] Virmani R, Burke AP, Kolodgie F. Morphological characteristics of coronary atherosclerosis in diabetes mellitus. Can J Cardiol 2006;22(Suppl B):81B–84B.

[72] Burchfiel CM, Reed DM, Marcus EB, et al. Association of diabetes mellitus with coronary atherosclerosis and myocardial lesions: an autopsy study from the Honolulu Heart Program. Am J Epidemiol 1993;137(12):1328–40.
[73] Rosen SD, Camici PG. The brain-heart axis in the perception of cardiac pain: the elusive link between ischaemia and pain. Ann Med 2000;32(5):350–64.
[74] Shakespeare CF, Katritsis D, Crowther A, et al. Differences in autonomic nerve function in patients with silent and symptomatic myocardial ischaemia. Br Heart J 1994;71(1):22–9.
[75] Wackers FJ, Young LH, Inzucchi SE, et al. Detection of Ischemia in Asymptomatic Diabetics investigators. Detection of silent myocardial ischemia in asymptomatic diabetic subjects: the DIAD study. Diabetes Care 2004;27(8):1954–61.
[76] Burgos LG, Ebert TJ, Asiddao C, et al. Increased intraoperative cardiovascular morbidity in diabetics with autonomic neuropathy. Anesthesiology 1989;70(4):591–7.
[77] Kitamura A, Hoshino T, Kon T, et al. Patients with diabetic neuropathy are at risk of a greater intraoperative reduction in core temperature. Anesthesiology 2000;92(5):1311–8.
[78] Milan Study on Atherosclerosis and Diabetes (MiSAD) Group. Prevalence of unrecognized silent myocardial ischemia and its association with atherosclerotic risk factors in non–insulin-dependent diabetes mellitus. Am J Cardiol 1997;79(2):134–9.
[79] Eagle KA, Guyton RA, Davidoff R, et al. ACC/AHA guidelines for coronary artery bypass graft surgery: a report of the American College of Cardiology/American Heart Association Task Force on practice guidelines (committee to revise the 1991 guidelines for coronary artery bypass graft surgery). American College of Cardiology/American Heart Association. J Am Coll Cardiol 1999;34(4):1262–347.
[80] Kharlip J, Naglieri R, Mitchell BD, et al. Screening for silent coronary heart disease in type 2 diabetes: clinical application of American Diabetes Association guidelines. Diabetes Care 2006;29(3):692–4.
[81] Cohen MC, Curran PJ, L'Italien GJ, et al. Long-term prognostic value of preoperative dipyridamole thallium imaging and clinical indexes in patients with diabetes mellitus undergoing peripheral vascular surgery. Am J Cardiol 1999;83(7):1038–42.
[82] De Lorenzo A, Lima RS, Siqueira-Filho AG, et al. Prevalence and prognostic value of perfusion defects detected by stress technetium-99m sestamibi myocardial perfusion single-photon emission computed tomography in asymptomatic patients with diabetes mellitus and no known coronary artery disease. Am J Cardiol 2002;90(8):827–32.
[83] Schinkel AF, Elhendy A, van Domburg RT, et al. Prognostic value of dobutamine-atropine stress myocardial perfusion imaging in patients with diabetes. Diabetes Care 2002;25(9): 1637–43.
[84] Berman DS, Kang X, Hayes SW, et al. Adenosine myocardial perfusion single-photon emission computed tomography in women compared with men: impact of diabetes mellitus on incremental prognostic value and effect on patient management. J Am Coll Cardiol 2003;41(7):1125–33.
[85] Pedone C, Schinkel AF, Elhendy A, et al. Incremental prognostic value of dobutamine-atropine stress 99mTc-tetrofosmin myocardial perfusion imaging for predicting outcome in diabetic patients with limited exercise capacity. Eur J Nucl Med Mol Imaging 2005;32(9): 1057–63.
[86] Scholte AJ, Bax JJ, Wackers FJ. Screening of asymptomatic patients with type 2 diabetes mellitus for silent coronary artery disease: combined use of stress myocardial perfusion imaging and coronary calcium scoring. J Nucl Cardiol 2006;13(1):11–8.
[87] Albers AR, Krichavsky MZ, Balady GJ. Stress testing in patients with diabetes mellitus: diagnostic and prognostic value. Circulation 2006;113(4):583–92.
[88] Hayat SA, Patel B, Khattar RS, et al. Diabetic cardiomyopathy: mechanisms, diagnosis and treatment. Clin Sci (Lond) 2004;107(6):539–57.
[89] Frustaci A, Kajstura J, Chimenti C, et al. Myocardial cell death in human diabetes. Circ Res 2000;87(12):1123–32.

[90] Galderisi M. Diastolic dysfunction and diabetic cardiomyopathy: evaluation by Doppler echocardiography. J Am Coll Cardiol 2006;48(8):1548–51.

[91] Piccini JP, Klein L, Gheorghiade M, et al. New insights into diastolic heart failure: role of diabetes mellitus. Am J Med 2004;116(Suppl 5A):64S–75S.

[92] Ritz E, Orth SR. Nephropathy in patients with type 2 diabetes mellitus. N Engl J Med 1999; 341(15):1127–33.

[93] Standard of Medical Care in Diabetes. Nephropathy screening and treatment. Diabetes Care 2007;30:S19–21.

[94] Gaede P, Vedel P, Larsen N, et al. Multifactorial intervention and cardiovascular disease in patients with type 2 diabetes. N Engl J Med 2003;348(5):383–93.

[95] Remuzzi G, Benigni A, Remuzzi A. Mechanisms of progression and regression of renal lesions of chronic nephropathies and diabetes. J Clin Invest 2006;116(2):288–96.

[96] Robertson RP, Davis C, Larsen J, et al. Pancreas and islet transplantation for patients with diabetes. Diabetes Care 2000;23(1):112–6.

[97] Robertson RP. Islet transplantation as a treatment for diabetes—a work in progress. N Engl J Med 2004;350(7):694–705.

[98] Kramer H, Molitch ME. Screening for kidney disease in adults with diabetes. Diabetes Care 2005;28(7):1813–6.

[99] Garg JP, Bakris GL. Microalbuminuria: marker of vascular dysfunction, risk factor for cardiovascular disease. Vasc Med 2002;7(1):35–43.

[100] Klausen K, Borch-Johnsen K, Feldt-Rasmussen B, et al. Very low levels of microalbuminuria are associated with increased risk of coronary heart disease and death independently of renal function, hypertension, and diabetes. Circulation 2004;110(1):32–5.

[101] Eknoyan G, Hostetter T, Bakris GL, et al. Proteinuria and other markers of chronic kidney disease: a position statement of the National Kidney Foundation (NKF) and the National Institute of Diabetes and Digestive and Kidney Diseases (NIDDK). Am J Kidney Dis 2003; 42(4):617–22.

[102] Hoepelman AI, Meiland R, Geerlings SE. Pathogenesis and management of bacterial urinary tract infections in adult patients with diabetes mellitus. Int J Antimicrob Agents 2003;22(Suppl 2):35–43.

[103] Nicolle LE. Urinary tract infection in diabetes. Curr Opin Infect Dis 2005;18(1):49–53.

[104] Mangano CM, Diamondstone LS, Ramsay JG, et al. Renal dysfunction after myocardial revascularization: risk factors, adverse outcomes, and hospital resource utilization. The Multicenter Study of Perioperative Ischemia Research Group. Ann Intern Med 1998; 128(3):194–203.

[105] Mehran R, Nikolsky E. Contrast-induced nephropathy: definition, epidemiology, and patients at risk. Kidney Int Suppl 2006;100:S11–5.

[106] Finn WF. The clinical and renal consequences of contrast-induced nephropathy. Nephrol Dial Transplant 2006;21(6):i2–10.

[107] Briguori C, Marenzi G. Contrast-induced nephropathy: pharmacological prophylaxis. Kidney Int Suppl 2006;100:S30–8.

[108] Marenzi G, Assanelli E, Marana I, et al. N-acetylcysteine and contrast-induced nephropathy in primary angioplasty. N Engl J Med 2006;354(26):2773–82.

[109] Koziel H, Koziel MJ. Pulmonary complications of diabetes mellitus: pneumonia. Infect Dis Clin North Am 1995;9(1):65–96.

[110] Ardigo D, Valtuena S, Zavaroni I, et al. Pulmonary complications in diabetes mellitus: the role of glycemic control. Curr Drug Targets Inflamm Allergy 2004;3(4):455–8.

[111] Cook CB, Tsui C, Ziemer DC, et al. Common reasons for hospitalization among adult patients with diabetes. Endocr Pract 2006;12(4):363–70.

[112] Antonelli Incalzi R, Fuso L, Pitocco D, et al. Decline of neuroadrenergic bronchial innervation and respiratory function in type 1 diabetes mellitus: a longitudinal study. Diabetes Metab Res Rev 2006;23(4):311–6.

[113] Ozsahin K, Tugrul A, Mert S, et al. Evaluation of pulmonary alveolo-capillary permeability in type 2 diabetes mellitus: using technetium 99mTc-DTPA aerosol scintigraphy and carbon monoxide diffusion capacity. J Diabetes Complications 2006;20(4):205–9.
[114] Benedetti A, Noacco C. Juvenile diabetic cheiroarthropathy. Acta Diabetol Lat 1976; 13(1–2):54–67.
[115] Khanna G, Ferguson P. MRI of diabetic cheiroarthropathy. AJR Am J Roentgenol 2007; 188(1):W94–5.
[116] Rosenbloom AL, Silverstein JH, Riley WJ, et al. Limited joint mobility in childhood diabetes: family studies. Diabetes Care 1983;6(4):370–3.
[117] Rao SR, Saltzman CL, Wilken J, et al. Increased passive ankle stiffness and reduced dorsiflexion range of motion in individuals with diabetes mellitus. Foot Ankle Int 2006;27(8): 617–22.
[118] Monnier VM, Bautista O, Kenny D, et al. Skin collagen glycation, glycoxidation, and crosslinking are lower in subjects with long-term intensive versus conventional therapy of type 1 diabetes: relevance of glycated collagen products versus HbA1c as markers of diabetic complications. DCCT Skin Collagen Ancillary Study Group. Diabetes Control and Complications Trial. Diabetes 1999;48(4):870–80.
[119] Erden V, Basaranoglu G, Delatioglu H, et al. Relationship of difficult laryngoscopy to long-term non–insulin-dependent diabetes and hand abnormality detected using the 'prayer sign.' Br J Anaesth 2003;91(1):159–60.
[120] Salzarulo HH, Taylor LA. Diabetic "stiff joint syndrome" as a cause of difficult endotracheal intubation. Anesthesiology 1986;64(3):366–8.
[121] Hogan K, Rusy D, Springman SR. Difficult laryngoscopy and diabetes mellitus. Anesth Analg 1988;67(12):1162–5.
[122] Kong MF, Horowitz M, Jones KL, et al. Natural history of diabetic gastroparesis. Diabetes Care 1999;22(3):503–7.
[123] Park MI, Camilleri M. Gastroparesis: clinical update. Am J Gastroenterol 2006;101(5): 1129–39.
[124] Abell TL, Bernstein VK, Cutts T, et al. Treatment of gastroparesis: a multidisciplinary clinical review. Neurogastroenterol Motil 2006;18(4):263–83.
[125] Camilleri M. Clinical practice: diabetic gastroparesis. N Engl J Med 2007;356(8):820–9.
[126] Joshi N, Caputo GM, Weitekamp MR, et al. Infections in patients with diabetes mellitus. N Engl J Med 1999;341(25):1906–12.
[127] Calvet HM, Yoshikawa TT. Infections in diabetes. Infect Dis Clin North Am 2001;15(2): 407–21.
[128] Benfield T, Jensen JS, Nordestgaard BG. Influence of diabetes and hyperglycaemia on infectious disease hospitalisation and outcome. Diabetologia 2007;50(3):549–54 [Epub 2006 Dec 23].
[129] Nielson CP, Hindson DA. Inhibition of polymorphonuclear leukocyte respiratory burst by elevated glucose concentrations in vitro. Diabetes 1989;38(8):1031–5.
[130] Gallacher SJ, Thomson G, Fraser WD, et al. Neutrophil bactericidal function in diabetes mellitus: evidence for association with blood glucose control. Diabet Med 1995;12(10): 916–20.
[131] Weekers F, Giulietti AP, Michalaki M, et al. Metabolic, endocrine, and immune effects of stress hyperglycemia in a rabbit model of prolonged critical illness. Endocrinology 2003; 144(12):5329–38.
[132] Turina M, Fry DE, Polk HC Jr. Acute hyperglycemia and the innate immune system: clinical, cellular, and molecular aspects. Crit Care Med 2005;33(7):1624–33.
[133] Turina M, Miller FN, Tucker C, et al. Effects of hyperglycemia, hyperinsulinemia, and hyperosmolarity on neutrophil apoptosis. Surg Infect (Larchmt) 2006;7(2):111–21.
[134] Mayrovitz HN, Sims N. Effects of support surface relief pressures on heel skin blood flow in persons with and without diabetes mellitus. Adv Skin Wound Care 2004;17: 197–201.

[135] Reynolds C. Management of the diabetic surgical patient: a systematic but flexible plan is the key. Postgrad Med 1985;77(1):265–9, 272–6, 279.

[136] Coutinho M, Gerstein HC, Wang Y, et al. The relationship between glucose and incident cardiovascular events: a meta-regression analysis of published data from 20 studies of 95,783 individuals followed for 12.4 years. Diabetes Care 1999;22(2):233–40.

[137] Norhammar AM, Ryden L, Malmberg K. Admission plasma glucose: independent risk factor for long-term prognosis after myocardial infarction even in nondiabetic patients. Diabetes Care 1999;22(11):1827–31.

[138] Capes SE, Hunt D, Malmberg K, et al. Stress hyperglycaemia and increased risk of death after myocardial infarction in patients with and without diabetes: a systematic overview. Lancet 2000;355(9206):773–8.

[139] Williams LS, Rotich J, Qi R, et al. Effects of admission hyperglycemia on mortality and costs in acute ischemic stroke. Neurology 2002;59(1):67–71.

[140] Pomposelli JJ, Baxter JK 3rd, Babineau TJ, et al. Early postoperative glucose control predicts nosocomial infection rate in diabetic patients. JPEN J Parenter Enteral Nutr 1998; 22(2):77–81.

[141] Thourani VH, Weintraub WS, Stein B, et al. Influence of diabetes mellitus on early and late outcome after coronary artery bypass grafting. Ann Thorac Surg 1999;67(4):1045–52.

[142] Furnary AP, Gao G, Grunkemeier GL, et al. Continuous insulin infusion reduces mortality in patients with diabetes undergoing coronary artery bypass grafting. J Thorac Cardiovasc Surg 2003;125(5):1007–21.

[143] Lazar HL, Chipkin SR, Fitzgerald CA, et al. Tight glycemic control in diabetic coronary artery bypass graft patients improves perioperative outcomes and decreases recurrent ischemic events. Circulation 2004;109(12):1497–502.

[144] Doenst T, Wijeysundera D, Karkouti K, et al. Hyperglycemia during cardiopulmonary bypass is an independent risk factor for mortality in patients undergoing cardiac surgery. J Thorac Cardiovasc Surg 2005;130(4):1144–50.

[145] Ouattara A, Lecomte P, Le Manach Y, et al. Poor intraoperative blood glucose control is associated with a worsened hospital outcome after cardiac surgery in diabetic patients. Anesthesiology 2005;103(4):687–94.

[146] Gandhi GY, Nuttall GA, Abel MD, et al. Intraoperative hyperglycemia and perioperative outcomes in cardiac surgery patients. Mayo Clin Proc 2005;80(7):862–6.

[147] Wilson M, Weinreb J, Soo Hoo GW. Intensive insulin therapy in critical care: a review of a dozen protocols. Diabetes Care 2007;30(4):1005–11.

[148] van den Berghe G, Wouters P, Weekers F, et al. Intensive insulin therapy in the critically ill patient. N Engl J Med 2001;345(19):1359–67.

[149] Clement S, Braithwaite SS, Magee MF, et al. American Diabetes Association Diabetes in Hospitals Writing Committee: management of diabetes and hyperglycemia in hospitals. Diabetes Care 2004;27(2):553–91.

[150] Langley J, Adams G. Insulin-based regimens decrease mortality rates in critically ill patients: a systematic review. Diabetes Metab Res Rev 2006;23(3):184–92.

[151] Krinsley JS. Effect of an intensive glucose management protocol on the mortality of critically ill adult patients. Mayo Clin Proc 2004;79(8):992–1000.

[152] Balkin M, Mascioli C, Smith V, et al. Achieving durable glucose control in the intensive care unit without hypoglycaemia: a new practical IV insulin protocol. Diabetes Metab Res Rev 2007;23(1):49–55.

[153] Schmeltz LR, Desantis AJ, Thiyagarajan V, et al. Reduction of surgical mortality and morbidity in diabetic patients undergoing cardiac surgery with a combined intravenous and subcutaneous insulin glucose management strategy. Diabetes Care 2007;30(4): 823–8.

[154] ACE/ADA Task Force on Inpatient Diabetes. American College of Endocrinology and American Diabetes Association Consensus statement on inpatient diabetes and glycemic control: a call to action. Diabetes Care 2006;29(8):1955–62.

[155] Inzucchi SE, Rosenstock J. Counterpoint. Inpatient glucose management: a premature call to arms? Diabetes Care 2005;28(4):976–9.

[156] Gandhi GY, Nuttall GA, Abel MD, et al. Intensive intraoperative insulin therapy versus conventional glucose management during cardiac surgery: a randomized trial. Ann Intern Med 2007;146(4):233–43.

[157] Gabriely I, Shamoon H. Hypoglycemia in diabetes: common, often unrecognized. Cleve Clin J Med 2004;71(4):335–42.

[158] Desouza C, Salazar H, Cheong B, et al. Association of hypoglycemia and cardiac ischemia: a study based on continuous monitoring. Diabetes Care 2003;26(5):1485–9.

[159] Robinson RT, Harris ND, Ireland RH, et al. Changes in cardiac repolarization during clinical episodes of nocturnal hypoglycaemia in adults with type 1 diabetes. Diabetologia 2004;47(2):312–5.

[160] Dronge AS, Perkal MF, Kancir S, et al. Long-term glycemic control and postoperative infectious complications. Arch Surg 2006;141(4):375–80.

[161] Tamai D, Awad AA, Chaudhry HJ, et al. Optimizing the medical management of diabetic patients undergoing surgery. Conn Med 2006;70(10):621–30.

[162] Kao J, Tobis J, McClelland RL, et al. Investigators in the prevention of restenosis with tranilast and its outcomes trial: relation of metformin treatment to clinical events in diabetic patients undergoing percutaneous intervention. Am J Cardiol 2004;93(11): 1347–50.

[163] Vreven R, De Kock M. Metformin lactic acidosis and anaesthesia: myth or reality? Acta Anaesthesiol Belg 2005;56(3):297–302.

[164] Holstein A, Stumvoll M. Contraindications can damage your health—is metformin a case in point? Diabetologia 2005;48(12):2454–9.

[165] Salpeter S, Greyber E, Pasternak G, et al. Risk of fatal and nonfatal lactic acidosis with metformin use in type 2 diabetes mellitus. Cochrane Database Syst Rev 2006;1:CD002967.

[166] Duncan AI, Koch CG, Xu M, et al. Recent metformin ingestion does not increase in-hospital morbidity or mortality after cardiac surgery. Anesth Analg 2007;104(1):42–50.

[167] Campbell IW, Duncan LJ, Munro JF. Acute diabetic abdomen. Br Med J 1976;2(6043): 1074.

[168] Johnston DG, Alberti KG. Diabetic emergencies: practical aspects of the management of diabetic ketoacidosis and diabetes during surgery. Clin Endocrinol Metab 1980;9(3): 437–60.

[169] Umpierrez G, Freire AX. Abdominal pain in patients with hyperglycemic crises. J Crit Care 2002;17(1):63–7.

[170] Koul PB, Sussmane JB. Metabolic hyperglycemic emergencies with acute pancreatitis in a child with known insulin-dependent diabetes mellitus. Eur J Emerg Med 2005;12(6): 309–11.

[171] Faglia E, Clerici G, Caminiti M, et al. The role of early surgical debridement and revascularization in patients with diabetes and deep foot space abscess: retrospective review of 106 patients with diabetes. J Foot Ankle Surg 2006;45(4):220–6.

[172] Umeh L. Preventing amputation in older adults with diabetes. Adv Nurse Pract 2006;14(7): 41–3, 70.

[173] Lipsky BA, Berendt AR, Deery HG, et al. Infectious Diseases Society of America: diagnosis and treatment of diabetic foot infections. Plast Reconstr Surg 2006;117(7 Suppl): 212S–38S.

ELSEVIER
SAUNDERS

Clin Podiatr Med Surg
24 (2007) 383–396

CLINICS IN
PODIATRIC
MEDICINE AND
SURGERY

Update on the Treatment of Diabetic Foot Infections

Mark A. Kosinski, DPM[a,b,*],
Warren S. Joseph, DPM, FIDSA[c]

[a] *Department of Medicine, New York College of Podiatric Medicine, 1800 Park Avenue, New York, NY 10035, USA*
[b] *Department of Surgery, New York Medical College, Valhalla, New York, NY 10595, USA*
[c] *Veterans Affairs Medical Center, 1400 Blackhorse Hill Road Coatesville, PA 19320, USA*

Up until the last 5 years or so, the entire topic of diabetic foot infections was poorly represented in the medical literature. Occasional original studies or review articles would be published, but, given the complexity of the problem and the number of patients involved, it did not receive the press that it warranted. This lack of attention has changed dramatically. The volumes of basic and clinical science articles have reached impressive highs with new manuscripts published monthly. New classification systems and validations thereof have been published. Antibiotic studies that specifically examine efficacy in the treatment of diabetic foot infections are now commonplace, with the US Food and Drug Administration (FDA) now granting worthy compounds specific indications for this unique condition. The controversial role of methicillin-resistant *Staphylococcus aureus* (MRSA) has been addressed specifically in these wounds, yet much still needs to be done. Osteomyelitis complicates a large percentage of diabetic foot infections, yet none of the newer antibiotics have been specifically studied for this condition. The FDA does not have "guidelines for industry" dealing with the investigation of bone infection and the role of antibiotics in its treatment. Even the question as to the relative roles of surgery versus antibiotics has yet to be clearly elucidated. Ancillary modalities including hyperbaric oxygen and local wound care need further evidence before definitive statements can be made suggesting one treatment over the other. The role of this article is not to be a definitive

* Corresponding author. Department of Medicine, New York College of Podiatric Medicine, 1800 Park Avenue, New York, NY 10035.
E-mail address: mkosins@nycpm.edu (M.A. Kosinski).

doi:10.1016/j.cpm.2007.03.009

treatise on the approach to diabetic foot infections but, rather, to bring the practicing clinician up to date on the current literature.

Classification of diabetic foot ulcers

Many attempts have been made to classify diabetic foot ulcerations. Probably the most commonly used system was introduced by Wagner [1]. This system, which originally addressed only the dysvascular foot, does not adequately address all diabetic foot ulcerations and infections. Most diabetic foot complications occur because of neuropathy not ischemia.

Few, if any, of the currently used ulcer classification systems are specific for infection. Although some may include infection as a comorbidity, most are more concerned with the width and depth of the lesion. One clinically validated system specific for infection has been proposed by the Guidelines Committee of the Infectious Diseases Society of America (IDSA) [2].

The IDSA Practice Guidelines for the Diagnosis and Treatment of Diabetic Foot Infections clearly define the clinical and laboratory features that distinguish a mild infection from a moderate or severe infection and have recently been validated as a useful tool for grading foot infections [3].

This system is particularly useful for predicting what organisms one can expect to find in a given situation, allowing one to institute appropriate empirical treatment before culture and sensitivity results are known. The guidelines also may assist in predicting patient outcomes with more severe infections leading to a higher rate of amputations and other complications.

Clean and noninfected ulcerations

Clean and noninfected ulcerations are just that, not infected. There is a good granulation tissue base and no sinus tracts that probe to bone. Clinical signs and symptoms of inflammation, such as erythema, edema, and heat, are absent. Because infection is primarily diagnosed by the clinical evidence of these signs of inflammation, their absence precludes the diagnosis. A common misconception is that patients with diabetes do not respond with cellulitis. Although there may be an altered response that mutes some of the symptoms, it is extremely unlikely that there would be no evidence of cellulitis at all; therefore, cellulitis is a reliable indicator of infection in all but the most arterially compromised patients.

Noninfected wounds do not require antibiotic therapy, and, to date, no study has conclusively proven that the use of systemic antibiotics either accelerates healing or prevents infection. The use of "precautionary" or "prophylactic" antibiotics to prevent infection from developing in these lesions, although a widespread practice, is not supported by medical evidence.

In a study by Chantelau and colleagues [4], 44 diabetic patients with noninfected Wagner grade I and II foot ulcers were randomized to an antibiotic (amoxicillin plus clavulanic acid) or placebo group. At the completion of the study, no benefit was seen in the antibiotic group, and there was no advantage to systemic antibiotic therapy as an adjunct to wound care and off-loading.

Colonization should be differentiated from contamination and infection. Contamination is defined as the presence of bacteria without multiplication; colonization is defined as the presence of bacteria with multiplication; and infection is defined as the presence of bacteria with multiplication and a host response.

Although virtually all ulcerations are colonized, usually with multiple organisms, there is little compelling evidence that this bioload inhibits healing. Routine culturing of these lesions should be avoided. Documentation of the nature of drainage (color, consistency, odor, amount) is extremely important. Serous drainage from an open lesion may be an entirely benign finding, whereas the presence of frank purulence is highly suggestive, although not necessarily diagnostic, of an infectious process. Although there are few, if any, good studies to show the efficacy of topical antimicrobials in diabetic foot ulcerations, most clinicians who treat these lesions seem to use something on the wound surface to decrease the colonization in the possibly misdirected hope of avoiding the subsequent development of infection.

Mupirocin is commonly used on ulcers, although it has only been studied and approved for treating impetigo and pyodermas. It is highly active against gram-positive organisms including MRSA, although increasing resistance has been reported.

Silver compounds are widely used in the wound care community. Although they are considered broad-spectrum antimicrobials, they are classified as antiseptics not antibiotics. Antibiotics selectively kill bacterial cells, whereas antiseptics kill all cells. It has been the thrust of product development to produce a silver-containing dressing that releases just enough silver over time to kill bacterial cells without harming an undue number of host cells. Nevertheless, most silver-containing products are supported by anecdotal case studies or have been studied in venous stasis ulcers and not the diabetic foot.

Another antiseptic, povidone-iodine, has been implicated as being "tissue toxic." Almost all of these studies were in vitro tissue culture work. There is little to no evidence to prove that povidone-iodine is toxic to wounds in vivo.

Fusidic acid is a potent anti-staphylococcal drug in topical and oral preparations. Although it is available in Europe and Canada, it is not currently approved for use in the United States.

Mild infection

In contradistinction to noninfected diabetic wounds, ulcers with a mild infection show at least two of the signs and symptoms of a host response. There is usually localized cellulitis around the wound that, by definition, extends less than 2 cm from the periphery of the ulcer. Pus may be present; however, the infection remains localized with no proximal spread. There is no lymphangitis or lymphadenopathy. There are no systemic signs or symptoms of infection, and the patient's white blood cell count and blood glucose are not above the usual range.

The belief that all diabetic foot infections are polymicrobial is changing. It was once thought that even mildly infected diabetic wounds harbored anaerobes, leading to across the board treatment with broad-spectrum antibiotics even with negative anaerobic cultures. We now know that mildly infected diabetic wounds harbor predominantly aerobic gram-positive cocci and not anaerobes. *Staphylococcus aureus* and Group B streptococcus are the most common pathogens in the infected diabetic foot with ulceration. Unfortunately, there is a serious concern about increasing rates of methicillin resistance in *S aureus* isolates.

Most of the literature on diabetic foot infection throughout the 1980s and into the early 1990s was based on studies from the 1970s that seemed to suggest that all diabetic foot infections were polymicrobial. This thinking started to change when a study by Lipsky and colleagues [5] showed that the majority of infections were caused by gram-positive organisms.

In a retrospective study by Armstrong and colleagues [6], the culture results of 112 admissions to a multidisciplinary diabetic foot care clinic with a primary diagnosis of infected diabetic pedal ulceration were examined. An average of 1.5 species per patient was isolated. Eighty-nine percent of wounds cultured grew two or fewer organisms. Anaerobic species were isolated in only 5% of all cultures.

Mildly infected diabetic wounds are treated no differently with respect to antibiotic choice than are similar wounds in non-diabetic patients. Anaerobic coverage is these wounds is unnecessary.

Moderate and severe infections

Moderate infections present with cellulitis extending more than 2 cm and have evidence of significant proximal spread. Lymphadenopathy and lymphangitis may be present. There is extension beneath superficial fascia to involve muscle, bone, or joint. The patient is systemically well and metabolically stable. There is an elevation of white blood cells, and the blood glucose is over and above the patient's usual values.

Severe infections are defined as moderate infections in a patient who is septic, has metabolic inbalance, or severe peripheral arterial insufficiency. Moderate infections are limb threatening; severe infections are life threatening.

Distinct from mild infections, moderate and severe infections tend to be polymicrobial. Gram-negative organisms and anaerobes are more commonly found. Although *Pseudomonas aeruginosa* and enterococcus are frequently cultured, there is evidence to cast doubt on their role as pathogens. The need to direct antibiotic therapy toward these organisms is debatable.

The role of *Pseudomonas aeruginosa* and MRSA in diabetic foot infections

In one of the largest studies of moderate-to-severe diabetic foot infection, the Study of Infections in Diabetic Feet Comparing Efficacy, Safety, and Tolerability of Ertapenem versus Piperacillin/Tazobactam (SIDESTEP), Lipsky and colleagues [7] recruited 576 patients to a randomized, double-blinded, multicenter trial. A total of 289 patients were assigned to receive 1 g daily of ertapenem, and 287 were assigned to receive 3.375 g four times daily of piperacillin/tazobactam. All of the patients had moderate-to-severe diabetic foot infections. By the end of intravenous therapy, the clinical success rates were 94.2% for the ertapenem group and 92.2% for the piperacillin/tazobactam group, with no difference in the incidence of drug-related adverse events. Based on this trial, ertapenem received an FDA indication for the treatment of diabetic foot infections.

Although it is an important pathogen in respiratory tract and urinary tract infections, there are data to suggest that therapy directed against *P aeruginosa* may not be necessary to effect a cure in diabetic lower extremity skin and skin structure infections. In the SIDESTEP study, clinical response rates for patients with *P aeruginosa* were similar for ertapenem and piperacillin/tazobactam (83.3% versus 70.0%). Because ertapenem has no activity against *P aeruginosa*, it appears this organism may not be as clinically important a pathogen in diabetic foot infections as once believed.

When cultured from skin and soft tissue infections, *P aeruginosa* may exist as a commensal rather than a true pathogen. The results found in SIDESTEP correlate with those found in an earlier pivotal trial on which basis ertapenem received an FDA indication for the treatment of complicated skin and skin structure infections. That study, published in 2002 by Graham, also compared the efficacy of once daily ertapenem with piperacillin/tazobactam given four times a day in 540 clinically evaluable patients. Not only were the outcomes similar between the two drugs, but, in patients who grew *P aeruginosa,* there was a positive clinical response 70% of the time with ertapenem compared with a 60% clinical response rate in the beta-lactamase inhibitor group [8].

Also noteworthy from SIDESTEP was the fact that clinical response rates for a small number of patients with MRSA infections were similar irrespective of whether the patient received concomitant vancomycin therapy. This finding is important because neither ertapenem nor piperacillin/tazobactam have activity against MRSA. Other investigators have noted similar outcomes with respect to MRSA and beta-lactam antibiotics [9].

In the largest study to date designed to evaluate the impact of antibiotic therapy on the outcome of patients with community acquired MRSA infections, investigators noted only a small difference in outcome between patients who received MRSA-active versus MRSA-inactive antimicrobial therapy. Ruhe and colleagues [10] performed a retrospective cohort study of 492 patients with 531 community acquired MRSA skin and soft tissue infections. Incision and drainage was performed for the majority of patients. Therapy was successful in 190 (87%) of 219 patients who did not receive an MRSA-active antibiotic compared with 296 (95%) of 312 patients who received an MRSA-active antibiotic.

This finding raises the question as to why some patients with MRSA infections improve while on an antibiotic that, by definition, has no activity against MRSA. The patient's immune response undoubtedly has a role. Before the advent of antibiotics, not every patient infected with *Staphylococcus aureus* succumbed to the infection. Especially in milder infections, incision and drainage may reduce the severity of the infection to a level manageable by the host defenses. The infection resolves spontaneously, and the patient gets better regardless of the antibiotic. There are data to suggest that a low pH (5.5) may suppress intrinsic resistance to methicillin in *S aureus* [11], causing MRSA to become as sensitive to beta-lactams as methicillin-susceptible *S aureus* (MSSA) in an acidic environment [12] An acidic pH does not affect the MRSA phenotype (mec A, PBP 2a) but may effect gene expression [13]. Although a pH in this range has been observed in the skin of hosts colonized by *S aureus*, there is no published study that validates these findings in vivo.

Bone infections in diabetic patients

Osteomyelitis complicates many diabetic wounds. Although the resection of infected bone often has a role in treatment, newer evidence suggests that, in some cases, antibiotics alone may be sufficient therapy [14].

There are instances when removal of infected bone is not an option, such as when surgery would cause an unacceptable loss of function, when surgery carries an unacceptable risk (the cure is worse than the disease), or when a patient is unwilling to undergo surgery or amputation.

New antibiotics with a high bioavailability have been introduced over the last few years, some of which have a high serum to bone ratio and can penetrate through biofilms and enter eukaryotic cells. Such advances have changed the way we think about treating chronic osteomyelitis and may make nonsurgical treatment feasible in some cases.

Poorly perfused bone is more susceptible to infection and more difficult to treat than viable, well-perfused bone. In many animal models, osteomyelitis is induced by creating a defect in healthy bone and injecting a large inoculum of pathogen; therefore, the clinical success rate of studies involving well-vascularized, non-human subjects may not reflect real world experience with diabetic patients with peripheral arterial disease.

Bone biopsy with culture is still considered the gold standard of diagnosis and is a safe procedure rarely associated with complications. Because osteomyelitis can be a focal disease, at least two to three specimens of bone should be taken. Systemic antibiotics should be discontinued for at least three drug half-lives. Bone should be sent for cultures, histology, and Gram stain.

A Gram stain of bone can be ordered at the time of the procedure or at a much later date. Diabetic patients with foot osteomyelitis and bone biopsy have been shown to have a better outcome than patients receiving broad-spectrum antibiotics directed against superficial culture samples (76.9% versus 45.8%) [15].

The initial event in bone infection is adhesion (acute osteomyelitis) followed by firm attachment (chronic osteomyelitis). Bacteria adhere to bone matrix by producing a polysaccharide capsule that forms a strong link between it and the solid surface. This slime layer protects bacterial colonies from antibiotics and from phagocytosis from macrophages. Synthesis begins shortly after adherence and stabilizes after 1 week. Surface proteins produced by *S aureus* are osteolytic, resulting in decreased bone matrix production. Infection spreads, and implants loosen.

Gradual exposure to antibiotics through a biofilm may promote resistance. Bacteria protected by biofilms can tolerate levels of antimicrobial agents that are 10 to 1000 times higher than their minimum inhibitory concentration (MIC90) [16]. It is well established that *S aureus* can exist as an intracellular pathogen and can infect and survive in osteoblasts. When osteoblasts die, viable bacteria are released to infect new osteoblasts. *S aureus* can exist intracellularly as small colony variants. Small colony variants of *S aureus* have a lower metabolic rate and can remain intracellular for indefinite periods. Osteomyelitis can thus remain latent for years.

In general, acute osteomyelitis and early chronic osteomyelitis are associated with the best treatment outcome. Treating an infection in well-perfused, viable bone carries a better prognosis than treating poorly perfused, necrotic bone.

If treatment fails, one should consider the following: Was the original diagnosis correct? Did antibiotics cover the pathogen? Is there residual necrotic bone or hardware that needs to be removed?

Antibiotic choice should be based on the bioavailability of the drug, the ability to penetrate biofilm, the ability to penetrate eukaryotic cells (specifically osteoblasts), and the activity against a bone biopsy–recovered pathogen. The length of treatment varies with the clinical situation (Table 1).

Antibiotics: new drugs and new indications

Many new antibiotics have recently been approved, received a new FDA indication, or are soon to be made available. Some are well known and have already been incorporated into clinical practice. It is outside the scope of this article to review all of the drugs that are available. Table 2 summarizes these antibiotics. Many of these newer antibiotics are first in their class and exploit novel mechanisms of action. The question is what place, if any, do these drugs have in the treatment of diabetic foot infections.

Table 1
Duration and route of antibiotic therapy for the treatment of diabetic foot osteomyelitis

Clinical situation	Route of therapy	Duration of therapy
No residual infected tissue (eg, post amputation)	Parenteral or oral	2–5 d
Residual infected soft tissue (but not bone)	Parenteral or oral	2–4 wk
Residual infected (but viable) bone	Initial parenteral, then consider oral switch	4–6 wk
No surgery, or residual dead bone postoperatively	Initial parenteral, then consider oral switch	>3 mo

Adapted from Lipsky B, Berendt A, Deery H, et al, Infectious Diseases Society of America. Guidelines for the diagnosis and treatment of diabetic foot infections. Clin Infect Dis 2004;39:901.

Linezolid

Linezolid, a first-in-class oxazolidinone, has 100% bioavailability after oral administration and is active against MRSA and vancomycin-resistant *Enterococcus faecalis*. Linezolid has no anaerobic activity. Although treatment failures and resistant strains of *Staphylococcus aureus* have been reported, linezolid remains a valuable antibiotic and has received an FDA indication for diabetic foot infections.

Table 2
Antibiotics used to treat moderate-to-severe diabetic foot infections

Drug	FDA indication	Class	MRSA activity	*B fragilis* activity
Ticarcillin/ clavulanate	cSSSI	Beta-lactam/ beta-lactamase inhibitor Cmpd	No	Yes
Piperacillin/ tazobactam	cSSSI/DFI	Beta-lactam/ beta-lactamase inhibitor Cmpd	No	Yes
Imipenem/ cilistatin	cSSSI	Carbapenem	No	Yes
Ertapenem	cSSSI/DFI	Carbapenem	No	Yes
Moxifloxacin	cSSSI	Quinolone	No	Yes
Daptomycin	cSSSI	Cyclic lipopeptide	Yes	No
Linezolid	cSSSI/DFI	Oxazolidinone	Yes	No
Tigecycline	cSSSI	Glycylcycline	Yes	Yes
Dalbavancin	Approval pending	Lipoglycopeptide	Yes	No
Ceftobiprole	Approval pending	Fifth-generation cephalosporin	Yes	No
Iclaprim	Approval pending	Diaminopyrimiadine	Yes	No

Abbreviations: Cmpd, compound; cSSSI, complicated skin and skin structure infections; DFI, diabetic foot infection.

In a randomized, open-label, multicenter study of diabetic foot infections of all types, Lipsky and colleagues [17] compared the efficacy and safety of parenteral and oral linezolid with parenteral ampicillin-sulbactam and intravenous and oral amoxicillin-clavulanate given for 7 to 28 days. Among 371 patients, clinical cure rates associated with linezolid and comparators were statistically equivalent (81% versus 71%, respectively) but were higher for linezolid-treated patients with infected foot ulcers (81% versus 68%) and for patients without osteomyelitis (87% versus 72%).

In a randomized, open-label trial involving 1200 adult patients hospitalized with complicated skin and soft tissue infections due to suspected or proven MRSA, Itani and colleagues [18] compared outcomes in patients treated with linezolid or vancomycin. When compared with vancomycin, linezolid was associated with a significantly shorter length of stay, decreased parenteral antibiotic duration, and higher discharge rates [18].

In an open-label comparative study, patients aged 18 years or older with proven MRSA-related complicated skin and soft tissue infections requiring surgical intervention were randomized to receive oral linezolid (n = 30) or intravenous vancomycin (n = 30) for 7 to 21 days. Linezolid was associated with greater rates of clinical cure and improvement, a 3-day shorter median length of stay, and reduced outpatient charges. Vancomycin therapy was associated with more treatment failures and subsequent lower extremity amputations [19].

Linezolid exhibits rapid penetration into bone, fat, and muscle. Mean concentrations at 90 minutes in cancellous bone are twice the MIC90 for staphylococci and streptococci [20].

Ertapenem

Ertapenem is a broad-spectrum carbapenem approved for the treatment of complicated skin and skin structure infections and has received FDA approval for complicated diabetic foot infections. It has a narrower spectrum of activity when compared with imipenem/cilastatin (Primaxin); good activity against MSSA, gram-negative organisms, and anaerobes; but no activity against *Pseudomonas aeruginosa* or MRSA [21].

Ertapenem's long half-life and once daily dosing make it particularly attractive for home intravenous therapy. In a prospective, randomized, double-blind trial comparing ertapenem (1 g once daily) with piperacillin-tazobactam (3.375 g every 6 hours) as parenteral treatment for 540 adults with complicated skin and skin structure infections, 82.4% of the patients who received ertapenem and 84.4% of those who received piperacillin-tazobactam were cured. The most common infections in the study were deep soft tissue abscess (18.9%), followed by diabetic lower extremity infection (18.1%). With the exception of MRSA, almost all of the predominant aerobic pathogens were susceptible to both study drugs. Of the 141 anaerobes tested, 97.2% were susceptible to ertapenem and 97.9% to piperacillin-tazobactam [7].

In a study by Jacqueline and colleagues [22], ertapenem in combination with linezolid showed in vitro synergy against MRSA. Using a rabbit endocarditis experimental model, linezolid plus ertapenem exhibited highly synergistic activity in vivo after 4 days of treatment. There are as yet no published human studies regarding ertapenem/linezolid synergy.

Moxifloxacin

A newer generation quinolone, moxifloxacin has shown good activity against MSSA, gram-negative organisms, and anaerobes. Moxifloxacin has no clinically useful activity against MRSA. As is characteristic of quinolones, it has high bioavailability after oral administration. Moxifloxacin received an FDA indication for complicated skin and skin structure infections in July of 2005. Moxifloxacin does not require dose adjustment for patients with renal impairment. The dose, regardless of serum creatinine, is 400 mg once daily.

In a study by Edmiston and colleagues [23], the in vitro activities of moxifloxacin, ciprofloxacin, levofloxacin, gatifloxacin, imipenem, piperacillin-tazobactam, clindamycin, and metronidazole against 900 surgical isolates were determined using National Committee for Clinical Laboratory Standards testing methods. Moxifloxacin exhibited good-to-excellent antimicrobial activity against most aerobic (90.8%) and anaerobic (97.1%) microorganisms. Moxifloxacin showed good activity against MSSA (MIC90 = 0.25 mg/L) and *Bacteroides fragilis* (MIC90 = 1.0 mg/L).

Tigecycline

Tigecycline is a first-in-class glycylcycline antibiotic. It received FDA approval in June of 2005 for the treatment of complicated skin and skin structure and intra-abdominal infections. Tigecycline is of interest because of its activity against MRSA, gram-negative organisms, and anaerobes, making it potentially useful as single agent therapy for moderate and severe diabetic foot infections.

In clinical trials, empiric monotherapy with tigecycline for the treatment of complicated skin and skin structure infections provided clinical cure rates comparable with those of combination therapy with vancomycin and aztreonam [24,25]. Unfortunately, the use of tigecycline may be overshadowed by its side effects. The most common treatment-emergent adverse events listed in the manufacturer's prescribing information were nausea (29.5%) and vomiting (19.7%) [26].

There are no published studies involving the use of tigecycline in the treatment of osteomyelitis in humans; however, animal studies by Yin and colleagues [27] have shown a 90% cure rate when used alone and a 100% cure rate when combined with rifampicin compared with an 81.8% cure rate for vancomycin alone and a 90% cure rate when vancomycin was combined with rifampicin.

Daptomycin

Daptomycin is a first-in-class lipopeptide. It is the only once daily agent approved for the treatment of MRSA-complicated skin and skin structure infections. Daptomycin is bactericidal and has activity against resistant gram-positive pathogens, including MRSA and vancomycin-resistant strains of *S aureus* [28]. It is available only in parenteral form. Although daptomycin should be considered for treating diabetic foot infections, its lack of gram-negative and anaerobic activity may necessitate combination therapy for moderate and severe diabetic foot infections if these organisms are a concern.

In a study comparing the effectiveness of daptomycin with semi-synthetic penicillins or vancomycin, Lipsky and Stoutenburgh concluded that, among 103 clinically evaluable patients, the clinical and microbiologic efficacy and safety of daptomycin were not statistically different from that of comparator antibiotics (66% versus 70%, respectively) for treating infected diabetic foot ulcers caused by gram-positive pathogens [29].

Dalbavancin

Dalbavancin is a novel, parenteral, lipoglycopeptide antibiotic with strong activity against gram-positive organisms including resistant staphylococci (MRSA). Its long half-life allows for once-a-week dosing. Still awaiting FDA new drug approval for the treatment of complicated skin and skin structure infections, dalbavancin should become available in 2007. As is true for daptomycin, combination therapy with an agent active against gram-negative organisms and anaerobes may be necessary in moderate-to-severe diabetic foot infections.

In a randomized, double-blind comparison of once weekly dalbavancin versus twice daily linezolid therapy, Jauregui and colleagues [30] found that two doses of dalbavancin (1000 mg given on day 1 followed by 500 mg given on day 8) were as well tolerated and as effective as linezolid given twice daily for 14 days for the treatment of patients with complicated skin and skin structure infections, including those infected with MRSA.

Telavancin, another antibiotic of the same class, has a similar spectrum of activity but with once daily rather than once weekly dosing.

Ceftobiprole

Ceftobiprole is a novel extended spectrum cephalosporin which some may classify as a fifth-generation cephalosporin. What makes ceftobiprole unique among cephalosporins is that it is the first cephalosporin to demonstrate activity against MRSA. Gram-negative coverage is similar to that of third-generation agents. Ceftobiprole has no activity against *Bacteroides fragilis*.

In a pivotal double-blind study, 784 patients with complicated skin and skin structure infections were randomized to receive ceftobiprole or vancomycin. A total of 397 were assigned to the ceftobiprole arm and 387 to the vancomycin arm. Patient demographics and backgrounds were similar in the two groups. Patients were randomly assigned to ceftobiprole, 500 mg every 12 hours, or vancomycin, 1g every 12 hours. Clinical cure rates were similar in the ceftobiprole and the vancomycin treatment groups. The most common treatment-emergent adverse event in the ceftobiprole group was nausea (14%) [31].

Iclaprim

Currently under development, iclaprim is a first-in-class diaminopyrimiadine antibiotic with activity against MRSA. When approved, it will be available in oral and parenteral forms. Like linezolid, serum levels after oral and parenteral administration are equivalent. An FDA new drug application for complicated skin and skin structure infections will be submitted in 2007. If approved, iclaprim will be the only oral agent besides linezolid that will have an FDA indication for MRSA-complicated skin and skin structure infections [32].

Summary

The once widely held belief that all diabetic foot infections are polymicrobial has been proven to be a myth. Mild infections in the diabetic patient can be treated identically to mild infections in the non-diabetic patient, namely, with an agent to cover *S aureus* and streptococcus. Anaerobic coverage is unnecessary. Although the incidence of MRSA is on the increase, there is evidence to show that, in uncomplicated skin infections at least, coverage with an MRSA-active agent may be superfluous to incision and drainage. Nonetheless, many exciting new compounds have been approved or are in the pipeline with excellent activity against MRSA, many of which will have a role in treating infections in the diabetic foot.

References

[1] Wagner FW. The dysvascular foot: a system for diagnosis and treatment. Foot Ankle 1981; 2(2):64–122.

[2] Lipsky BA, Berendt AR, Deery HG, et al. Infectious Diseases Society of America. Diagnosis and treatment of diabetic foot infections. Clin Infect Dis 2004;39(7):885–910.

[3] Lavery LA, Armstrong DG, Murdoch DP, et al. Validation of the Infectious Diseases Society of America's diabetic foot infection classification system. Clin Infect Dis 2007;44(4):562–5.

[4] Chantelau E, Tanudjaja T, Altenhofer F, et al. Antibiotic treatment for uncomplicated neuropathic forefoot ulcers in diabetes: a controlled trial. Diabet Med 1996;13(2):156–9.

[5] Lipsky BA, Pecoraro RE, Larson SA, et al. Outpatient management of uncomplicated lower-extremity infections in diabetic patients. Arch Intern Med 1990;150(4):790–7.

[6] Armstrong DG, Liswood PJ, Todd WF. 1995 William J. Stickel Bronze Award. Prevalence of mixed infections in the diabetic pedal wound: a retrospective review of 112 infections. J Am Podiatr Med Assoc 1995;85(10):533–7 [erratum in: J am Podiatr Med Assoc 1995 Nov85(11); 695].

[7] Lipsky BA, Armstrong DG, Citron DM, et al. Ertapenem versus piperacillin/tazobactam for diabetic foot infections (SIDESTEP): prospective, randomised, controlled, double-blinded, multicentre trial. Lancet 2005;366(9498):1695–703.

[8] Graham DR, Lucasti C, Malafaia O, et al. Ertapenem once daily versus piperacillin-tazobactam 4 times per day for treatment of complicated skin and skin-structure infections in adults: results of a prospective, randomized, double-blind multicenter study. Clin Infect Dis 2002; 34(11):1460–8.

[9] Moran GJ, Krishnadasan A, Gorwitz RJ, et al. Methicillin-resistant *Staphylococcus aureus* infections among patients in the emergency department. N Engl J Med 2006;355: 666–74.

[10] Ruhe JJ, Smith N, Bradsher RW, et al. Community-onset methicillin-resistant *Staphylococcus aureus* skin and soft-tissue infections: impact of antimicrobial therapy on outcome. Clin Infect Dis 2007;44(6):777–84.

[11] Sabath LD, Wallace SJ, Gerstein DA. Suppression of intrinsic resistance to methicillin and other penicillins in *Staphylococcus aureus*. Antimicrob Agents Chemother 1972;2(5):350–5.

[12] Lemaire S, Van Bambeke F, Mingeot-Leclercq M, et al. Carbapenems are active against intracellular MRSA poster A-1832. Presented at the 45th Interscience Conference on Antimicrobial Agents and Chemotherapy. Washington, DC, December 16–19, 2005.

[13] Weinrick B, Dunman PM, McAleese F, et al. Effect of mild acid on gene expression in *Staphylococcus aureus*. J Bacteriol 2004;186(24):8407–23.

[14] Jeffcoate WJ, Lipsky BA. Controversies in diagnosing and managing osteomyelitis of the foot in diabetes. Clin Infect Dis 2004;39(Suppl 2):S115–22.

[15] Senneville E, Michele A, Lombart M, et al. Bone biopsy for foot osteomyelitis complicating diabetes [poster 337]. Presented at the 43rd Annual Meeting of the Infectious Diseases Society of America. San Francisco (CA), October 6–9, 2005.

[16] Jefferson K, Goldmann D, Pier G. Use of confocal microscopy to analyze the rate of vancomycin penetration through *Staphylococcus aureus* biofilms. Antimicrob Agents Chemother 2005;49(6):2467–73.

[17] Lipsky BA, Itani K, Norden K. Treating foot infections in diabetic patients: a randomized, multicenter, open-label trial of linezolid versus ampicillin-sulbactam/amoxicillin-clavulanate. Clin Infect Dis 2004;38(1):17–24.

[18] Itani KM, Weigelt J, Li JZ, et al. Linezolid reduces length of stay and duration of intravenous treatment compared with vancomycin for complicated skin and soft tissue infections due to suspected or proven methicillin-resistant *Staphylococcus aureus* (MRSA). Int J Antimicrob Agents 2005;26(6):442–8.

[19] Sharpe JN, Shively EH, Polk HC Jr. Clinical and economic outcomes of oral linezolid versus intravenous vancomycin in the treatment of MRSA-complicated, lower-extremity skin and soft-tissue infections caused by methicillin-resistant *Staphylococcus aureus*. Am J Surg 2005; 189(4):425–8.

[20] Rana B, Butcher I, Grigoris P, et al. Linezolid penetration into osteo-articular tissues. J Antimicrob Chemother 2002;50(5):747–50.

[21] Goldstein EJ, Citron DM, Merriam CV, et al. General microbiology and in vitro susceptibility of anaerobes isolated from complicated skin and skin-structure infections in patients enrolled in a comparative trial of ertapenem versus piperacillin-tazobactam. Clin Infect Dis 2002;35(Suppl 1):S119–25.

[22] Jacqueline C, Caillon J, Grossi O, et al. In vitro and in vivo assessment of linezolid combined with ertapenem: a highly synergistic combination against methicillin-resistant *Staphylococcus aureus*. Antimicrob Agents Chemother 2006;50(7):2547–9.

[23] Edmiston CE, Krepel CJ, Seabrook GR, et al. In vitro activities of moxifloxacin against 900 aerobic and anaerobic surgical isolates from patients with intra-abdominal and diabetic foot infections. Antimicrob Agents Chemother 2004;48(3):1012–6.

[24] Breedt J, Teras J, Gardovskis J, et al. Safety and efficacy of tigecycline in treatment of skin and skin structure infections: results of a double-blind phase 3 comparison study with vancomycin-aztreonam. Antimicrob Agents Chemother 2005;49(11):4658–66.

[25] Ellis-Grosse EJ, Babinchak T, Dartois N, et al, Tigecycline 300 cSSSI Study Group, Tigecycline 305 cSSSI Study Group. The efficacy and safety of tigecycline in the treatment of skin and skin-structure infections: results of 2 double-blind phase 3 comparison studies with vancomycin-aztreonam. Clin Infect Dis 2005;41(Suppl 5):S341–53.

[26] TYGACIL (tigecycline) Prescribing Information. Philadelphia: Wyeth Pharmaceuticals; 2007.

[27] Yin LY, Lazzarini L, Li F, et al. Comparative evaluation of tigecycline and vancomycin, with and without rifampicin, in the treatment of methicillin-resistant *Staphylococcus aureus* experimental osteomyelitis in a rabbit model. J Antimicrob Chemother 2005;55(6):995–1002.

[28] Bosso JA. The antimicrobial armamentarium: evaluating current and future treatment options. Pharmacotherapy 2005;25(9):55S–62S.

[29] Lipsky BA, Stoutenburgh U. Daptomycin for treating infected diabetic foot ulcers: evidence from a randomized, controlled trial comparing daptomycin with vancomycin or semi-synthetic penicillins for complicated skin and skin-structure infections. J Antimicrob Chemother 2005;55(2):240–5.

[30] Jauregui LE, Babazadeh S, Seltzer E, et al. Randomized, double-blind comparison of once-weekly dalbavancin versus twice-daily linezolid therapy for the treatment of complicated skin and skin structure infections. Clin Infect Dis 2005;41(10):1407–15.

[31] Noel G, Strauss R, Pypstra R. Successful treatment of skin and skin structure infections due to staphylococci including methicillin-resistant *Staphylococcus aureus* with ceftobiprole [poster L1212]. Presented at the 46th Interscience Conference on Antimicrobial Agents and Chemotherapy. San Francisco (CA), September 27–30, 2006.

[32] Appelbaum PC, Jacobs MR. Recently approved and investigational antibiotics for treatment of severe infections caused by gram-positive bacteria. Curr Opin Microbiol 2005;8(5):510–7.

ELSEVIER
SAUNDERS

Clin Podiatr Med Surg
24 (2007) 397–424

CLINICS IN
PODIATRIC
MEDICINE AND
SURGERY

Medical Imaging of the Diabetic Foot

Rebecca A. Loredo, MD*, Glenn Garcia, MD, Samir Chhaya, MD

Department of Radiology, University of Texas Health Science Center, 7703 Floyd Curl Drive, San Antonio, TX 78229-3900, USA

Despite the awareness of distinguishing radiographic features, confident differentiation between neuroarthropathy, osteomyelitis, and septic arthritis in the diabetic foot remains a difficult task. The differentiation of cellulitis from underlying osteomyelitis and the early detection of abscesses remain important diagnostic issues. Unfortunately, there is not yet "one best imaging test" for evaluation of the diabetic foot. Nevertheless, several diagnostic tests are useful in the assessment of this common diagnostic dilemma.

Imaging modalities used in the evaluation of the diabetic foot include conventional radiography, CT, nuclear medicine scintigraphy, MRI, ultrasonography, and a newcomer, positron emission tomography combined with CT scanning. Angiography is another diagnostic imaging modality used to evaluate the diabetic foot and is discussed elsewhere in this issue.

Conventional radiography

Conventional radiography or plain radiographs have been the mainstay for evaluation of the diabetic foot. This modality remains a valuable means of documenting major structural changes.

Neuroarthropathy

Distal symmetric neuroarthropathy, a classic form of diabetic neuroarthropathy, leads to destruction, fragmentation, and deformity of the bones and joints. The forefoot and midfoot are the most frequent sites of involvement [1]. The intertarsal and tarsometatarsal joints undergo osseous fragmentation with osteosclerosis or osteolysis and joint subluxation or

* Corresponding author.
E-mail address: loredo@uthscsa.edu (R.A. Loredo).

0891-8422/07/$ - see front matter
doi:10.1016/j.cpm.2007.03.010

dislocation (Fig. 1A, B). The metatarsophalangeal joint shows osseous resorption, flattening, and fragmentation of the metatarsal head (Fig. 2). Abnormalities of the interphalangeal articulations are less common, and the ankle is infrequently involved (Fig. 3).

Diabetic neuropathic disease represents a spectrum of pathology ranging from painful mild alterations resembling degenerative arthritis to the extreme of complete articular disorganization following a pattern of Lisfranc fracture-dislocation or involving Chopart's joint with the development of a "rocker-bottom" deformity (Fig. 4) [2]. Progression of the destructive process of neuroarthropathy may be followed with conventional radiography as it rapidly evolves over days or a few weeks or slowly progresses over months to years.

Conventional radiographs are useful for the identification and documentation of neuropathic disease; however, the early subtle changes of neuroarthropathy such as microfractures may not be obvious [3], and soft tissue problems such as cellulitis, fasciitis, pyomyositis, sinus tracts, and abscesses are not as easily appreciated.

Infection

The predominant types of infection that involve the diabetic foot are nonsuppurative cellulitis and deep soft tissue abscess that can lead to osteomyelitis. Dorsal cellulitis presents as swelling of the dorsum of the foot and usually is secondary to surface infection in the nails, toes, or web spaces.

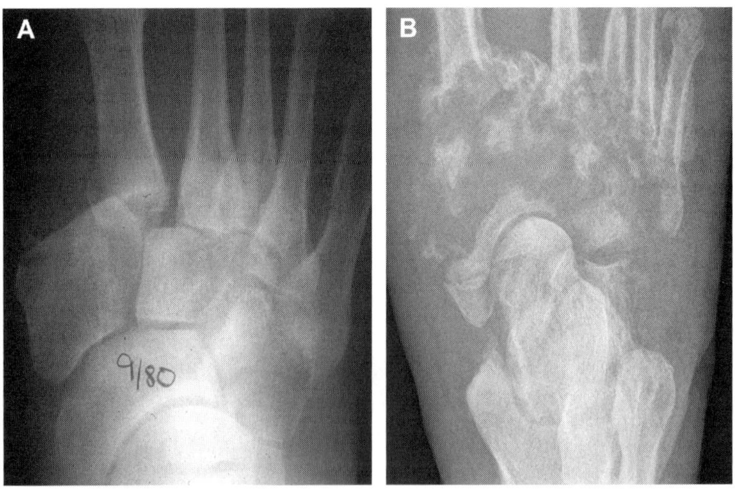

Fig. 1. Neuropathic arthropathy involving the tarsus and proximal metatarsus. (*A, B*) Anteroposterior views of the feet in two different patients demonstrating homolateral Lisfranc level dislocation and striking osteolysis with midfoot and proximal metatarsus joint destruction, respectively.

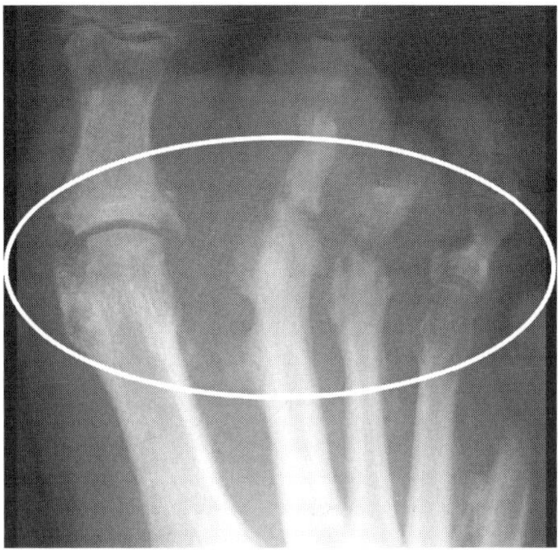

Fig. 2. Neuroarthropathy affecting the forefoot. Anteroposterior radiograph showing osseous resorption, flattening, and fragmentation of the metatarsal heads and adjacent proximal phalanges (*circle*).

Frequent sites of abscess formation are the toes, web spaces, flexor sheaths, plantar spaces, and heel [4]. Osteomyelitis is usually associated with local abscess, and the most common sites are the first, fifth, and second rays [2]. Calcaneal involvement also may occur; however, the other tarsal bones are infrequently affected.

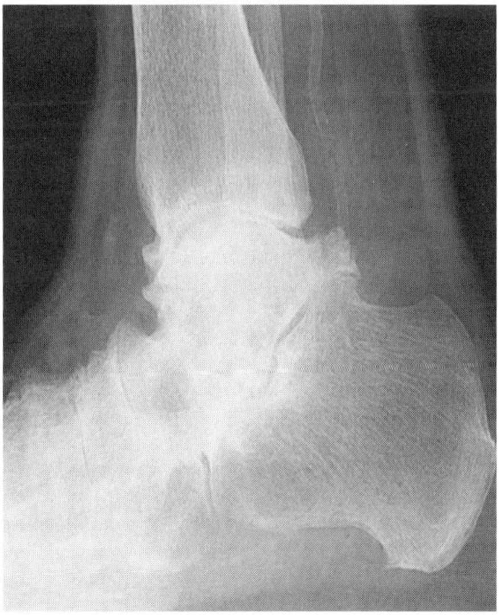

Fig. 3. Neuropathic changes involving the ankle joint and subtalar joint. Lateral radiograph of the ankle and hindfoot demonstrating tibiotalar greater than subtalar joint space narrowing, subcortical sclerosis, and osteophytosis, consistent with neuroarthropathy. Limited view of the talonavicular and intertarsal joints shows concomitant neurarthropathic changes.

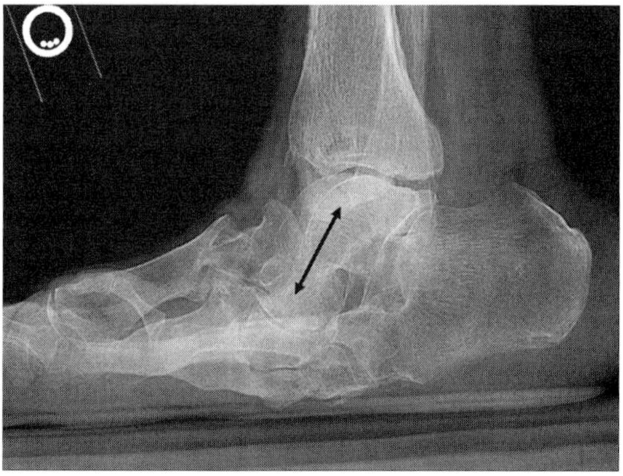

Fig. 4. Marked neuropathic changes with rocker-bottom deformity. Lateral weight-bearing radiograph demonstrating complete osseous and articular disorganization involving Lisfranc and Chopart's joints with marked talar plantar flexion (*near vertical line*) and development of rocker-bottom deformity.

Radiographically, soft tissue infection is seen as diffuse or focal swelling with or without soft tissue gas (Fig. 5). Focal demineralization is a classic manifestation of early osteomyelitis (Fig. 6). Periostitis, osteosclerosis, and cortical thickening are other radiographic signs [5]. Unfortunately, osteomyelitis usually produces no radiographic changes until the late stages of destruction, sclerosis, or periosteal reaction occur (Fig. 7) [3]. In a large number of cases, the early, often subtle, radiographic changes of osteomyelitis may be obscured by the chronic destructive process of neuroarthropathy.

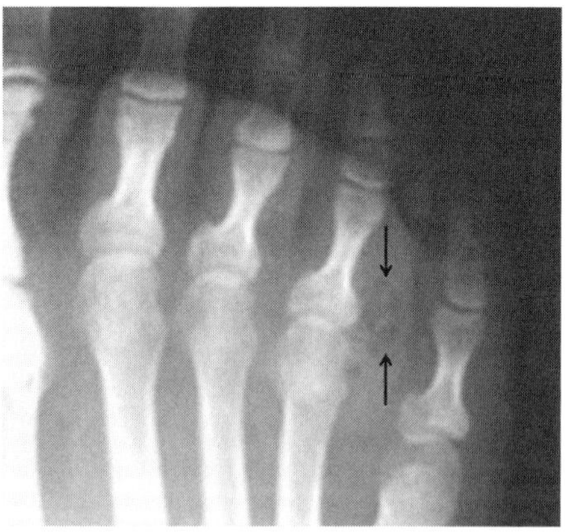

Fig. 5. Soft tissue gas in a soft tissue abscess. Magnified anteroposterior view of the forefoot showing soft tissue gas in the fourth-fifth web space (*arrows*) associated with an abscess. No focal abnormality is seen in the adjacent bone or joint.

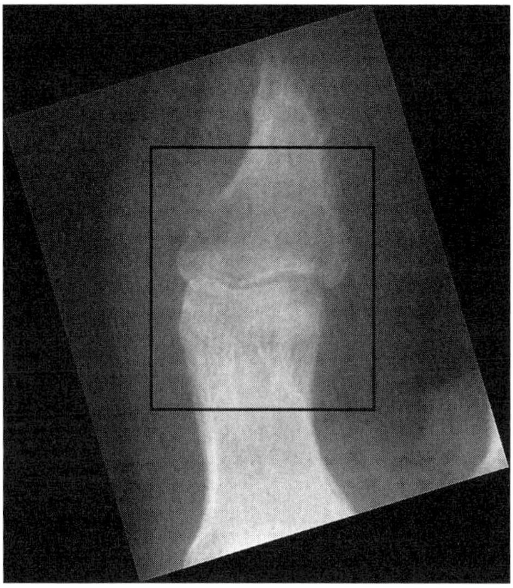

Fig. 6. Early osteomyelitis. Anteroposterior view of the hallux of the right foot demonstrating focal periarticular demineralization in the base of the distal phalanx and head of the proximal phalanx associated with distal interphalangeal joint space narrowing and overlying soft tissue swelling, consistent with septic arthritis and osteomyelitis (*rectangle*).

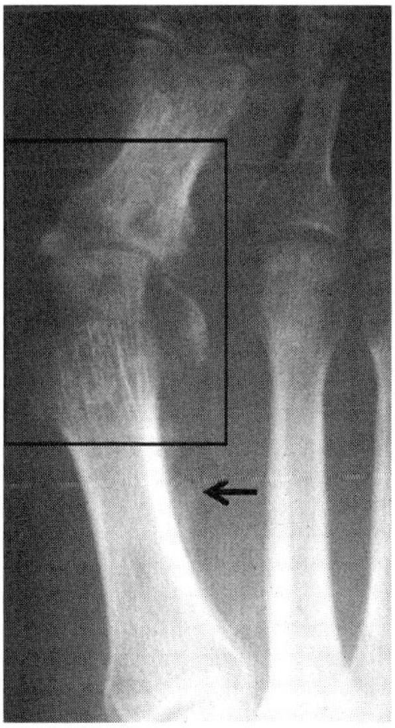

Fig. 7. Periostitis in a setting of subacute osteomyelitis. Anteroposterior view of the hallux demonstrating periostitis (*arrow*) about the metatarsal (*arrow*), with areas of cortical and trabecular bone destruction about the metatarsophalangeal joint (*rectangle*). (*From* Loredo R, Metter D. Imaging of the diabetic foot. Emphasis on nuclear medicine and magnetic resonance imaging. Clin Podiatr Med Surg 1997;14:241; with permission.)

Computed tomography

CT is associated with optimal spatial resolution. In comparison with plain films, CT offers improved three-dimensional understanding and much better tissue contrast. In comparison with plain films and MRI, CT is more sensitive and specific for the identification of subtle cortical erosions, small sequestra, foreign bodies, soft tissue gas, and calcification (Figs. 8–10) [6].

In the diagnosis of osteomyelitis or soft tissue abscess, CT may be used effectively. Compartmental anatomy can be well demonstrated, and early infection tends to involve the compartments that are adjacent to skin ulcers. Eventual extracompartmental involvement may be detected.

CT findings correlate well with the extent of infection; however, CT cannot contribute to the precise location of the boundary between normal and abnormal tissue [7]. At times, CT does not provide clear bone marrow visualization in the small bones of the feet due to beam-hardening artifact caused by the adjacent cortical bone [8]; however, the advancement of CT technology to multidetector capability has improved diagnostic image quality in the small bones of the feet (Fig. 11A).

Multidetector CT (MDCT) uses a two-dimensional array of detector elements that replace the linear array of detector elements used in typical CT scanners. The two-dimensional array permits CT scanners to acquire multiple slices or sections simultaneously. This capability greatly increases the speed of CT image acquisition and provides thin-slice images (<1 mm) with improved image resolution (Fig. 11B).

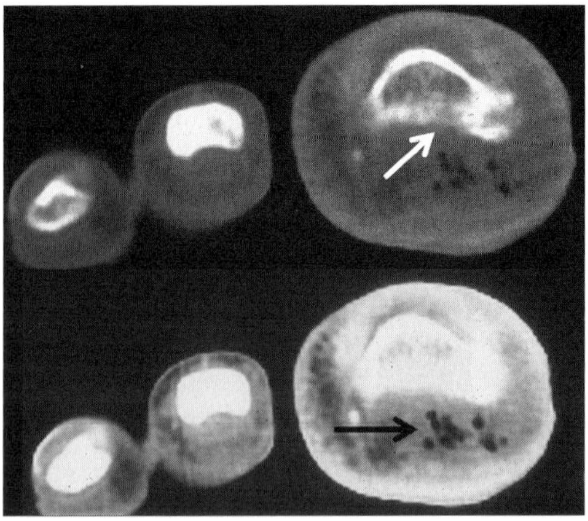

Fig. 8. Cortical changes and soft tissue gas. Bone window (*top*) and soft tissue window (*bottom*) axial CT images demonstrating small cortical erosion (*top arrow*) and soft tissue gas (*bottom arrow*) (*From* Loredo R, Metter D. Imaging of the diabetic foot. Emphasis on nuclear medicine and magnetic resonance imaging. Clin Podiatr Med Surg 1997;14:241; with permission.)

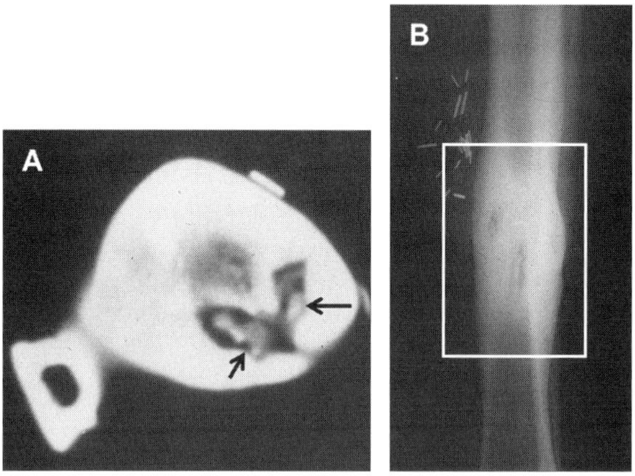

Fig. 9. Chronic osteomyelitis with multiple sequestra. (*A*) Axial CT scan demonstrating multiple sequestra (*arrows*). (*B*) Correlative lateral view of the tibia shows cortical thickening with sequestra formation (*rectangle*). (*From* Loredo R, Metter D. Imaging of the diabetic foot. Emphasis on nuclear medicine and magnetic resonance imaging. Clin Podiatr Med Surg 1997;14:241; with permission.)

Nuclear medicine

Nuclear medicine scintigraphy provides physiologic information and improved diagnostic sensitivity when compared with conventional radiography. Well-known procedures that are often used in evaluation of the diabetic foot include technetium 99m methylene diphosphonate bone scans, indium 111–labeled leukocyte scans, gallium 67 scintigraphy, and technetium 99m sulfur colloid studies [3,9,10]. These different studies vary in sensitivity and specificity. The ideal radionuclide method for localizing infection would entail only one study; however, multitracer studies have

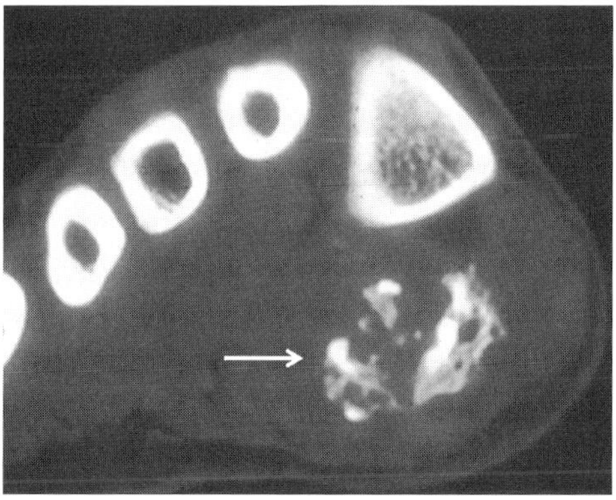

Fig. 10. Calcification in soft tissue. Axial CT scan characterizing mineralization in the plantar soft tissues of the foot (*arrow*) in a patient with a benign cartilaginous tumor.

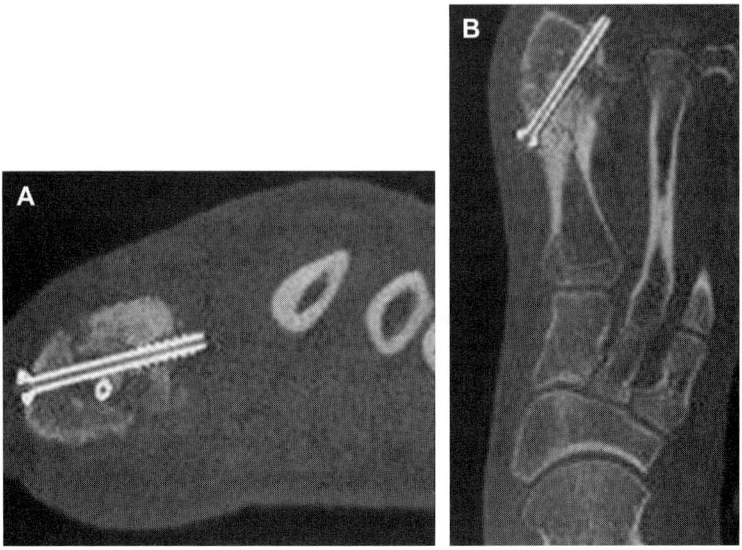

Fig. 11. MDCT images. (*A, B*) Axial and coronal foot MDCT images demonstrating superior image quality despite reconstruction of the coronal image from raw data.

been found to be more accurate than a single-tracer study, primarily due to improved specificity.

Technetium 99m methylene diphosphonate bone scan

In the diabetic foot, the bone scan is clinically invaluable in detecting and localizing abnormal bone with an accuracy of 90%, sensitivity of 94%, and specificity of 95% [11,12]. This modality is particularly notable for the diagnosis of osteomyelitis in nonviolated bone that has not been affected by underlying conditions. In complicated cases in which there is bone remodeling (neuroarthropathy, tumor, trauma, or surgery), this specificity is markedly reduced to 33% while the sensitivity remains high at 95% [12]. In a setting of osteomyelitis, within 48 to 72 hours following the onset of symptoms, a three-phase positive bone scan will demonstrate hyperemia in the first (angiographic, immediate, dynamic) phase, increased activity in the second (blood pool, static) phase, and increased focal uptake in the third (delayed, 3–4 hour bone) phase (Fig. 12A–C). Four-phase bone scan imaging (24 hour) is an additional method that has been used to enhance the specificity of the radionuclide diagnosis of osteomyelitis (Fig. 13A–C).

The principle of extending the three-phase study to the four-phase study is that, while the uptake of diphosphonates in normal bone ceases by 4 hours after tracer injection, the uptake in woven (immature) bone found in osteomyelitis continues for several hours [13]. In osteomyelitis, tracer uptake in infected bone should be greater at 24 hours (fourth phase) than at

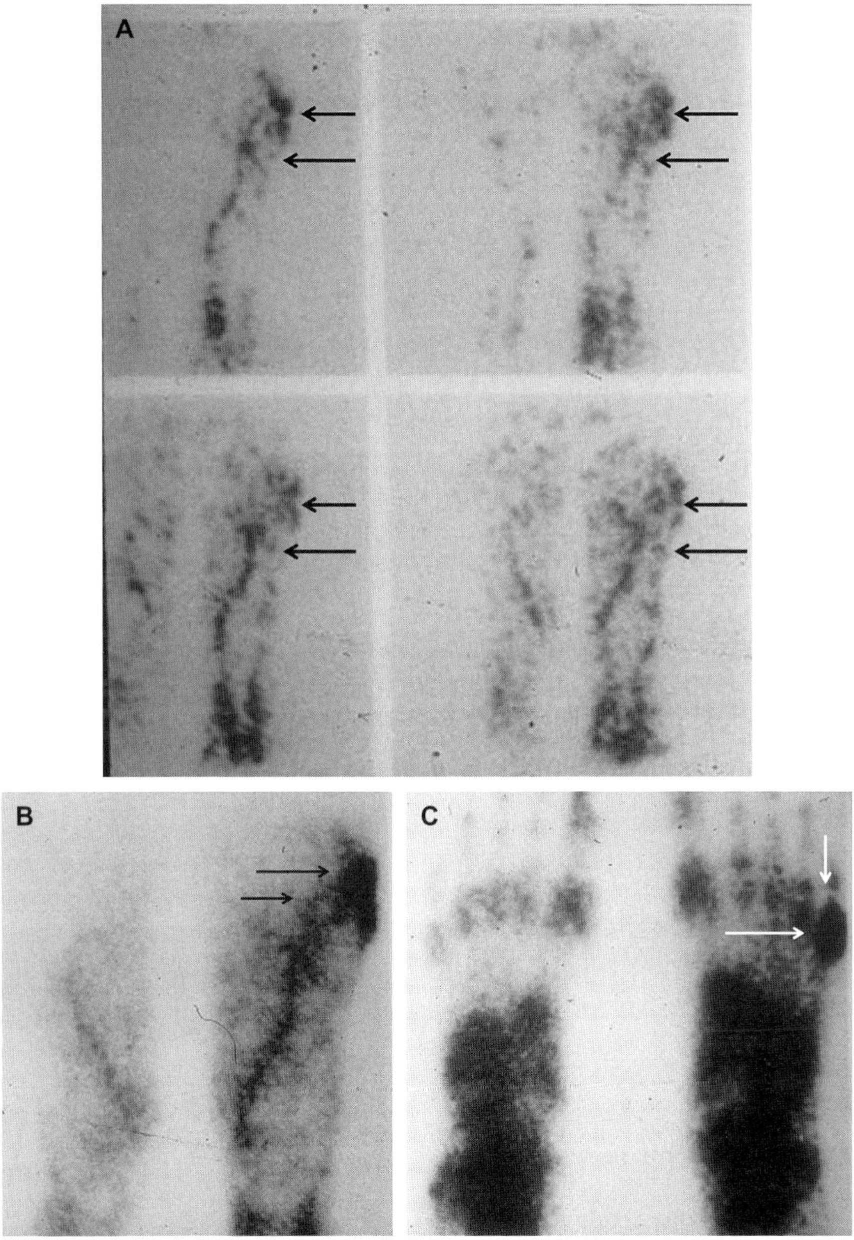

Fig. 12. A positive three-phase bone scan for osteomyelitis of the fifth metatarsal. (*A*) Initial dynamic phase showing asymmetric increased flow toward the lateral aspect of the right foot (*arrows*). (*B*) Second phase, blood pool image demonstrating increased uptake along the lateral foot (*arrows*). (*C*) Delayed phase showing persistent, more focal increased uptake in the fifth metatarsal, consistent with osteomyelitis (*arrows*).

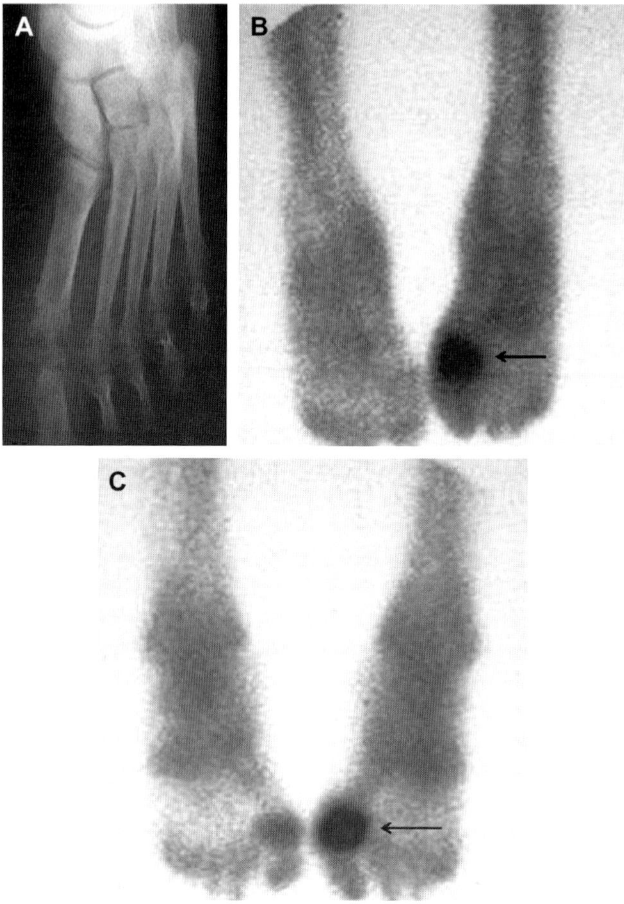

Fig. 13. Positive 24-hour bone scan for osteomyelitis of the hallux compared with 3-hour scan. (*A*) Anteroposterior radiograph of the foot demonstrating osseous destruction of the hallux metatarsal head and adjacent proximal phalangeal base. (*B*) Third (3–4 hour) phase of bone scan showing abnormal uptake in the hallux (*arrow*). (*C*) The fourth (24-hour) phase shows increased target-to-background focal uptake in the symptomatic hallux (*arrow*). (*Courtesy of* Dr. Kamal Singh, WHMC, San Antonio, Texas.)

3 to 4 hours (third phase), thereby increasing the target-to-background ratio and the conspicuity of abnormal foci of increased activity. Nonetheless, the utility of fourth phase imaging in the diabetic foot is questioned. The extended fourth phase of the examination has been shown to be of value in the assessment of osteomyelitis in patients with peripheral vascular disease [14]; however, more recently, Tronco and colleagues [13] showed that, although it is more specific than three-phase imaging and visual interpretation of the fourth phase of bone scans, the accuracy of a semiquantitative four-phase study was well below the 85% to 90% reported for dual-tracer studies

such as combined labeled leukocyte scans and bone scans and combined labeled leukocyte scans and sulfur colloid marrow scans. In this latter study, they concluded that the four-phase imaging procedure had no role in the radionuclide evaluation of osteomyelitis.

In a patient who has cellulitis (versus osteomyelitis), the bone scan demonstrates increased flow during the first (angiographic) phase and in the second (blood pool) phase. On the delayed third phase, the increased soft tissue activity (hyperemia) in a setting of cellulitis clears owing to renal excretion of the tracer. In cases complicated by neuroarthropathy, tumor, trauma, or surgery, the bone scan alone can give significant false-positive results, and supplemental imaging with radiolabeled leukocyte studies can aid in improving diagnostic specificity.

Indium 111 oxine leukocyte scan and Technetium 99m hexamethylpropyleneamine oxime leukocyte scan

Indium 111 leukocyte scintigraphy and technetium 99m leukocyte scintigraphy have proven to be clinically useful for diagnosing infections, especially in patients who have bone or joint involvement [15]. The superiority of labeled leukocytes resides in the ability to detect infection at sites of bone remodeling with an accuracy of approximately 80% in cases of diabetic pedal osteomyelitis [16]. The clinical indications for white blood cell scintigraphy are fever of unknown origin, the postoperative patient (>2 weeks) with fever, osteomyelitis (other than vertebral), diabetic foot infection, and vascular graft infection (Fig. 14A–C). There are several disadvantages of indium 111 leukocyte labeling. It is expensive; the radionuclide is not always readily available; the procedure of cell labeling may take up to 2.5 hours; there is a risk of handling blood products; and the lengthy total examination time is 24 hours. False-positive results are described in the setting of recent fracture, recent surgery, acute arthritis, neuropathic joints, and in metastatic carcinoma [7].

Clinical studies with technetium 99m hexamethylpropyleneamine oxime (HMPAO) leukocyte scanning have found the overall accuracy for the detection of infection to be similar to that of indium 111 leukocyte studies. The advantages of technetium 99m HMPAO studies are faster imaging (within 2 hours), higher energy photons for better images, the ability to perform single-photon emission CT (SPECT) imaging to increase contrast resolution (optimal in the feet and hands), and a lower dose to the spleen. The findings are similar to those of indium 111 leukocyte scans [17].

Indium 111 oxine leukocytes localize in predominantly neutrophil-mediated inflammatory processes such as bacterial infection within bone marrow. Some difficulty remains in separating bone and soft tissue infection; however, one study has demonstrated high sensitivity and specificity of indium 111 leukocytes in a small group of patients with neuropathic joint disease [9].

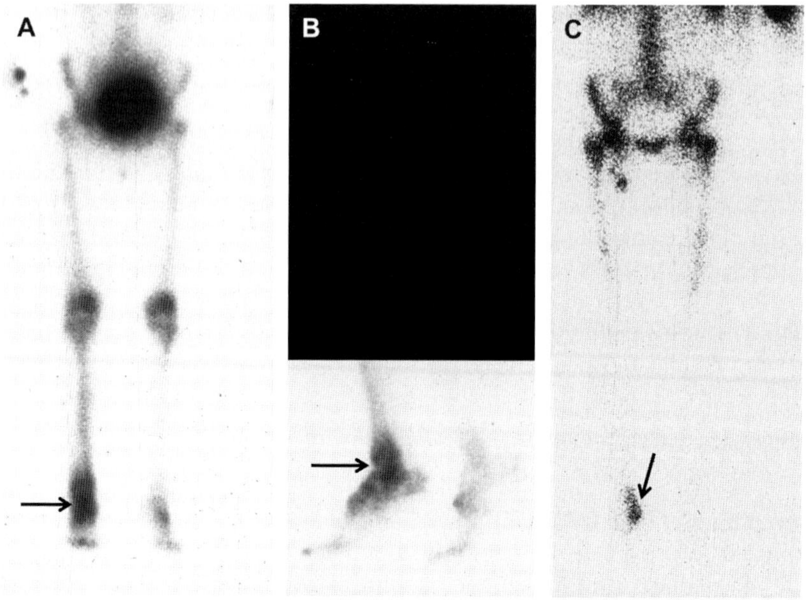

Fig. 14. Dual-study (technetium 99m bone scan and indium 111 white blood cell scan) evaluation of osteomyelitis. (*A, B*) Three-phase bone scan images showing uptake within the right ankle (*arrows*). (*C*) Indium 111 white blood cell scan shows more focal uptake at the medial malleolus (*arrow*). (*From* Loredo R, Metter D. Imaging of the diabetic foot. Emphasis on nuclear medicine and magnetic resonance imaging. Clin Podiatr Med Surg 1997;14:241; with permission.)

Technetium 99m sulfur colloid bone marrow scan

A combined evaluation using leukocyte scintigraphy and bone marrow imaging has been shown to be useful in diagnosing osteomyelitis in patients with underlying neuroarthropathy [10]. Sites of infection incite uptake of labeled leukocytes and by the same mechanism will displace or infarct normal marrow elements, leading to reduced accumulation of the bone marrow scanning agent. On the nuclear medicine images, increased uptake of labeled leukocytes alone in the absence of a corresponding uptake of radiocolloid is consistent with infection. Technetium 99m sulfur colloid labeled bone marrow imaging combined with indium-labeled leukocyte imaging improves the accuracy of the diagnosis of osteomyelitis in the diabetic foot and its differentiation from cellulitis. The sensitivity of this combination is 92%, with a specificity of 100% [10].

Gallium 67 citrate scan

Gallium 67 imaging in combination with bone scintigraphy is occasionally used. The addition of a gallium scan has been shown to increase specificity, although the diagnostic accuracy is not usually high. The diminished accuracy is possibly related to false-positive results secondary to recent bone fractures or neuroarthropathy.

Although there is evidence that gallium 67 uptake can be seen in areas of sterile bone remodeling and neuropathic change, this radiopharmaceutical is sensitive in the detection of osteomyelitis, particularly acute exacerbation of chronic osteomyelitis [18]. Assessment of the gallium 67 study necessitates a comparison of the distribution and the intensity of uptake with that seen on the preceding technetium 99m bone scan. If the gallium 67 scan is normal, osteomyelitis can be excluded [19]. When the gallium 67 uptake is more intense and focal than that seen on the bone scan, there is an increased likelihood of bone infection [20]. In acute osteomyelitis, bone scans and gallium 67 scans have been used to monitor the response to therapy [21]. A gallium 67 study is associated with added cost, additional radiation exposure, and extended time (48 hours) before completion of the study. It can be useful in unraveling the diagnostic problems associated with the diabetic foot; however, it should be reserved for patients in whom there is a high clinical suspicion of disease not clearly defined by the standard bone scan (Fig. 15A–C) [20].

Nuclear medicine studies on the horizon

The primary nuclear medicine method of detection of infection is indium 111 leukocyte scans; however, due to the limitations associated with indium 111 use (less availability, high cost, lengthy ex vivo cell labeling procedure, and false-positive results), other methods for the detection of infection have been studied. Antibody labeling [22,23], labeling of recombinant human interleukin-8 [24], and the use of combined SPECT studies and CT imaging [25] have been investigated.

An alternative technique of white blood cell scintigraphy involves antigranulocyte Fab' fragment antibody in vivo scintigraphy (LeukoScan, Sulesomab). This study has been shown to be effective in diagnosing infection

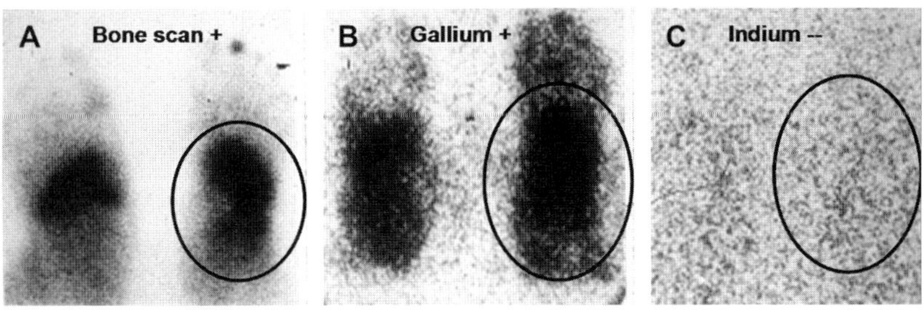

Fig. 15. Triple-study examination in a patient with a history of neuropathic changes and suspicion of osteomyelitis in the foot. (*A*) Three-phase bone scan demonstrating positive uptake in the symptomatic foot (*circled*). (*B*) Gallium scan showing positive uptake with questionable wider distribution in the same region (*circle*). (*C*) Indium scan showing no abnormal uptake (*circled area*), consistent with a negative study. The diagnosis is a Charcot joint. (*Courtesy of* Dr. Darlene Metter, UTHSC, San Antonio, Texas.)

[26]. A review of the literature shows that, in general, the results in detecting osteomyelitis obtained with LeukoScan (Sulesomab) scintigraphy produce a sensitivity and specificity comparable with that of ex vivo labeled leukocytes [27–31]. It is a fast and simple examination that is promoted for the ease of labeling, no ex vivo handling of blood, low radiation, and the provision of a rapid diagnosis [26]. Unfortunately, this type of white blood cell imaging is not yet available for clinical use in the United States.

Fluorine 18 fluorodeoxyglucose (FDG) positron emission tomography (PET) is currently used as a valuable clinical tool for assessing malignancies and for cardiac and brain imaging; however, fluorine 18 FDG is a nonspecific tracer of increased intracellular glucose metabolism and it accumulates in sites of infection and inflammation as well. The hybrid PET-CT technology provides precise registration of metabolic and structural imaging data obtained in the same session on a single device and may improve the diagnosis and localization of infection. Fluorine 18 FDG leukocyte PET-CT scanning is an additional method of imaging infection that is on the horizon [32]. Two recent investigations into the use of PET-CT imaging combined with leukocyte radiolabeling have been conducted using diabetic patient populations in Israel and Belgium. Both studies found that fluorine 18 FDG PET could be used for investigation of diabetic wounds and diagnosis of diabetes-related infection (Fig. 16A–D). The conclusion in both studies was that the precise anatomic localization of increased fluorine 18 FDG uptake provided by PET-CT enabled accurate differentiation between osteomyelitis and soft tissue infection [32,33].

The problem is that fluorine 18 FDG PET is expensive and not yet approved by Medicare as a reimbursable diagnostic test for the evaluation of infection. It is successfully used for the detection of prosthetic infection but is not yet reimbursable for this use either. Medicare reimburses PET studies according to a certain list of disorders, and infection is not yet on the list. Nonetheless, the study may be approved for use in the detection of infection on a case-by-case basis when a physician makes a special request for approval and can show that the condition is not adequately demonstrated by any other radiologic test or nuclear medicine test.

Magnetic resonance imaging

MRI has been advocated in the evaluation of the diabetic foot because it offers excellent anatomic detail and visualization of bone marrow, superior soft tissue contrast, and multiplanar imaging capability. MRI has been shown to have high sensitivity and specificity in the detection of osteomyelitis in diabetic patients [34].

MRI techniques usually include T1-weighted and T2-weighted (fluid-sensitive) sequences in multiple planes with the addition of a gadolinium-enhanced T1-weighted sequence when investigating infection or neoplasms. T1-weighted and T2-weighted images provide a combination of excellent

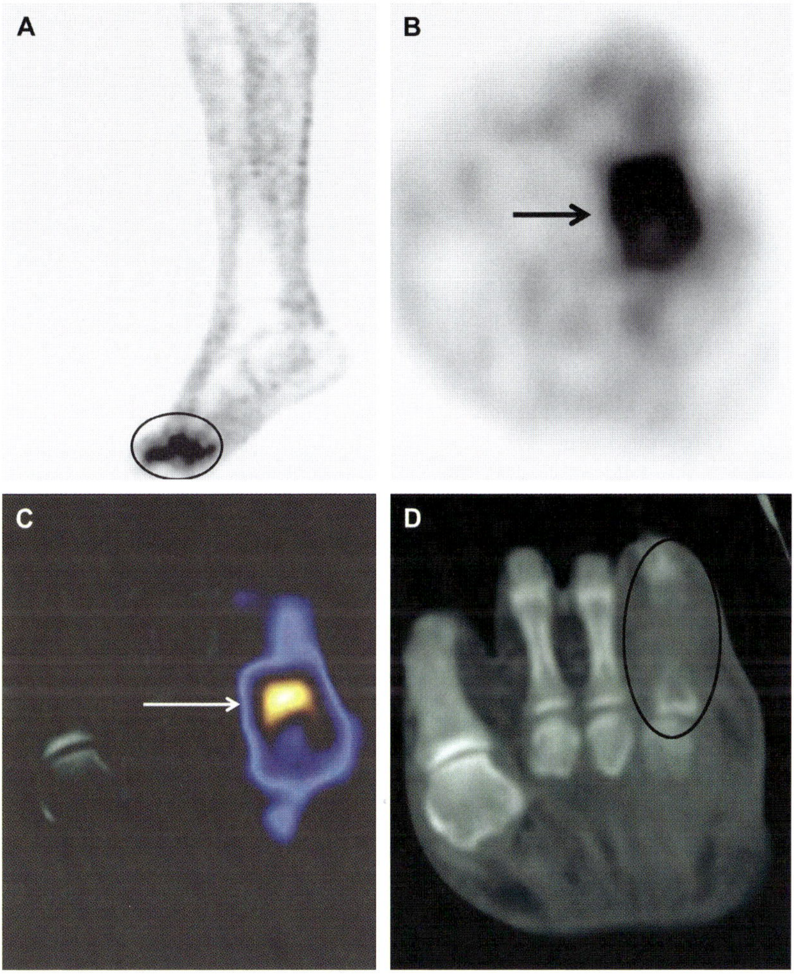

Fig. 16. PET-CT leukocyte-labeled imaging of osteomyelitis in a diabetic foot of a 50-year-old man with a nonhealing forefoot wound. (*A, B*) Fluorine 18 FDG sagittal and axial PET images showing an area of increased uptake in the forefoot (*circle*) that is lateral in location (*arrow*). (*C*) PET-CT fluorine 18 FDG leukocyte-labeled image localizing abnormal uptake in the region of the head of the fourth proximal phalanx (*arrow*). (*D*) Traditional CT image showing destruction of bone in the corresponding area (*circle*). (*Adapted from* Reidar Z, Militianu D, Melamed E, et al. The diabetic foot: initial experience with F-18-FDG PET/CT. J Nucl Med 2005;46(3):447; with permission.)

anatomic detail and demonstrate areas of abnormal signal intensity in bone marrow and soft tissue. Short tau inversion recovery (STIR) images are sensitive in the detection of subtle water changes in the marrow caused by osteomyelitis [34]. In diabetic pedal abnormalities, MRI has the ability to reveal numerous pathologic processes that are not detectable or are not as obvious with other imaging methods.

Soft tissue problems

Diffuse high T2-weighted (or STIR) signal intensity related to edema in the soft tissues is one of the most frequent positive findings when imaging the diabetic foot [5]. The edema most frequently involves the plantar foot and less frequently involves the dorsal subcutaneous soft tissues [5]. In the absence of infection, edema may be secondary to vascular insufficiency or peripheral neuropathy alone versus a combined effect of these common problems. With clinically suspected soft tissue infection, the presence of edema is nonspecific and cannot be differentiated from cellulitis by MRI alone. Areas of cellulitis enhance in a diffuse pattern. At times, focal cellulitis may be seen as abnormal signal intensity tracking from an ulcer or a region of osteomyelitis (Fig. 17A, B).

High T2-weighted signal intensity in the deep soft tissues may be secondary to inflammation, infection, neuropathy, or vascular insufficiency. Pyomyositis is seen as muscular high T2-weighted signal intensity related to edema and inflammation with small areas of intramuscular rim enhancement following intravenous gadolinium. An abscess may be distinguished from edema or focal cellulitis because of its smooth margin, focal higher/brighter T2-weighted signal intensity (pus) than the surrounding edema, and rim enhancement (wall enhances) following administration of intravenous gadolinium contrast (Fig. 18). MRI may be beneficial in the presurgical evaluation of patients with known or suspected multifocal abscesses

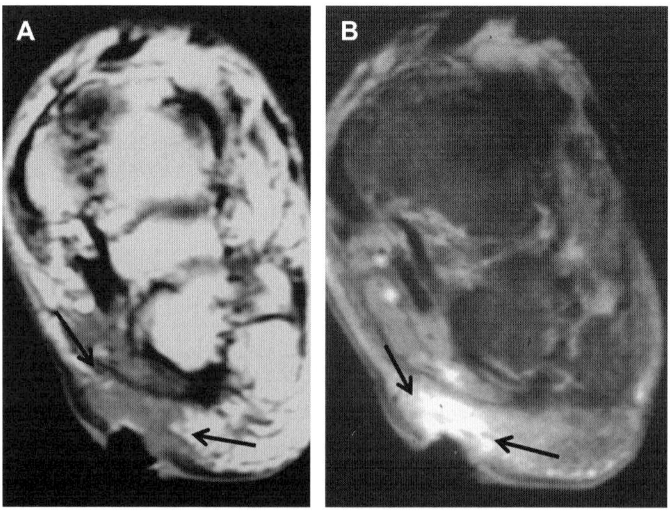

Fig. 17. Focal cellulitis extending from a plantar ulcer. (*A*) Focal intermediate signal intensity is seen adjacent to the ulcer on an axial T1-weighted MR image (*arrows*). (*B*) The corresponding T1-weighted image, following administration of gadolinium, shows high signal intensity enhancement in the area of inflammation (*arrows*).

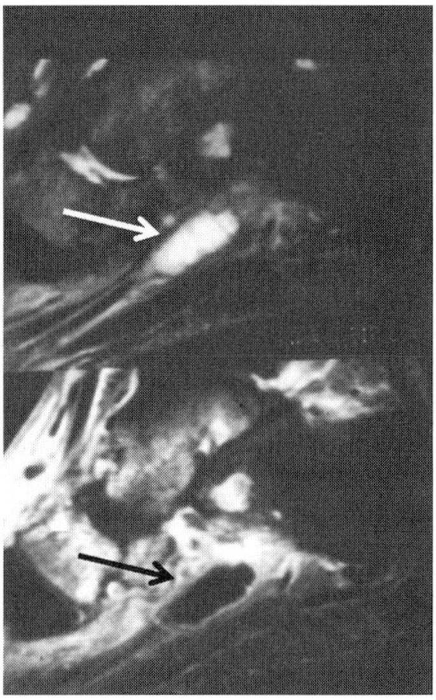

Fig. 18. A soft tissue abscess within the plantar foot. Fat-suppressed sagittal T2-weighted (*top*) and T1-weighted post intravenous contrast (*bottom*) MR images demonstrating focal high T2-weighted signal intensity (*arrow*) and post contrast wall enhancement (*arrow*) without central enhancement of pus. (*Courtesy of* Dr. William B. Morrison, Jefferson University, Philadelphia, PA). (*From* Loredo R, Metter D. Imaging of the diabetic foot. Emphasis on nuclear medicine and magnetic resonance imaging. Clin Podiatr Med Surg 1997;14:241; with permission.)

because it provides information regarding the precise location and number of collections (Fig. 19) [35].

A sinus tract may appear as low signal intensity on a T1-weighted image with high T2-weighted signal intensity in the tract with enhancement of the wall of the tract following administration of intravenous gadolinium (Fig. 20A, B).

One other localized soft tissue problem is fluid within tendon sheaths. A small quantity of fluid in a tendon sheath is frequently observed and nonspecific. Infected tenosynovitis may be suspected if there is gross distention or abnormal signal intensity in or about a tendon sheath (Fig. 20B) located adjacent to an ulceration, or if other clinical signs of an infection exist. In general, infected fluid cannot be distinguished from uninfected fluid with MRI because both appear as high T2-weighted signal intensity.

Bone and joint infection

Small joint effusions are common in diabetic patients and may be present with or without infection, perhaps as a manifestation of peripheral neuropathy [5,34]. The most common clinical request for MRI in the diabetic patient is related to the detection of osteomyelitis. MRI evaluation may be requested as a search for undiagnosed disease or as documentation of

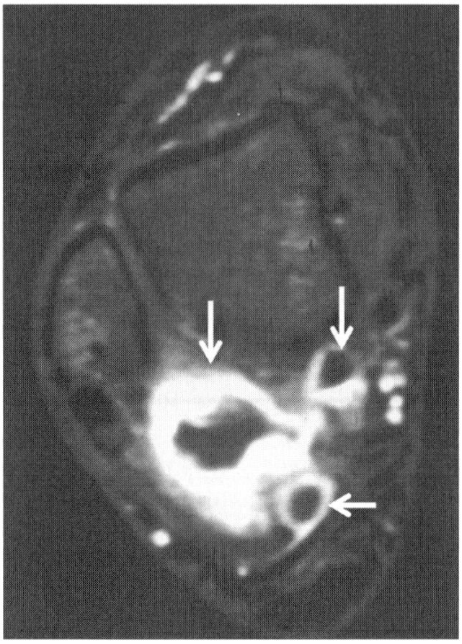

Fig. 19. Multiple rim-enhancing abscesses within the posterior preachilles region. Axial T1-weighted, fat-suppressed MR image post contrast demonstrating three abscess collections (*arrows*). (*Courtesy of* William B. Morrison, MD, Philadelphia, PA). (*Adapted from* Harkless, editor. Clin Podiatr Med Surg 1997;14(2):258; with permission.)

healing or progression of infection. Owing to the excellent soft tissue contrast and anatomic detail afforded by MRI, a separation of soft tissue edema or fluid collections from underlying osseous infection is possible, particularly with the use of intravenous gadolinium. On the MR images, osteomyelitis appears as decreased T1-weighted signal intensity and increased T2-weighted signal intensity within the intramedullary space with enhancement of the infected region (Fig. 21A–C). The literature shows that the resection of infected bone, as demonstrated by MRI, leads to healing [36]; hence, foot-sparing surgery is made possible. Intravenous administration of gadolinium improves the specificity of MRI, allowing for the identification of intraosseous abscesses (Fig. 22A, B) and sequestra. Unfortunately, postsurgical changes, trauma, and adjacent septic arthritis can cause false-positive results [37,38].

Morrison and colleagues [39] evaluated the clinical accuracy, surgical utility, and cost-effectiveness of MRI of diabetic feet in the evaluation of osteomyelitis. Comparisons were made among contrast-enhanced MRI, three-phase technetium 99m methylene diphosphonate bone scans, gallium 67 scans, and indium 111 leukocyte scans. With MRI, there was comparatively good sensitivity and specificity, with rates of 82% and 80%, respectively, in diabetic patients and 89% and 94%, respectively, in non-diabetic patients. Using cost analysis techniques, they found that MRI was competitively priced when one takes into account the high costs associated with

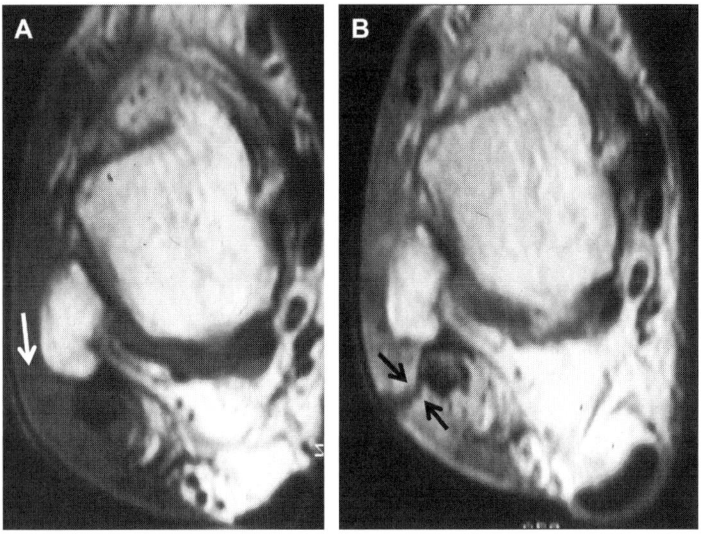

Fig. 20. Sinus tract with enhancing wall. (*A*) Axial T1-weighted MR image showing low signal intensity in the lateral superficial soft tissues and encircling the peroneal tendons (*arrow*). (*B*) Axial T1-weighted contrast-enhanced image illustrating enhancement of the wall of the sinus tract (*arrows*) and the adjacent infected sheath of the thickened, disrupted peroneal tendons. (*From* Loredo R, Metter D. Imaging of the diabetic foot. Emphasis on nuclear medicine and magnetic resonance imaging. Clin Podiatr Med Surg 1997;14:241; with permission.)

multistudy preoperative scintigraphy, costs that are related to the combined cost of multiple studies and the additional days of preoperative hospitalization required for the performance of the tests [39].

Neuroarthropathy

The changes of acute or rapidly progressive neuroarthropathy are observed as osseous inhomogeneous low T1-weighted signal intensity and high T2-weighted signal intensity, often observed in the tarsus and proximal metatarsus. Frequently, the areas of involvement are some distance from ulcers or other sites of infection such as abscesses or sinus tracts. The soft tissue about the osseous neuropathic region demonstrates little or no abnormal signal intensity on the T2-weighted images, less signal intensity than may be seen in cellulitis and osteomyelitis (Fig. 23A–D) [3].

As neuroarthropathy progresses, multiple fractures and dislocations result in complete collapse of the longitudinal and transverse arches. Even in the absence of infection, there may be scattered areas of abnormal bone marrow signal intensity, loss of the normal foot architecture, and gross bone fragmentation (Fig. 23) [3]. Nevertheless, the bone marrow signal intensity and amount of surrounding abnormal soft tissue signal intensity

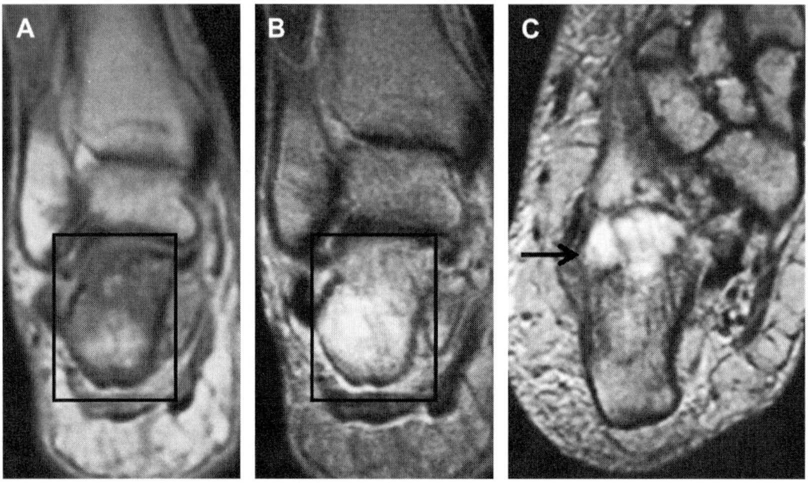

Fig. 21. Osteomyelitis of the calcaneus. (*A, B*) Coronal T1-weighted and T2-weighted MR images demonstrating low and high marrow signal intensity (*rectangles*). (*C*) Following administration of intravenous gadolinium contrast, the corresponding axial T1-weighted image showing abnormal calcaneal enhancement (*arrow*). (*Courtesy of* Dr. Robert Daehler, San Antonio, Texas.)

should be less in the neuropathic joint than in the infected one. Chronic neuroarthropathy may demonstrate ununited fractures with low signal intensity fracture lines and adjacent normal or mildly increased T2-weighted marrow signal intensity [3].

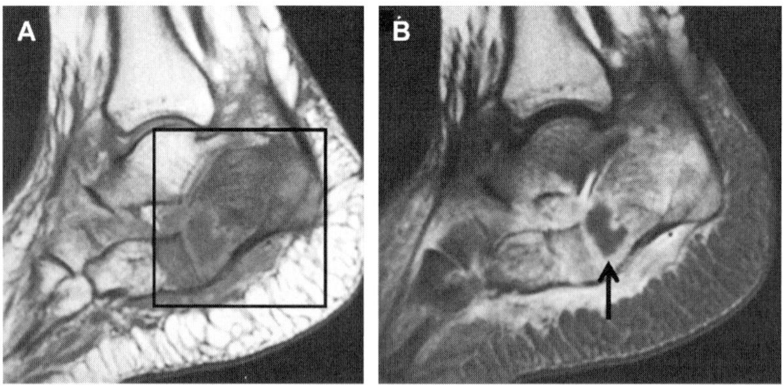

Fig. 22. Intraosseous calcaneal abscess. (*A*) T1-weighted sagittal MR image illustrating low calcaneal marrow signal intensity (*square box*). (*B*) Corresponding T1-weighted image after intravenous gadolinium contrast showing focal rim enhancement of the abscess (*arrow*) and marked surrounding marrow and soft tissue enhancement in areas of inflammation. (*Courtesy of* Dr. Robert Daehler, San Antonio, Texas.)

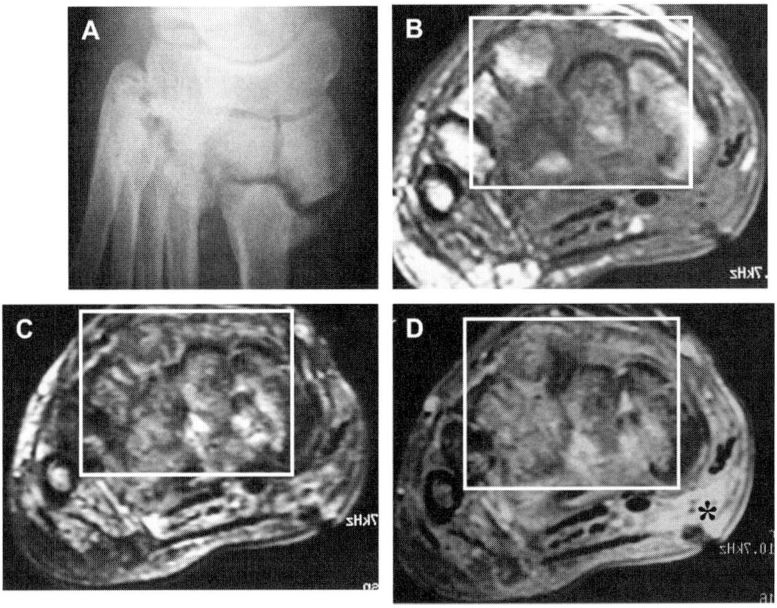

Fig. 23. Neuroarthropathy. (*A*) Anteroposterior view of the midfoot and proximal metatarsus showing the degree of neuroarthropathic changes and Lisfranc dislocation. (*B*) T1-weighted axial MR image demonstrating low signal intensity marrow within the cuneiforms (*rectangle*). (*C, D*) Fat-suppressed, T2-weighted and T1-weighted images, post intravenous contrast, showing only mildly increased marrow signal intensity and enhancement, respectively (*rectangle*). The increase in signal intensity on the latter sequences is even less than the adjacent focal cellulitis (*) about a plantar ulcer.

Posterior tibialis dysfunction

Posterior tibialis tendon dysfunction (PTTD) is the most common cause of acquired flatfoot deformity in adults [40]. The condition can be attributed to ischemic and mechanical factors [41].

On plain radiographs, posterior tibialis tendon failure is best illustrated by analyzing weight-bearing and non–weight-bearing lateral radiographs of the foot. The weight-bearing images will show collapse of the midfoot with the talar head plantar flexed in relation to the midfoot (Fig. 24). MRI is used to evaluate the integrity of tendon tissue. The axial plane is the most accurate for evaluating posterior tibialis tendon pathology [42]. The normal posterior tibialis tendon is dark in signal intensity on all the sequences and should be no larger than twice the size of the adjacent flexor digitorum longus and flexor hallucis longus tendons. Tendon disease or tendinopathy, whether ischemic or mechanical, can be manifested on MRI as increased T1- and T2-weighted signal intensity within the tendon, a change in tendon size, or fluid in the tendon sheath

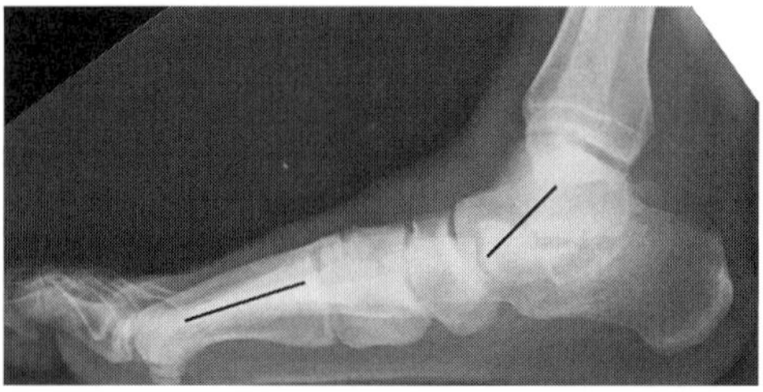

Fig. 24. Midfoot collapse with posterior tibialis dysfunction. Lateral radiograph demonstrating midfoot collapse with plantar flexed talus.

(Fig. 25A, B). One must closely scrutinize the tendon at the level of the medial malleolus and just proximal to the navicular insertion for the changes described, as these are the typical locations for PTT lesions to occur.

In conjunction with a thorough physical examination, lateral weight-bearing radiographs of the foot along with MRI can markedly increase the diagnostic accuracy for posterior tibialis tendon disorders. Undetected and untreated dysfunction often results in total collapse of the longitudinal arch and severe osteoarthritis of the ankle or hindfoot [40].

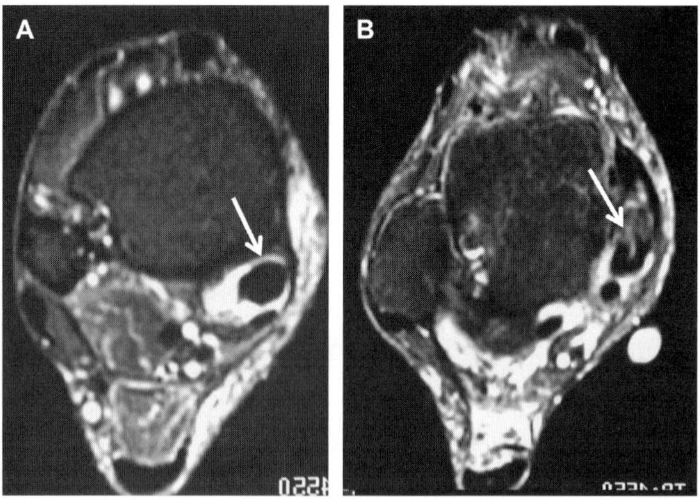

Fig. 25. Posterior tibialis tendon tenosynovitis and tear. (*A*) Axial fat-suppressed, T2-weighted MR image above the medial malleolus illustrating an enlarged posterior tibialis tendon (*arrow*) with increased synovial sheath high signal intensity fluid (tenosynovitis). (*B*) Axial image showing tendon disruption (*arrow*) just beneath the medial malleolus.

Surgical changes

Knowledge of any previous surgical, traumatic, or iatrogenic manipulation is essential information when interpreting MR images of a diabetic patient's foot. Amputation sites are prone to ulcer formation and infection. MR images can be useful in documenting the progression of disease or healing of these postoperative complications. The differentiation between osteomyelitis and cellulitis at an amputation site can be extremely difficult; however, gadolinium enhancement of the bone marrow in osteomyelitis assists in making the distinction.

Ultrasonography

Ultrasonography can provide structural and functional information in the diabetic foot. Imaging with ultrasound is operator dependent; however, radiologists, technologists, and even non-radiology clinicians are becoming competent in imaging the extremities. Ultrasonography is noninvasive, involves no ionizing radiation, and is generally well tolerated by patients. Structural information comes from gray-scale imaging. Functional information is initially derived from the dynamic evaluation of structures during motion and secondly from Doppler evaluation of the vasculature and vascularity.

The use of high-frequency ultrasound transducers with frequencies in excess of 7 MHz allows evaluation of superficial structures. With respect to the foot, even the plantar musculature may be visualized. Ultrasound is excellent at differentiating fluid from solid structures/lesions and is therefore used for evaluating joint effusions, soft tissue fluid collections, and abscesses

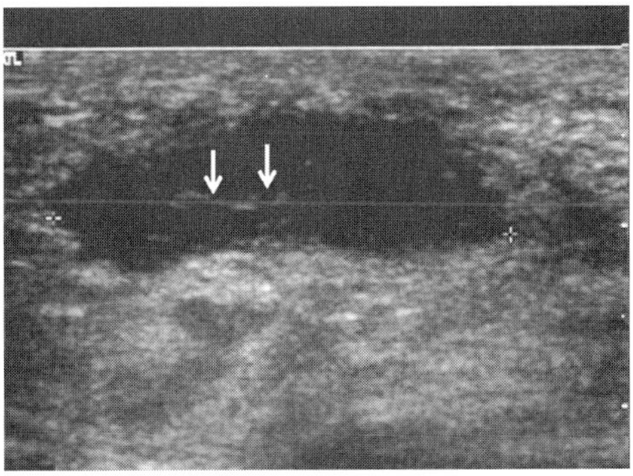

Fig. 26. Abscess in the plantar foot. A 12-MHz linear array transducer images a hypoechoic (dark) ill-defined lesion containing internal echoes (*arrows*), which demonstrate motion and swirling on compression. The uppermost aspect of the image represents the probe in contact with the skin surface. Note that the tissues deep to the abscess appear brighter, a phenomenon seen when imaging through a fluid-filled structure, confirming the fluid nature of the lesion.

without the need for contrast enhancement in CT and MRI. Sonography is reliably able to distinguish synovial hypertrophy from joint effusion and phlegmonous solid masses or granulation tissue from fluid collections. The appearance of simple fluid is characteristic and appears black on ultrasound imaging with an absence of echoes. Debris, internal particulate matter, or septations within a fluid collection are easily seen. Pus is characteristically fluid containing multiple internal echoes but is seen to move and swirl on compression and is also reliably diagnosed with ultrasound (Fig. 26).

The soft tissues may be evaluated from the level of the superficial skin to the deep bone. The tendons are better seen at the level of the ankle by sonography than by any other imaging modality. The fibrillar tendinous structure is easily seen, and evaluation of the echotexture of the tendon together with its size will provide an accurate assessment of tendinosis (Fig. 27) and tendon tears, both partial and complete. Intrasubstance partial tendon disruption is difficult to distinguish from tendinosis on sonography; however, this observation is no different from the findings in other cross-sectional imaging modalities, including CT and MRI. Sonography is more sensitive at detecting these tendon pathologies than the other modalities. Complete tendon tears are also well evaluated, and the end of

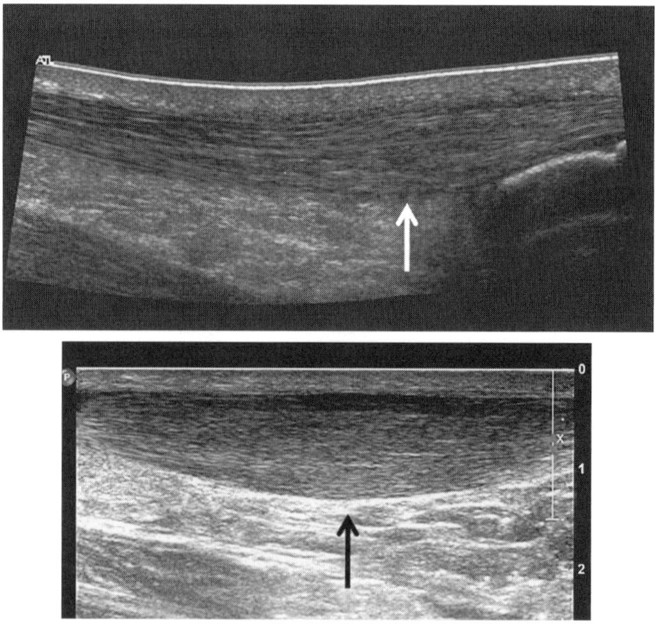

Fig. 27. Achilles tendinosis in two patients. Longitudinal sagittal views showing distal (*top*) Achilles tendon fusiform thickening (*arrow*) at the calcaneal insertion and more proximal (*bottom*) fusiform thickening (*arrow*). The normal Achilles tendon should be seen as a straplike structure of uniform thickness.

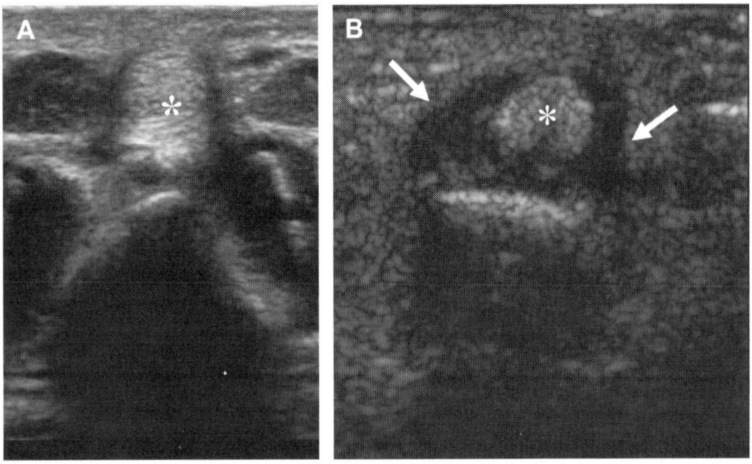

Fig. 28. Tenosynovitis and synovial hypertrophy. (*A*) Image on left demonstrates a normal flexor tendon in axial section using a linear array 12-MHz transducer. The tendon (*asterisk*) appears uniformly echogenic and has no surrounding synovial hypertrophy or soft tissue edema. (*B*) Image on the right demonstrating marked tenosynovitis with a central echogenic tendon (*asterisk*) surrounded by a halo of hypoechoic material (*arrows*) representing edematous and thickened synovium.

a retracted tendon can be located and marked before operative intervention. The tibialis posterior and peroneus longus tendons become more difficult to visualize as they pass more distal to the navicular bone and the inferolateral cuboid margin, respectively. The ability to dynamically assess tendons by passive and active movements during imaging allows for a reliable assessment of tendon integrity. Tendon subluxation is best evaluated using sonography. The static location of tendons may be imaged and tendon motion may be evaluated by performing provocative maneuvers. Sonographic imaging may be recorded as a series of static images and as cine movies, allowing effective documentation of such dynamic pathologies. Tenosynovitis is well visualized, and, as is true for other areas of synovial hypertrophy (Fig. 28A, B), the vascularity of the synovium may be evaluated by use of Doppler sonography.

Summary

This article has focused on the utility of multiple diagnostic modalities that are available and beneficial for imaging of the diabetic foot. There is not yet "one best test" for sorting out the diagnostic dilemmas that are commonly encountered. Confirmation or exclusion of the frequent diagnosis of osteomyelitis often requires multiple studies, which are complementary. Understanding the utility of these studies is important if one is to plan and accomplish foot-sparing surgery when necessary.

Acknowledgments

The authors thank Dr. Darlene Metter, Associate Professor of Radiology, University of Texas Health Science Center (UTHSC), San Antonio, Texas, for her expert guidance regarding nuclear medicine imaging and her literary proficiency; Dr. Umber A. Salman, Assistant Professor of Radiology, UTHSC, San Antonio, Texas, for her expert guidance regarding nuclear medicine imaging; and Patricio Hernandez, Jr., for his patience and assistance with the preparation of this manuscript.

References

[1] Resnick D. Disorders of other endocrine glands and of pregnancy. In: Resnick D, Niwayama G, editors. Diagnosis of bone and joint disorders. 2nd edition. Philadelphia: WB Saunders; 1988. p. 2292–317.

[2] Zlatkin MB, Pathria M, Sartoris DJ, et al. The diabetic foot. Radiol Clin North Am 1987;25: 1095–105.

[3] Moore TE, Yuh WTC. Magnetic resonance imaging of the diabetic foot. In: Bloem JL, Sartoris DJ, editors. MRI and CT of the musculoskeletal system, a text-atlas. Baltimore (MD): Williams & Wilkins; 1992. p. 207–16.

[4] Nguyen VD. The radiologic spectrum of abnormalities of the foot in diabetic patients. Can Assoc Radiol J 1992;43:333–9.

[5] Moore TE, Yuh WTC, Kathol MH, et al. Abnormalities of the foot in patients with diabetes mellitus: findings on MR imaging. AJR Am J Roentgenol 1991;157:813–6.

[6] Murphy WA, Totty WG, Destouet JM, et al. Musculoskeletal system. In: Lee JKT, Sagel SS, Stanley RJ, editors. Computed body tomography with MRI correlation. New York: Raven Press; 1989. p. 899–987.

[7] Abreu SH. Skeletal uptake of indium-111 labeled white blood cells. Semin Nucl Med 1989; 19:152–5.

[8] Spaeth HJ, Dardani M. Magnetic resonance imaging of the diabetic foot. Magn Reson Imaging Clin N Am 1994;2(1):123–30.

[9] Maurer AH, Millmond SH, et al. Infection in diabetic osteoarthropathy: use of indium-labeled leukocytes for diagnosis. Radiology 1986;161:221–5.

[10] Palestro CJ, Mehta HH, Patel M, et al. Marrow versus infection in the Charcot joint: indium-111 leukocyte and technetium-99m sulfur colloid scintigraphy. J Nucl Med 1998;39: 346–50.

[11] Love C, Din AS, Tomas MB, et al. Radionuclide bone imaging: an illustrative review-1. Radiographics 2003;23:341–58.

[12] Schauwecker DS. The scintigraphic diagnosis of osteomyelitis. AJR 1992;158:9–18.

[13] Tronco G, Tomas MB, Palestro CJ. Four-phase bone scintigraphy and osteomyelitis: a reevaluation. Clin Nucl Med 1999;24(3):216.

[14] Alazraki N, Dries D, Datz F, et al. Value of a 24-hour (four-phase bone scan) in assessing osteomyelitis in patients with peripheral vascular disease. J Nucl Med 1985;26:711–7.

[15] Devillers A, Miosan A, Jean S, et al. Tecnetium-99m-HMPAO leukocyte scintigraphy for the diagnosis of bone and joint infections: a retrospective study in 116 patients. Eur J Nucl Med 1995;22:302–7.

[16] Palestro CJ, Tomas MB. Scintigraphic evaluation of the diabetic foot. In: Freeman LM, editor. Nuclear medicine annual 2000. Philadelphia: Lippincott Williams & Wilkins; 2000. p. 143–72.

[17] Ziessman H, O'Malley JP, Thrall JH. Infection and inflammation. In: Ziessman H, editor. Nuclear medicine—the requisites in radiology. Philadelphia: Elsevier Mosby; 2006. p. 384–418.
[18] Graham GD, Lundy NM, Fredrick FJ, et al. Scintigraphic detection of osteomyelitis with Tc-99m MDP and Ga-67 citrate. J Nucl Med 1983;24:1019–22.
[19] Datz FL, Patch GG, Arias JM, et al. Skeletal. In: Scott J, editor. Nuclear medicine teaching file. St. Louis (MO): Mosby; 1992. p. 21–58, 189, 206.
[20] Van der Wall H. Assessment of infection. In: Murray IPC, Ell PJ, editors. Nuclear medicine in clinical diagnosis and treatment. New York: Churchill Livingstone; 1994. p. 963–81.
[21] Alazraki N. Radionuclide techniques. In: Resnick D, editor. Diagnosis of bone and joint disorders. Philadelphia: Saunders; 1995. p. 430–74.
[22] Hotze AL, Briele B, Overbeck B, et al. Technetium-99m labeled antigranulocyte antibodies in suspected bone infections. J Nucl Med 1992;33:526–31.
[23] Seybold D, Frey LD, Locher J. Immunoscintigraphy of infections using I-123 and Tc-99m labeled monoclonal antibodies: advanced experiences in 230 patients. Angiology 1992;43:85–90.
[24] Gross MD, Shapiro B, Fig LM, et al. Imaging of human infection with I-131 labeled recombinant human interleukin-8. J Nucl Med 2001;42(11):1656–9.
[25] Filippi L, Schillaci O. Usefulness of hybrid SPECT/CT in Tc-99m HMPAO-labeled leukocyte scintigraphy for bone and joint infections. J Nucl Med 2006;47(12):1908–13.
[26] Delcourt M, Huglo D, Prangere T, et al. Comparison between LeukoScan (Sulesomab) and gallium-67 for the diagnosis of osteomyelitis in the diabetic foot. Diabetes Metab 2005;31: 125–33.
[27] Rubello D, Casara D, Maran A, et al. Role of anti-granulocyte Fab' fragment antibody scintigraphy (LeukoScan) in evaluating bone infection: acquisition protocol, interpretation criteria and clinical results. Nucl Med Commun 2004;25(1):39–47.
[28] Locher JT, Seybold K, Andres RY, et al. Imaging of inflammatory and infectious lesions after injection of radioiodinated monoclonal anti-granulocyte antibodies. Nucl Med Commun 1986;7:659–70.
[29] Joseph K, Hoffken H, Bosslet K, et al. Imaging of inflammation with granulocytes labeled in vivo. Nucl Med Commun 1988;9:763–9.
[30] Becker W, Bair J, Behr T, et al. Detection of soft-tissue infections and osteomyelitis using a technetium-99m-labeled anti-granulocyte monoclonal antibody fragment. J Nucl Med 1994;35:1436–43.
[31] Harwood SJ, Valdivia S, Hung GL, et al. Use of Sulesomab, a radiolabeled antibody fragment, to detect osteomyelitis in diabetic patients with foot ulcers by leukoscintigraphy. Clin Infect Dis 1999;28:1200–5.
[32] Dumarey N, Egrise D, Blocklet D, et al. Imaging infection with F-18-FDG-labeled leukocyte PET/CT: initial experience in 21 patients. J Nucl Med 2006;47:625–32.
[33] Reidar Z, Militianu D, Melamed E, et al. The diabetic foot: initial experience with F-18-FDG PET/CT. J Nucl Med 2005;46(3):444–9.
[34] Yuh WTC, Corson JD, Baraniewski HM, et al. Osteomyelitis of the foot in diabetic patients: evaluation with plain film, 99mTc-MDP bone scintigraphy, and MR imaging. AJR Am J Roentgenol 1989;152:795.
[35] Durham JR, Lukens ML, Campanini DS, et al. Impact of magnetic resonance imaging in the management of diabetic foot infections. Am J Surg 1991;162:150–3.
[36] Weinstein D, Wang A, Chambers R, et al. Evaluation of magnetic resonance imaging in the diagnosis of osteomyelitis in diabetic foot infections. Foot Ankle 1993;14:18–22.
[37] Unger E, Moldofsky P, Gatenby R, et al. Diagnosis of osteomyelitis by MR imaging. AJR 1988;150:605–10.
[38] Erdman WA, Tamburro F, Jayson HT, et al. Osteomyelitis: characteristics and pitfalls of diagnosis with MR imaging. Radiology 1991;180:533–9.
[39] Morrison WB, Schweitzer ME, Wapner KL, et al. Osteomyelitis in feet of diabetics: clinical accuracy, surgical utility, and cost-effectiveness of MR imaging. Radiology 1995;196:557–64.

[40] Simonsen OH, Revald P, Kjaer IL, et al. Tibialis posterior tendon dysfunction: an often neglected cause of painful adult flatfoot. Ugeskr Laeger 2006;168(47):4113.

[41] Mann RA, Thompson FM. Rupture of the posterior tibialis tendon causing flat foot. J Bone Joint Surg Am 1985;67:556–61.

[42] Mengiardi B, Pfirrmann C, Zanetti M. MR imaging of tendons and ligaments of the midfoot. Semin Musculoskelet Radiol 2005;9:187–98.

ELSEVIER
SAUNDERS

Clin Podiatr Med Surg
24 (2007) 425–448

CLINICS IN
PODIATRIC
MEDICINE AND
SURGERY

Diabetic Neuropathy: Medical and Surgical Approaches

A. Lee Dellon, MD, PhD[a,b,c,*]

[a] *Department of Neurosurgery and Division of Plastic Surgery, Johns Hopkins University, Suite 370, 3333 North Calvert Street, Baltimore, MD 21218, USA*

[b] *Division of Plastic Surgery, Neurosurgery and Anatomy, University of Arizona, Tucson, AZ, USA*

[c] *Dellon Institutes® for Peripheral Nerve Surgery, Baltimore, MD, USA*

Writing about the medical and surgical management of patients with diabetic neuropathy offers the possibility to bring these concepts into focus in the era of evidence-based medicine. Today, when most people begin a medical writing assignment, they go to PubMed, the official site of the National Library of Medicine and the National Institutes of Health, and type into the search engine the key words [1]. If you type in "diabetic neuropathy," you will retrieve about 12,500 references [1]. Surely all we will ever need to know is contained therein! If you subdivide this search into "diabetic neuropathy medical" and "diabetic neuropathy surgical," about 2000 references for each are identified. There are about 1950 references for "diabetic neuropathy treatment review." The purpose of this article is to establish the most critical, practical, and successful treatment options and their controversies for the practicing clinician caring for the patient with symptomatic diabetic neuropathy from the available literature.

Medical management of the patient with diabetic neuropathy is now standardized based on the research of the past four decades and is outlined in Box 1. For most patients with the most common form of diabetic neuropathy, a symmetrical, diffuse, distal, polyneuropathy (DPN), who do not have a pain component, the bulwark of treatment is to provide a euglycemic state, with a glycosylated hemoglobin (HbA_{1c}) in the range of less than 7.0 mg/dL. This approach involves diet, exercise, and an oral agent or insulin to control the blood sugar. Currently, there is no known medicine to reverse or prevent diabetic neuropathy in the symptomatic patient. When one reviews

Dr. Dellon owns a proprietary interest in the Pressure-Specified Sensory Device and the company Sensory Management Services, LLC.

* Johns Hopkins University, Suite 370, 3333 North Calvert Street, Baltimore, MD 21218.
E-mail address: aldellon@dellon.com

0891-8422/07/$ - see front matter
doi:10.1016/j.cpm.2007.03.003

Box 1. Medical management of diabetic neuropathy

1. Strive for euglycemic control
2. Relieve pain
   a) Tricyclic antidepressants
      Amitriptyline
      Desipramine
   b) Calcium channel regulators
      Pregabalin (Lyrica)
      Neuroapentin (Neurontin)
   c) Serotonin and norepinephrine uptake inhibitors
      Duloxetine (Cymbalta)
      Venlafaxine (Effexor)
   d) Opioids
      Tramadol (Ultram)
      Oxycodone CR
      Methadone
      Hydromorphone (Dilaudid)
3. Foot care*
   a) Clean feet daily using warm water and mild soap, dry with soft towel
   b) Inspect feet and toes twice daily for cuts, blisters, redness
   c) Moisturize feet with lotion, avoiding interdigital spaces
   d) File calluses, corns with pumice stone
   e) Cut toenails regularly
   f) Do not go barefoot; wear slippers or thick socks
   g) Wear well-fitted shoes; check inside shoe before use

* http://diabetes.niddk.nih.gov/dm/pubs/neuropathies and http://ndep.nih.gov/materials/pubs/feet/feet.htm.

the extensive experience of Dyck [2] from the Mayo Clinic from 1968 through 2005 [3], it is clear that there has been little, if any, change in the basic concepts of the pathophysiology of DPN. Although traditional neurology reviews suggest the prevalence of painful DPN is 10%, the most recent estimate is 50% [4]. For this important subgroup, there is the established pain management approach leading from neuropathic pain medications such as tricylic antidepressants to serotonin uptake inhibitors to opiods (Box 1). Dosage and success rates for the many drug options have been discussed recently in detail [4]. This costly approach often leaves cognitive function impaired and the patient drug dependent and impoverished.

Despite many successful basic science models and phase I and II clinical trials, a 2005 review by the world's most respected diabetologists led by Boulton and colleagues [5] of Manchester, England, demonstrated that the randomized clinical trial approach has failed to identify the hoped for pharmacologic agent to reverse or prevent DPN. Drug types reviewed included aldose reductase inhibitors, myoinositol, alpha-lipoic acid, vasodilators, protein kinase C inhibitors, C-peptide, nerve growth factors (NGF, BDNF), acetyl-1-carnitine, gama-linolenic acid, and others. Indeed, when writing in the orthopedic surgery literature in 2005 about DPN, Rather and Boulton [6] stated, "to date no treatment that prevents or reverses its development and progression has been identified."

Surgical management can be divided into two approaches. The classic involvement of the surgeon in DPN is to debride wounds, drain infection, and amputate necrotic tissues [7]. This approach comprises the majority of the literature on the surgical management of DPN. Beginning in 1988, a theoretical editorial suggested that there was an "optimism" for diabetic neuropathy if one could identify peripheral nerve entrapments in the patient with diabetes [8]. Since the first clinical series of patients with DPN and nerve compressions in the lower extremity was reported in 1992 [9], there has been a continuing increase in peer-reviewed scientific publications, especially in the past 2 years, confirming these initial clinical observations (Table 1). These studies consistently demonstrate that decompression of sites of chronic nerve entrapment in the patient with DPN can relieve symptoms, which means that a surgical approach can relieve pain and restore sensation if (when) the medical approach fails [9–28]. These studies demonstrate consistently that the incidence of ulceration and amputation can be changed, which means that a surgical approach can prevent the sequelae of DPN if (when) the medical approach fails [9–29].

This article reviews the evidence that demonstrates that, by identifying and surgically releasing compressed lower extremity peripheral nerves, the natural history of diabetic neuropathy can be reversed, and its associated morbidity can be greatly reduced.

The references listed in Table 1 do not suggest that every diabetic patient with neuropathy should have decompression of peripheral nerves; rather, the literature suggests that if a nerve compression is identified in the patient with diabetic neuropathy, decompression of that nerve can relieve symptoms. The symptoms of chronic nerve compression can be identical to those of neuropathy. The failure to appreciate this critical point of emphasis has caused misinterpretation of the available literature by neurologists [30,31].

Diagnosis of peripheral neuropathy

As they have every year for more than a decade [32,33], the January 2007 Guidelines of the American Diabetes Association, published as a supplement to *Diabetes Care*, document that the standard of care for management of the foot in the patient with diabetes is to evaluate sensibility of the feet [34]. The

Table 1
Results of Dellon triple nerve decompression in diabetic patients

Study	Number of nerves	Preoperative number		Results improved (%)		New or recurrent ulceration/ amputation (%)
		Ulcers	Amputations	Pain	Touch	
Dellon, 1992 [9]	31	0	0	85	72	0
Wieman, 1995 [10]	33	13	0	92	72	7
Chaffe, 2000 [11]	58	11	6	86	50	0
Aszmann, 2000 [12]	16	0	0	NA	69	0
Tambwekr, 2001 [13]	10	6	4	NA	80	0
Wood, 2003 [14]	33	0	0	90	67	0
Biddinger, 2004 [15]	22	0	0	86	80	0
Lee, 2004 [16]	46	0	0	92	92	NA
Aszmann, 2004 [17]	50	0	0	NA	NA	0
Valdivia, 2005 [18]	60	0	0	87	85	0
Rader, 2005 [19]	49	0	0	90	75	0
Yong, 2005 [20]	90	0	0	94	90	0
DiNucci, 2005 [21]	72	0	0	80	80	0
Steck, 2005 [22]	25	0	0	84	72	0
Siemionow, 2006 [23]	36	0	0	90	90	0
Yuksel, 2006 [24]	22	0	0	89	85	0
Shaffiroff, 2006 [25]	300	0	0	85	80	0
Nelson, 2007 [26]	9	0	0	88	88	0
Massa, 2007 [27]	20	0	0	80	86	0
Maloney, 2007 [28]	95	0	0	86	83	0
Bae, 2007 [29]	33	0	0	75	72	0

Abbreviation: NA, not available.

goal is to identify the presence of neuropathy and to follow its progressive "loss of protective sensation," with its attendant risk of ulceration, infection, and amputation. The guidelines suggest that some form of quantitative sensory testing be performed to obtain the cutaneous perception thresholds for temperature, vibration, or pressure. The exact measurement devices to be used are not specified. If abnormal measurements are identified by screening that suggest the presence of neuropathy, the test should be repeated every 3 to 6 months. Previously, the performance of traditional "nerve conduction" testing was recommended at least once in the diabetic patient with symptoms of neuropathy, but this has now been changed to "electrophysiological testing is rarely ever needed, except in situations where the clinical features are atypical" [34].

A 2005 Mayo Clinic continuing medical education publication elucidated an approach to documenting peripheral nerve function [35]. Quantitative sensory testing was described as a "computer-based, non-invasive, psychophysical and semi-objective measure of thermal, vibratory or thermal-evoked pain thresholds, not specific to peripheral nerve function," and required specialized equipment. Nerve conduction velocity (amplitude was not described) was "useful to exclude other causes of neuropathy, decreases gradually in DPN, is effected by glycemic control, but does not correlate with severity of neuropathy, speed of onset of neuropathy, or clinical symptoms of neuropathy, and is unrelated to the painful component of neuropathy."

This recommendation sets the "pay for performance" stage for 2007, envisioning that the foot care specialist, internist, endocrinologist, diabetologist, or wound healing specialist should perform screening tests with Semmes-Weinstein nylon monofilaments, using the 5.07 filament as the cutoff for loss of protective sensation, or with vibrometry, using the 25 V cutoff for loss of protective sensation, so that appropriate foot care can be instituted to protect the insensate foot [36]. It also recommends that the person with symptoms of neuropathy be referred for a definitive computer-assisted evaluation of the sensibility of the foot. Currently available equipment uses the CASE IV approach, which measures one-point static touch threshold, thermal thresholds, and the vibratory threshold to a 128-Hz stimulus, or the Pressure-Specified Sensory Device (PSSD), which measures the one- and two-point moving and static-touch pressure thresholds. There have been extensive reports of the reliability and validity of the PSSD in diabetic patients with and without neuropathy, and with and without ulceration [14–16,18,19,21–25,27,28,37–54]. In a report from 2005, the PSSD was shown to have a sensitivity of 95% compared with a sensitivity for the Semmes-Weinstein monofilaments of 56% and for vibrometry of 21% in identifying the presence of abnormal tibial nerve function in the big toe pulp [54]. The best available nonpainful method to document and stage the presence and degree of neuropathy is the PSSD. It is appropriate to refer patients with diabetes and symptoms of neuropathy for this definitive non-screening test. Decisions can then be made regarding the best medical foot care available [33,55–57], or, once nerve degeneration is documented, a referral can be made to determine whether the patient is a candidate for decompression of superimposed chronic peripheral nerve compressions.

Can medical management prevent neuropathy?

I would like to emphasize two recent critically important outcome studies. In essence, these studies demonstrate that, regardless of achieving the best possible medical management of the underlying diabetes, symptomatic neuropathy will occur anyway in a significant percentage of diabetic patients.

In 2006, the results of an 8-year study were published in the United Kingdom [58]. The study subjects were 300 diabetic patients, 100 of whom had neuropathy. Neuropathy was defined as a vibratory perception threshold greater than 25 V. An earlier study by this group had demonstrated that subclinical neuropathy could be identified if a vibratory threshold of 12 V were used [59]. At the onset of the study, the HbA_{1c} was 9.1 in the neuropathy group and 8.6 in the diabetic patients without neuropathy. From 1995 through

2002, despite modest improvements in glycemic control (HbA_{1c} was 8.6 in the neuropathy group and 8.4 in the control group), neuropathy became worse ($P < .001$) in the neuropathy group and remained unchanged in the control group. This study demonstrates again that diabetic neuropathy is progressive and irreversible even under the best medical management for diabetes.

In 2006, a "final" outcome study was published from the Diabetes Comprehensive Control Trial (DCCT) 8 years after that study ended [60]. There were 624 patients in the "usual control" and 633 patients in the "strict control" group. By 8 years after the completion of the DCCT, neuropathy was present in 17.8% of patients who had been on strict glycemic control and in 28% of the patients in the usual control group. The prevalence of neuropathy was based on a physical examination. This difference was significant at the $P < .001$ level, demonstrating that tight glycemic control reduces, but does not prevent, neuropathy. Importantly, there were ulcerations in both groups of patients (4 versus 11) and amputations in both groups (2 versus 5).

Although this knowledge is sobering and perhaps discouraging, it should serve as the step-off point to ask whether there is another approach to the prevention and treatment of the consequences of DPN than purely attempting to control blood sugar and masking the neuropathy symptoms with mind-altering polypharmacopia.

A proactive surgical approach to symptomatic diabetic peripheral neuropathy

To appreciate the magnitude of the educational task ahead of us, it is helpful to consider the September/October 2006 issue of the *Journal of Foot & Ankle Surgery*, a supplement entitled "Diabetic foot disorders: a clinical practice guideline (2006 revision)" [61]. Despite the fact that this issue was authored by 13 of the most distinguished podiatric foot and ankle surgeons in the United States, not one of the 569 references in this clinical practice guideline refers to the possibility that there is a surgical approach, a change for optimism, for this progressive and irreversible problem. Considering that most of these contributing authors know well the concept of decompression of lower extremity nerves in the patient with diabetic neuropathy and nerve compressions, why this public denial?

The task for a surgical educator like myself is, indeed, huge. And this is just the educational task related to all medical professions. Medical doctors may think that it is not appropriate to operate on the diabetic foot electively. Neurologists [30] may (1) fail to accept that this optimism is based on quantifying and staging the degree of neuropathy, which remains a challenge using traditional electrodiagnostic techniques, (2) fail to identify nerve compression in the presence of neuropathy with traditional electrodiagnostic techniques, or (3) fail to examine the patient for a positive Tinel sign to identify the presence of a chronic nerve entrapment at known sites of anatomic narrowing.

The controversy begins with the classic teaching in medical schools that diabetic neuropathy is progressive and irreversible. It follows immediately that there is no role for surgery in the treatment of this painful condition. Furthermore, diabetic neuropathy occurs in a stocking and glove distribution, consistent with a systemic metabolic disease. This concept also leads to the immediate conclusion that there should be no role for surgery in this debilitating condition; however, my clinical experiences challenged this traditional teaching. The history of this controversial approach to treating the symptoms of diabetic neuropathy relates to my training in plastic surgery, which is really an approach to problem solving.

When I finished my plastic surgery training, which included a hand surgery fellowship, it was natural for patients with diabetes to be referred to me for the treatment of carpal tunnel syndrome. The similarities of the symptoms of chronic nerve compression and those of diabetic neuropathy were very close and, in many patients, were identical. When the thumb, index, and middle finger felt "normal" after carpal tunnel decompression in the diabetic patient but the little and ring fingers still felt numb, tingling, or burning or cold, it seemed reasonable to consider that these symptoms in the diabetic patient might represent cubital tunnel syndrome. If I could identify a positive Tinel sign over the ulnar nerve in the postcondylar groove, it was possible that there was nerve compression at this location. Although traditional ulnar nerve transposition has varied success depending on the degree of nerve compression [62], an approach to submuscular transposition of the ulnar nerve was developed that included a lengthening of the flexor/pronator muscle mass [63–65]. This approach was associated with excellent relief of symptoms despite advanced degrees of nerve compression. The technique relieved these symptoms in the diabetic patient and restored strength to the hand. The patient would still have numbness and burning over the dorsal radial aspect of their hand, which was presumed to be due to their diabetic neuropathy. In 1986, compression of the radial sensory nerve in the forearm was described [66], and, thereafter, decompression of this nerve was added to my approach to the diabetic patient with painful upper extremity complaints, with the result that these symptoms could be relieved. At this point, my clinical considerations of three different sites of nerve compression in the arm suggested that decompression of these three peripheral nerves resulted in relief of pain symptoms that were in a glove distribution.

Patients with diabetes who had been referred for the treatment of upper extremity nerve symptoms and who found relief after nerve decompression would ask me, "Could you do the same thing for my feet?" I used to answer, "No, we don't do feet." One day, when in a more contemplative mode instead of the mode that just regurgitates what we have been taught classically, I responded to this same question by saying, "Maybe we can, because the nerves should behave the same way in the lower extremity as they do in the upper extremity." I went to the anatomy laboratory and identified the sites of compression for the nerves of the lower extremity.

Although compression of the common peroneal nerve at the fibular head was described as early as 1897 in a patient who had been in the lithotomy position for a gynecologic procedure [67], decompression of this nerve is still not commonly reported [68,69]. Decompression of the tarsal tunnel for compression of the posterior tibial nerve was not reported until 1962 [70,71]. In general, this procedure is not commonly done because it has not been reported to give excellent results; however, work by the author and his colleagues identified four separate tunnels that needed to be decompressed, not just one, to achieve relief of symptoms in the medial ankle [39,72]. Furthermore, our work identified a new site of distal compression of the deep peroneal nerve over the dorsum of the foot [73]. The implication of these observations is that decompression of multiple peripheral nerves in the lower extremity can restore sensation in a stocking distribution. Technical details of these procedures have been published for the upper and the lower extremities [74].

My first clinical experience with decompression of nerves in the upper and lower extremities in diabetic patients with peripheral neuropathy was published in 1992 [9]. Overall, 80% of the patients improved to the good or excellent level. This improvement was documented electrophysiologically in 68% of the patients. Perhaps most importantly, none of the patients who were operated on had progression of their neuropathy, whereas 50% of the patients had progression of their neuropathy in an extremity that was not decompressed. These first clinical observations set the stage for (1) basic scientific research to elucidate the underlying mechanisms that made this new proactive surgical approach work, and (2) basic science and clinical work to demonstrate that the natural history of diabetic neuropathy could be changed by this new proactive approach.

The nerve in diabetes is susceptible to compression

Ample evidence in the medical and surgical literature suggests that the patient with diabetes has a high incidence of chronic nerve compression. This incidence has been reported to be as high as 33%, with the most common nerve compressions in the upper extremity being the median nerve at the wrist, the ulnar nerve at the elbow, and the radial sensory nerve in the forearm. In the lower extremity, the most common nerve compressions are the tibial nerve in the tarsal tunnel and the common peroneal nerve at the fibular head [75–81]. Researchers agree that traditional electrodiagnostic studies cannot easily identify these entrapments in the presence of an underlying metabolic neuropathy, and that physical examination is essential in identifying these compressions. The presence of a positive Tinel sign over the tibial nerve in the tarsal tunnel, for example, has been demonstrated to have a 92% positive predictive value in identifying neuropathy patients who will have a good-to-excellent result from nerve decompression in the lower extremity [16].

Two metabolic changes in the peripheral nerves of diabetic patients render the nerves susceptible to chronic compression. The most critical is the increased water content within the nerve as the result of glucose being metabolized into sorbitol [82,83]. This increased water content causes the nerve to have an increased volume. The second metabolic change is a decrease in the slow anterograde component of axoplasmic flow [84,85]. This component of axoplasmic flows transports the lipoproteins necessary to maintain and rebuild the nerve. The peripheral nerve, as it crosses a known area of anatomic narrowing like the carpal tunnel at the wrist, the cubital tunnel at the elbow, the fibular tunnel at the outside of the knee, or the tarsal tunnel at the ankle, passes through a region of increased external pressure. Because the peripheral nerve in the diabetic patient has an increased volume owing to its water content, there is an increased pressure on the nerve in each of these anatomic regions. This increased external pressure creates an increased intraneural pressure that decreases blood flow [86,87]. The decreased blood flow results in a relative ischemic condition for the peripheral nerve. The neurophysiologic consequence of decreased blood flow in a peripheral nerve is the perception of paresthesias, interpreted centrally as numbness and tingling. The chronic pathophysiologic result of this area of increased pressure along a peripheral nerve is demyelination [88]. The peripheral nerve with decreased axoplasmic flow, such as in the diabetic patient, cannot transport sufficient protein structures to rebuild itself.

A third mechanism that may render the peripheral nerve in the diabetic patient susceptible to chronic compression is the fact that advanced glycosylation end products (AGE) build up within the nerve. Although the biomechanical properties of the peripheral nerve in the diabetic patient have not been studied yet, the presence of these AGE within the nerve theoretically should make the nerve more stiff, decreasing nerve gliding with joint motion. The non-enzymatic binding of glucose to the collagen within the nerve and in the epineurium is the basis for this decreased elasticity. This decreased elasticity in the peripheral nerve combined with the nerve's normal physiologic requirement to stretch as it glides across joints increases the stress and strain of the peripheral nerve within areas of known anatomic narrowing. This increasing tension along the nerve further decreases blood flow within the nerve [86,87].

The hypothesis that the peripheral nerve in the diabetic patient has an increased susceptibility to compression has been tested in the rat model [89]. Rats were made diabetic by being given streptozocin. Silicone bands were placed about the sciatic nerve in these rats and also in a group of non-diabetic, age-matched rats. Electrophysiology was tested in both groups after 6 months of banding, which had been demonstrated to be sufficient time to develop electrophysiologic and histologic changes consistent with chronic nerve compression in this model. The diabetic rat had a statistically significant lower conduction velocity and a statistically significant lower amplitude for the sciatic nerve measured across the region of compression than did the non-diabetic banded rat, confirming that the peripheral nerve had an increased susceptibility to chronic nerve compression in diabetes.

The most critical basic science study was conducted in the streptozocin model of the diabetic rat. Two groups of rats were made diabetic with blood sugars of 400 mg/dL. One group of rats had the compression sites along the tibial nerve in the tarsal and plantar tunnels released, creating a group of rats that did not have a distal site for nerve compression. They were evaluated by walking track analysis monthly for one full year. At the end of the year, the rats that had an intact tarsal tunnel had developed a neuropathic walking track pattern. In contrast, the group that had no known site of compression walked with a pattern that was not different than that in normal weight-matched non-diabetic rats [90,91]. In the absence of an anatomic site for peripheral nerve compression, neuropathy did not develop in these diabetic rats. These seminal basic science studies have been duplicated by surgical scientists in Turkey [92] and the Cleveland Clinic [93].

Success and the tarsal tunnels

When the first publications relating to tibial nerve compression at the ankle were published, they were focused on the site of compression being within the tarsal tunnel, similar to the median nerve being compressed at the carpal tunnel, both by a flexor retinaculum. Approaching the compression site in the foot by dividing this single compartment gave disappointing results, with many studies reporting 15% to 50% excellent results (Table 2) [94–107] compared with a more than 90% rate of good-to-excellent results expected by hand surgeons. What was the difference?

From the first patient referred to me around 1980, I began to compare the anatomic relationships in the medial ankle region with those in the hand. It became clear that there were a set of homologies [72] that implied that the proper approach to the symptoms in the foot would require releasing four separate medial ankle tunnels. Furthermore, in the hand, two of these tunnels were separated by a bone process, the hook of the hamate, which for painful non-unions is removed; therefore, I developed an operation that included release of the four medial ankle tunnels and removal of the septum between the medial and lateral plantar tunnels (Table 3) (Fig. 1). In my first series of patients in whom the four medial ankle tunnels were decompressed and the septum between the medial and lateral plantar tunnels removed, there was an 82% rate of excellent results and an 11% rate of good results [108]. When this technique was reported in 1992 for my first series of patients with diabetic neuropathy, who also had tibial nerve compression in the tarsal tunnel, the success rate was 69% good-to-excellent results [9]. In my last reported series of patients with diabetic neuropathy and tarsal tunnel syndrome, the success rate was 92% good-to-excellent results [16]. This improvement was attributed to patients being referred to me at an earlier stage of their nerve compression and neuropathy than in my first series of patients.

Table 2
Summary of "therapeutic level 4" tarsal tunnel studies

Study	Number of patients	NCV/ EMG[a]	Tinel positive	Tunnels released	Immobilized postoperatively	Results (%) Excellent	Good	Fair	Poor
Lam, 1967 [94]	13	No	Yes	3?	NA	86	7	7	0
Edwards et al, 1969 [95]	16	33%	Yes	1	Cast, time?	88	6	0	6[c]
Linscheid et al, 1970 [96]	24	100%	Yes	1	NA	0	50	30	20
Mann, 1974 [97]	9	90%	Yes	3	3 weeks	78	0	11	11
Stern and Joyce, 1989 [98]	15	40%	Yes	4	10 d	54	20	20	6
Byank and Curtis, 1992 [99]	49	100%	Yes	1	NA	26	53	12	9
Sammarco et al, 1993 [100]	5	100%	Yes	4	NA	20	80	0	0
Pfeiffer and Cracchiolo, 1994 [101]	32	100%	Yes	3	10 d	15	29	23	33
Mahan et al, 1996 [102]	45	NA	Yes	3	NA	24	36	11	29
Turan et al, 1997 [103]	18	0%	Yes	4	2 weeks	61	22	0	17
Baba et al, 1997 [104]	34	100%	Yes	3	3 weeks	70	16	8	6
Bailie and Kelitian, 1998 [105]	36	80%	Yes	3[e]	2 weeks	57	16	11	16
Kohno et al[b], 2000 [106]	12	40%	Yes	1	NA	50	34	8	8
Gondring et al[b], 2003 [107]	68	100%	Yes	2?	3 weeks	51[d]	0	0	49
Mullick and Dellon, 2007 [108]	87	50%	Yes	4+[e]	None	82	11	5	2

Abbreviations: NA, not available; NCV/EMG, nerve conduction velocity/electromyography.

[a] Percentage of patients in series who had electrodiagnostic testing. For Pfeiffer/Cracchiolo series, 81% were positive. For Linscheid et al, 68% were positive. For Baile and Kelikian, 81% were positive. In none of these studies did the NCV/EMG result correlate with surgical outcome.

[b] A pneumatic tourniquet was not used.

[c] Follow-up was just 3 to 4 months.

[d] Outcome: patient-reported improvement. Rates of surgeon-reported pain relief: 85% relief of pain and 15% no relief of pain.

[e] The intertunnel septum was excised.

Table 3
Homologies between the carpal and tarsal tunnels and sites for nerve compression

Ankle	Wrist
Tarsal tunnel	Distal forearm
Medial plantar tunnel	Carpal tunnel
Lateral plantar tunnel	Guyon's canal
Calcaneal tunnel	Tunnel for the palmar cutaneous branch of median nerve
Intertunnel septum	Hook process of hamate

I believe that if we call tibial nerve compression at the ankle "tarsal tunnels" instead of "tarsal tunnel syndrome," it will focus on the need to decompress four medial ankle tunnels and remove the septum between the medial and lateral plantar tunnels, as illustrated in Fig. 1. This figure and a patient-oriented brochure entitled "Tarsal Tunnels Syndrome" can be downloaded from the Dellon.com Web site.

Back to changing the future

If one looks back 10 to 15 years ago, one sees the agreement that diabetic neuropathy is progressive and irreversible [109], and these same statements are being made today [4,6]. If one looks back about a decade, one sees the emphasis on using vibration and pressure thresholds to identify patients at risk for loss of protective sensation [110–112], which is now codified into the standards of care for the diabetic foot [34,57,61]. This traditional approach has led to well-known costs to the health care system. Ulceration occurs owing to neuropathy, infection in the diabetic foot occurs owing to ulceration, the majority of amputations in the diabetic patient are performed owing to neuropathy, and the loss of balance from neuropathy is associated with attendant wrist and hip fractures owing to falls. Little, if any, change has occurred in this overall morbidity and the costs for neuropathic pain medications.

E. J. Barett, MD, in the presidential address to the American Diabetes Association in 2004 [113], stated the following, "It is estimated that the cost of caring for people with diabetes and obesity will, as the population ages, be a dominant factor in bankrupting the Medicare trust fund by the year 2019." A 2007 review predicts for the future. The number of diabetic persons worldwide will increase from 171 million in the year 2000 to 366 million by 2030, constituting a pandemic. In addition, the present number of 197 million people worldwide with impaired glucose intolerance will increase to 420 million people by 2025 [114]. If 10% to 50% of these people develop neuropathy depending on their glycemic control, the prevalence of neuropathy worldwide due to diabetes only will be enormous.

How can we work together to impact and diminish the burden of this morbidity? One way would be for different medical specialties to have

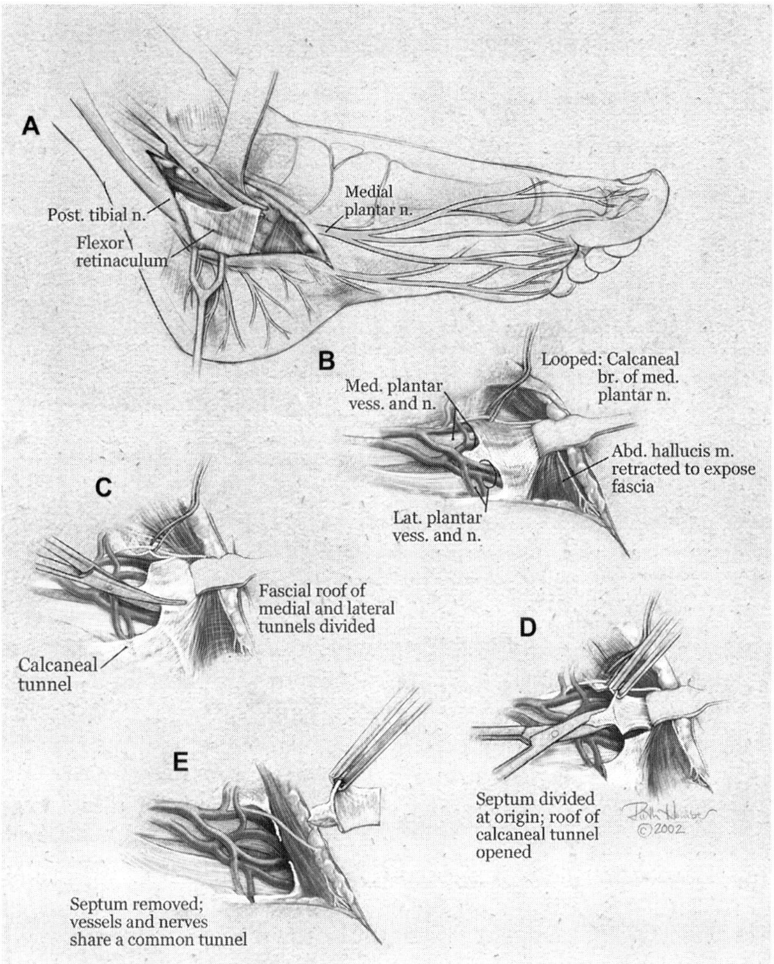

Fig. 1. The medial ankle tunnels are depicted in this drawing. (*A*) The tarsal tunnel is illustrated with its flexor retinaculum. This is not the site of pressure-causing symptoms but is necessary to open to identify the anatomy and its variations. (*B*) The abductor hallucis muscle is retracted, and the frequently present branch from the medial plantar nerve to the medial calcaneal region is identified and preserved. The roof of the medial and lateral plantar tunnels is identified. (*C*) The roof of the medial plantar tunnel has been incised. The roof of the lateral plantar tunnel is being incised. (*D*) The calcaneal tunnel has been incised, and the septum between these two tunnels is being incised longitudinally. (*E*) The septum is removed, completing Dellon's technique for the tarsal tunnels syndrome (*Courtesy of* A. Lee Dellon, MD, Baltimore, MD; Available at: Dellon.com/brochures).

respect for each other. Over the past 20 years, I have found that surgeons who examine their patients, who observe surgery to decompress lower extremity nerves, and who evaluate patient outcomes from this surgery are encouraged at the relief their patients express to them and are impressed with the objective reduction in morbidity when compared with the ulcers and amputations these patients experienced before. Although it may be said that the relief of pain is subjective and the surgeon biased, the patient, not the surgeon, is the one who supplies the number for the visual analogue scale. Although it may be said that improvement in sensation is subjective, it is someone other than the surgeon who makes this measurement. Measures such as the presence or absence of ulceration or amputation are clearly objective outcomes and are beyond the criticism of placebo effect. In contrast, neurologists have taken an extremely adverse approach to the surgical concepts expressed thus far in this article. Why are neurologists so opposed to this surgical approach, and where can we identify errors in their reasoning?

This very week, as I complete the writing of this article, a "Commentary" has been published in the February 2007 issue of *Diabetes Care* [31]. The lead author is Cornblath [115], a neurologist from my own university, Johns Hopkins, who has known of my work in this field since its inception, who has authored one article with me on the electrophysiologic status of the peripheral nerves in an aged diabetic rhesus monkey, and who has done experimental animal research with me that included electrodiagnostic testing in the cynomolgus monkey with multiple sites of silicon tube compression of nerves (David Cornblath, unpublished data, 1988). Cornblath and colleagues' [31] commentary is an extension of the Therapeutics and Technology Assessment Subcommittee of the American Academy of Neurology's 2004 statement [30] on the "Utility of surgical decompression for treatment of diabetic neuropathy." The lead author on that report is Chaudhry [30], also a neurologist at my university, and with whom I have spent time discussing the underlying assumptions that have been spelled out herein. The former chief of neurology at Johns Hopkins Hospital, for whom both Cornblath and Chaudhry worked before he retired last year, has known of my work for more than a decade, and knows that my hypothesis is that decompression of compressed nerves in the diabetic patient is the approach I am taking, and that I am not advocating decompression of all nerves in all diabetic patients.

Both Drs. Chaudhry and Cornblath know perfectly well that the hypothesis I am expounding, and have expounded, is that if there is a nerve compression in the diabetic patient with neuropathy, then a portion and perhaps most of the patient's symptoms are related to that compression, and, if that is true, then the nerve compression should be decompressed. As a surgeon I can change compression; clearly, no surgeon can change the metabolism of the underlying neuropathy by decompression of a nerve. Interestingly, Cornblath and colleagues' commentary [31] has no direct reference to any of my peer-reviewed work. Cornblath and colleagues [31] have included in their commentary so many misrepresentations of my work that it raises questions about their own objectivity. For example, they state that I am advocating decompression of the peroneal nerve in the "anterior tarsal tunnel,....the sural nerve in the distal posterior calf, ...and the radial nerve in the radial tunnel." I have never written this. Indeed, as noted previously,

I have written about the radial sensory nerve in the forearm [66], not the radial nerve at the elbow, and I have written about the deep peroneal nerve over the dorsum of the foot [73], distal to the anterior tarsal tunnel, and have never decompressed the sural nerve in the calf. Cornblath and colleagues [31] state, "entrapment cannot explain sensory or motor symptoms or signs above the anatomic levels of the 'entrapped' nerves," and that my approach is related to the "peroneal nerve at the fibular head causing foot drop." This is an amazing statement, because the sensory symptoms that extend above the ankle laterally clearly can come from compression above the ankle, from this very common peroneal nerve. Indeed, as the electrophysiologist within him should remind him, often, electrically, the sensory evidence of compression is identified before the motor, and it is rare that a diabetic patient with neuropathy has ever come to me for foot drop in the absence of true trauma. Furthermore, it is within everyone's experience that patients with carpal tunnels syndrome complain of shoulder pain [116], or is this because there is an occult C6 radiculopathy, a double crush?

With regard to multiple sites of entrapment along a peripheral nerve, Cornblath and colleagues [31] do attribute correctly to me the application of the 1973 Double Crush Theory of Upton and McComas to the clinical diabetic neuropathy problem. Because the neurologists have decided to pursue this subject against my work, and in an effort to understand why the neurologists may feel so threatened by my work, please consider the following two conversations (although, by definition, these are anecdotal evidence at best). I had the privilege of discussing this concept with two preeminent electrophysiologists. Kimura [117], who in 1979 reported the now universally used "inching technique" to identify the site of median nerve compression at the wrist, was with me at an international meeting on nerve repair and regeneration in Cannes, France, in 1988. The second conversation was with Gilliatt and Thomas [118], two of the pioneers in the 1960s of identifying sites of nerve compression and of evaluating diabetic neuropathy electrophysiologically [119]. Dr. Gilliatt was with me in Washington, DC, in 1990 at the meeting of the Plastic Surgery Research Council. Also with me were the initial group that went on to found the American Society for Peripheral Nerve Surgery, of which I am past president. Dr. Gilliatt had retired from his post in London and was, at the time I met with him, the Senior Consultant to the National Institute of Neurologic Disorders and Stroke at the National Institutes of Health. I asked Drs. Kimura and Gilliatt on those two separate occasions the same question, that is, whether electrodiagnostic testing could distinguish between an axonal neuropathy and multiple sites of compression along the course of a nerve. Each gave me the same answer, "No." To put their answer into context, consider the analogy of the radiologist reading a chest radiograph with a white spot in the lung field. A differential diagnosis is given. In the patient with diabetes, when the neurologist reports certain measurements of the peroneal and tibial nerve bilaterally to be consistent with an axonal loss, it might be appropriate for their report to say, "These findings are consistent with a diffuse symmetrical polyneuropathy, but superimposed multiple nerve compressions may be present and cannot be excluded by this study. Clinical correlation is advised." Would that type of report not be more honest?

As another example of the many misrepresentations in the commentary by Cornblath and colleagues [31], they state that "the actual frequency of peripheral nerve entrapment in diabetic individuals is small," when, in fact, one of their co-authors, Vinik [80], has written that as many of one third of diabetic patients have nerve entrapment. Dr. Vinik refers his own patients to one of the co-authors of that article, a plastic surgeon, for peripheral nerve decompression.

Because Dr. Cornblath and neurologists in general are advocates of electrodiagnostic testing, which has obvious financial benefit to themselves, they continue to suggest, as do Chaudhry and colleagues [30], that in Cornblath and colleagues' [31] words, "The proponents of the subjective Tinel sign ignore the proven value of electrodiagnostic studies, and objective tests of nerve function." Yet neurologists themselves ignore the almost universal disappointment and frustration of non-neurologist medical physicians and surgeons with the inability of electrodiagnostic studies to give a diagnosis and guide patient care for even the most simple of chronic nerve entrapments, carpal tunnel syndrome. In fact, an article essentially never quoted by neurologists, their own assessment committee report, suggests that there are 33% false-negative results with electrodiagnostic testing in patients with carpal tunnel syndrome [120]. In other words, 33% of the patients that insurance companies spend money on to evaluate the most common nerve compression in the hand have false-negative results.

Surgical decompression of the chronically compressed nerve is one of the most successful surgical procedures of all time, and this success has been documented throughout the world for upper and lower extremity nerves. The success rate in general approaches 80%. Cornblath and colleagues [31] ignore the sophisticated report by a University of Toronto leading expert in neurology, Vera Bril, MD, who, when writing with a diabetologist from the Joslin Clinic in Boston and a statistician from Harvard University, concluded that with regard to the presence of carpal tunnel syndrome in the presence of diabetic neuropathy, "electrodiagnostic parameters are not significant predictors of the presence of carpal tunnel syndrome" and that "therapeutic decisions for carpal tunnel syndrome can be made independently of electrodiagnostic findings" [75]. Her group found that, by history and physical examination, 30% of the patients with diabetic peripheral neuropathy had carpal tunnel syndrome, clearly not "the small number" that Cornblath and colleagues [31] would have us believe. Their report means we must rely on the Tinel sign.

I would like to call attention to what Dyck [121], Professor of Neurology at the Mayo Clinic, wrote in the September 22, 2006 issue of *Neurology* as correspondence to address the conclusions of Chaudhry and colleagues

[30]. Dr. Dyck wrote, "It should be emphasized that it is decompression of leg nerves at anatomical sites not known to be entrapped that is being discussed (which may not have been sufficiently emphasized in the Advisory)." In other words, Dr. Dyck recognized that my work, and that of the other surgical scientists who have trained with me and who have either written about or have presented on this subject [9,12–29], is about a localized nerve entrapment identified by the presence of a positive Tinel sign. He was pointing out to the neurologists reading this correspondence (but unfortunately not to those who would only read Chaudhry and colleagues' [30] June advisory) that the advisory only made conclusions about surgery on the general group of patients with diabetic neuropathy, which is not my hypothesis.

The neurology reports [30,31] call for randomized clinical trials of the work reported in Table 1. Certainly, there are appropriate uses for randomized clinical trials. That use is to compare different diagnostic methods or different treatment methods; however, not all patient care needs to based on this type of clinical research. For example, just this month Lavery and colleagues [122] reported the results of a physician-blinded randomized trial comparing identification of the foot at risk for ulceration. They concluded that using an infrared temperature system versus standard or structured foot therapy reduced recurrent ulceration from 17 of 58 and 17 of 56 in the control groups to 5 of 59 in the "experimental" group. The incidence was reduced significantly ($P = .003$) from 30% to 9% in a study that only lasted 15 months. In a multicentered prospective study (available online at neuropathyregistry.com), researchers evaluated the results of tibial nerve decompression in the medial ankle tunnels. A recurrence or new ulcer was seen in 2% of 50 patients at 1 year, in 4% of 49 patients at 1.5 years, and in 6% of 49 patients at 3.5 years (neuropathyregistry.com). Although these two studies were not performed on the same cohort of patients, when evaluating a disease like diabetic neuropathy, which has been proven to be progressive and irreversible without any change in its pathophysiology or morbidity for about 40 years, I believe it is appropriate to learn from these two concurrent studies even though no patients were randomized. Ulceration is an objective endpoint and is not at risk for misinterpretation for what Cornblath and colleagues [31] call the "unblinded surgeons, ...placebo effect."

In another example of a concurrent comparison of the progressive and irreversible disease of diabetic neuropathy, consider the report by Armstrong and colleagues [123]. They used hospitalization for foot infection as the outcome and evaluated the results of ideal foot care in the United States. Among the 1666 patients with diabetic neuropathy followed up for 2 years, 155 or 9.5% were admitted to the hospital with infection. From the multicentered prospective study available online (neuropathyregistry.com), of the patients with diabetic neuropathy who had evidence of tibial nerve compression in the medial ankle and who had decompression by surgeons trained by myself, only 0.9% of 817 patients were admitted to the hospital over a 5.5-year observation period. Hospital admission for foot infection is an objective outcome and is not subject to the "blinded surgeon's" bias.

Because there is no accepted treatment of diabetic neuropathy except glycemic control and neuropathic pain medication, there is no treatment group to use as a control group for a prospective blinded study of the effect of decompression of compressed lower extremity peripheral nerves in the patient with diabetic neuropathy. Both Chaudhry and colleagues [30] and Cornblath and colleagues [31] suggest a sham surgery control group. I am skeptical if an ethics committee would include such a group simply to control for a presumed surgery placebo effect. The diabetic patient has an increased risk for cardiovascular events and wound healing problems, and an ethics committee must weigh this against the benefit of a sham surgical control. Even if sham surgery were to have a placebo effect of a magnitude of 30%, the observed 80% effect in Box 1 would easily create the situation for statistical significance in favor of the surgery, even with a small cohort of patients. I believe it is unethical to withhold decompression of a nerve chronically compressed in a person with or without diabetes, with or without neuropathy, if that patient has not responded to the best nonsurgical care and the degree of compression is such that axonal loss is documented. I am not against any prospective study the neurologists would like to propose, and I would be happy to ensure that the surgeon working with them has the appropriate training to perform the surgery safely and effectively; however, I believe it is unethical to withhold care that has been shown by surgeons in 43 states within the Unites States and in 18 other countries to be effective and reproducible.

Summary

We can change the future if we can but learn from the past as follows:

- Appreciate that the patient with diabetes is likely to have chronic nerve compressions in the upper and lower extremities, and that these compressions can give symptoms in a stocking and glove distribution [80].
- Appreciate that surgical approaches to decompress the peroneal nerve at the knee, in the leg, and at the dorsum of the foot, and to decompress the tibial nerve in the four medial ankle tunnels have been developed, and that these procedures can be done safely in the patient with diabetes as long as there is adequate circulation to the foot and the surgeon has been trained appropriately.
- Appreciate that if a patient with diabetes has had a successful release of the carpal tunnel to treat symptoms of nerve compression in the hand, there is an 88% positive predictive value that decompression of nerve entrapments in the lower extremity, as described herein, will result in good-to-excellent relief of pain and restoration of sensation to the foot in that same patient [124].

Appreciate that chronic nerve compression in the presence of a metabolic neuropathy like diabetes is difficult to diagnose with traditional electrodiagnostic techniques, and that the physical examination must include an evaluation of the Tinel sign at known sites of anatomic narrowing in the lower extremity to identify the presence of these chronic nerve compressions [16,75].

Appreciate that animal studies and human studies have demonstrated that decompression of a peripheral nerve in the diabetic patient with symptoms of neuropathy and superimposed nerve compression can change the natural history of diabetic neuropathy by reversing its symptoms and preventing progression on the decompressed side, while the neuropathy progresses in the control group or in the nonoperated side [17,90–93].

Apply these new appreciations to your next patient with symptoms of neuropathy. If the symptoms or the screening test suggest the presence of neuropathy, document this with definitive measurements of cutaneous sensibility by measuring the cutaneous pressure threshold at which one from two points can be distinguished, because this will become abnormal before the one-point static threshold (which is estimated by the nylon monofilament). If the physical examination demonstrates a positive Tinel sign at one of the above known sites of compression, understand that there is about an 80% chance that the pain can be relieved and the sensibility restored. Know that if sensibility is restored, the risk of ulceration and amputation will approach zero, balance will be improved, and the risk of admission to the hospital for infection will be greatly diminished.

Know that if you do what you understand to be true for your own patient's care, if you have taken a history and actually examined your patient, if you have documented medical necessity, and if you have informed your patient appropriately, you will have demonstrated the secret to caring for your patient, which is caring for your patient. You will prevail against all those who rail against you. Your patient will thank you and become your advocate.

References

[1] Available at: http://www.ncbi.nlm.nih.gov/entrez/query.fcgi?DB=pubmed. Accessed March 1, 2007.

[2] Dyck PJ. Peripheral neuropathy: changing concepts, differential diagnosis, and classification. Med Clin North Am 1968;52:895–90.

[3] Sinnreich M, Taylor BV, Dyck PJ. Diabetic neuropathies, classification, clinical features and pathophysiologic basis. Neurologist 2005;11:63–79.

[4] Argoff Ce, Backonja M, Belgrade MJ, et al. Consensus guidelines: treatment planning and options. Mayo Clin Proc 2006;81(4 Suppl):S12–25.

[5] Boulton AJM, Vinik AI, Arezzo JC, et al. Diabetic neuropathies: a statement by the American Diabetes Association. Diabetes Care 2005;28:956–62.

[6] Rather HM, Boulton AJM. Recent advances in the diagnosis and management of diabetic neuropathy. J Bone Joint Surg 2005;87B:1605–10.
[7] Sanders LJ. Johns Hopkins Medical Institution CME Lectures Series, best practices in podiatry: improving screening and management strategies for diabetic peripheral neuropathy. 2005;5(12):8–10.
[8] Dellon AL. A cause for optimism in diabetic neuropathy. Ann Plast Surg 1988;20:103–5.
[9] Dellon AL. Treatment of symptomatic diabetic neuropathy by surgical decompression of multiple peripheral nerves. Plast Reconstr Surg 1992;89:689–97.
[10] Wieman TJ, Patel VG. Treatment of hyperesthetic neuropathic pain in diabetics: decompression of the tarsal tunnel. Ann Surg 1995;221:660–5.
[11] Chafee H. Decompression of peripheral nerves for diabetic neuropathy. Plast Reconstr Surg 2000;106:813–5.
[12] Aszmann OA, Kress KM, Dellon AL. Results of decompression of peripheral nerves in diabetics: a prospective, blinded study. Plast Reconstr Surg 2000;106:816–22.
[13] Tambwekar SR. Extended neurolysis of the posterior tibial nerve to improve sensation in diabetic neuropathic feet. Plast Reconstr Surg 2001;108:1452–3.
[14] Wood WA, Wood MA. Decompression of peripheral nerves for diabetic neuropathy in the lower extremity. J Foot Ankle Surg 2003;42:268–75.
[15] Biddinger KR, Amend KJ. The role of surgical decompression for diabetic neuropathy. Foot Ankle Clin 2004;9:239–54.
[16] Lee CH, Dellon AL. Prognostic ability of Tinel sign in determining outcome for decompression surgery in diabetic and nondiabetic neuropathy. Ann Plast Surg 2004;53: 523–7.
[17] Aszmann O, Tassler PL, Dellon AL. Changing the natural history of diabetic neuropathy: incidence of ulcer/amputation in the contralateral limb of patients with a unilateral nerve decompression procedure. Ann Plast Surg 2004;53:517–22.
[18] Rader AJ. Surgical decompression in lower-extremity diabetic peripheral neuropathy. J Am Podiatr Med Assoc 2005;95:446–50.
[19] Valdivia JM, Maloney CM, Dellon AL, et al. Surgical treatment of peripheral neuropathy: outcomes from 100 consecutive decompressions. J Am Podiatr Med Assoc 2005;95:451–4.
[20] Yao Y, Wang R-Z. Peripheral nerve decompression (Dellon procedure) and diabetic neuropathy. Chinese Journal of Medicine 2005;10:1756–8.
[21] DiNucci K. Results of decompression of multiple lower extremity peripheral nerves in diabetics with symptomatic neuropathy. Presented at the American College of Foot and Ankle Surgery meeting. New Orleans (LA), March 22, 2005.
[22] Steck J. Results of decompression of lower extremity peripheral nerve for treatment of symptomatic neuropathy. Presented at the American Society of Peripheral Nerve meeting. Puerto Rico, January 12, 2005.
[23] Sienionow M, Alghoul M, Molski M, et al. Clinical outcome of nerve decompression in diabetic and non-diabetic peripheral neuropathy. Ann Plast Surg 2006;57:385–90.
[24] Yuksel F. Lower extremity nerve decompression in diabetic neuropathy. Presented at the American Society of Peripheral Nerve meeting. Tucson (AZ), January 14, 2006.
[25] Shafiroff B. Decompression of lower extremity nerves in neuropathy. Presented at the Lower Extremity of Peripheral Nerve Surgery meeting. Sante Fe (NM), October 14, 2006.
[26] Nelson SC, Little ER Jr. Pilot study of the use of the SF 36 questionnaire outcome evaluation for multiple lower extremity nerve decompressions in diabetic peripheral neuropathy. J Am Podiatr Med Assoc 2007;97:121–5.
[27] Massa E. Diabetic neuropathy: decompression of compressed lower extremity nerves. Presented at the International Diabetes Federation meeting. Cape Town, South Africa, January, 2007.
[28] Maloney CT, Valdivia JV, Weinand M. Nerve decompression results in a consecutive series of 165 patients with neuropathy. Neurol Surg, in press.

[29] Bae S, Biddinger K, Shon L. Independent, retrospective review of surgical nerve decompression for diabetic neuropathy. Presented at the American Academy of Orthopedic Surgery and Foot & Ankle Society meeting. San Diego (CA), February 22, 2007.
[30] Chaudhry V, Stevens JC, Kincaid J, et al. Practice advisory: utility of surgical decompression for treatment of diabetic neuropathy. Report of the Therapeutics and Technology Assessment Subcommittee of the American Academy of Neurology. Neurology 2006;66:1805–8.
[31] Cornblath DR, Vinik A, Feldman E, et al. Commentary: surgical decompression for diabetic sensorimotor polyneuropathy. Diabetes Care 2007;30:421–2.
[32] Asbury AK, Porte D Jr. American Diabetes Association Clinical Practice Recommendations 1995: consensus statement on standardized measures in diabetic neuropathy. Diabetes Care 1995;18(Suppl 1):59–82.
[33] Clinical Practice Recommendations 1997: S31. Foot care in patients with diabetes mellitus. Diabetes Care 1997;19(Suppl 1):580–1.
[34] American Diabetes Association. Standards of medical care in diabetes—2007. Diabetes Care 2007;30(Suppl 1):S22–4.
[35] Argoff CE, Cole BE, Fishbain DA, et al. Diabetic peripheral neuropathic pain: clinical and quality of life issues. Mayo Clinic Proceedings 2006;81(4 Suppl):S2–11.
[36] Armstrong DA. Detection of diabetic peripheral neuropathy: strategies for screening and diagnosis. In: Saudek CD, editor. Best practices in podiatry: improving screening and management strategies for diabetic peripheral neuropathy. Johns Hopkins Medical Institutions CME 2005;5(12):8–12.
[37] Tassler PL, Dellon AL, Sheffler N. Cutaneous pressure thresholds in ulcerated and non-ulcerated diabetic feet, measured with the pressure-specified sensory device. Journal of the American Podiatric Medical Society 1995;85:679–84.
[38] Tassler PL, Dellon AL. Correlation of measurements of pressure perception using the pressure-specified sensory device with electrodiagnostic testing. J Occup Med 1995;37:862–6.
[39] Dellon AL. Computer-assisted sensibility evaluation and surgical treatment of tarsal tunnel syndrome. Advances in Podiatry 1996;2:17–40.
[40] Tassler PL, Dellon AL. Pressure perception in the normal lower extremity and in tarsal tunnel syndrome. Muscle Nerve 1996;19:285–9.
[41] Lee RH, Dellon AL. Insulin resistance: does it play a role in peripheral neuropathy? Diabetes Care 1999;22:1914–5.
[42] Dellon AL. Somatosensory testing and rehabilitation. Baltimore (MD): Institute for Peripheral Nerve Surgery; 2000.
[43] Barber MA, Conolley J, Spaulding CM, et al. Evaluation of pressure threshold prior to foot ulceration: one versus two-point static touch. J Am Podiatr Med Assoc 2001;91:508–14.
[44] Dellon AL. Clinical grading of peripheral nerve problems. Neurosurg Clin N Am 2001;12:229–40.
[45] Cohen MD, Dellon AL. Computer-assisted sensorimotor testing documents neural regeneration after ulnar nerve repair at the wrist: case report. Plast Reconstr Surg 2001;107:501–5.
[46] Dellon AL. Deciding when heel pain is of neural origin. J Foot Ankle Surg 2001;40:341–5.
[47] Coert JH, Meek MF, Gibeault D, et al. Documentation of post-traumatic nerve compression in patients with normal electrodiagnostic studies. J Trauma 2004;56:239–44.
[48] Dellon AL, Swier P, Levingood M, et al. Cisplatin/Taxol neuropathy: treatment by decompression of peripheral nerve. Plast Reconstr Surg 2004;114:478–83.
[49] Ducic I, Dellon AL, Short KW. Relationship between loss of pedal sensibility, balance, and falls in patients with peripheral neuropathy. Ann Plast Surg 2004;52:535–40.
[50] Seiler DK, Wilton JP, Dellon AL. Detection of neuropathy due to *Mycobacterium leprae* using non-invasive neurosensory testing of susceptible peripheral nerves. Ann Plast Surg 2005;55:633–7.

[51] Wood WA, Wood MA, Werter S, et al. Cross-sectional study relating loss of protective sensation to testing methodology in patients with foot ulceration. J Am Podiatr Med Assoc 2005;95:469–74.
[52] Dellon AL. Post-arthroplasty palsy and systemic neuropathy: a peripheral nerve management algorithm. Ann Plast Surg 2005;55:638–42.
[53] Ducic I, Taylor NS, Dellon AL. Relationship between peripheral nerve decompression, gain of pedal sensibility and balance in patients with peripheral neuropathy. Ann Plast Surg 2006;56:145–50.
[54] Radoiu H, Rosson GD, Andonian G, et al. Comparison of measures of large-fiber nerve function in patients with chronic nerve compression and neuropathy. J Am Podiatr Med Assoc 2005;95:438–45.
[55] Caputo GM, Cavanagh PR, Ulbrecht JS, et al. Assessment and management of foot disease in patients with diabetes. N Engl J Med 1994;331:854–60.
[56] Uccioli L, Faglia E, Monticone G, et al. Manufactured shoes in the prevention of diabetic foot ulcers. Diabetes Care 1995;18:1376–8.
[57] Singh N, Armstrong DG, Lipsky BA. Preventing foot ulcers in patients with diabetes. J Am Med Assoc 2005;293:217–28.
[58] Coppini DV, Spruce MC, Thomas P, et al. Established diabetic neuropathy seems irreversible despite improvements in metabolic and vascular risk markers: a retrospective, case-control study in a hospital patient cohort. Diabet Med 2006;23:1016–20.
[59] Coppini DV, Wellmer A, Weng C, et al. The natural history of diabetic peripheral neuropathy determined by a 12 year prospective study using vibration perception thresholds. J Clin Neurosci 2001;8:520–4.
[60] Martin CL, Albers J, Herman PC, et al. Neuropathy among the diabetes control and complications trial cohort 8 years after trial completion. Diabetes Care 2006;29:340–4.
[61] Frykberg RG, Zgonis T, Armstrong DG, et al. Diabetic foot disorders: a clinical practice guideline (2006 revision). J Foot Ankle Surg 2006;45(Suppl):S1–64.
[62] Dellon AL. Review of treatment results for ulnar nerve entrapment at the elbow. J Hand Surg [Am] 1989;14:688–700.
[63] Dellon AL. Operative technique for submuscular transposition of the ulnar nerve. Contemp Orthop 1988;16:17–24.
[64] Dellon AL. Techniques for successful management of ulnar nerve entrapment at the elbow. Neurosurg Clin N Am 1991;2:57–73.
[65] Dellon AL, Coert JH. Technique of musculofascial lengthening for treatment of ulnar nerve compression at the elbow. J Bone Joint Surg Am 2004;86:169–79.
[66] Dellon AL, Mackinnon SE. Radial sensory nerve entrapment in the forearm. J Hand Surg [Am] 1986;11:199–205.
[67] Pershing HT. Pressure neuritis caused during surgical operations. Medical News, New York, 1897:71, 329.
[68] Mont MA, Dellon AL, Chen F, et al. Operative treatment of peroneal nerve palsy. J Bone Joint Surg Am 1996;78:863–9.
[69] Dellon AL, Ebmer J, Swier P. Anatomic variations related to decompression of the common peroneal nerve at the fibular head. Ann Plast Surg 2002;48:30–4.
[70] Keck C. The tarsal tunnel syndrome. J Bone Joint Surg [Am] 1962;44:180–2.
[71] Lam SJS. A tarsal tunnel syndrome. Lancet 1962;2:1354–5.
[72] Mackinnon SE, Dellon AL. Homologies between the tarsal and carpal tunnels: implications for treatment of the tarsal tunnel syndrome. Contemp Orthop 1987;14:75–9.
[73] Dellon AL. Entrapment of the deep peroneal nerve on the dorsum of the foot. Foot and Ankle 1990;11:73–80.
[74] Mackinnon SE, Dellon AL. Surgery of the peripheral nerve. New York: Thieme; 1988.
[75] Perkins BA, Olaleye D, Bril V. Carpal tunnel syndrome in patients with diabetic polyneuropathy. Diabetes Care 2002;25:565–9.

[76] Dimitrakoudis D, Bril V. Comparison of sensory testing on different toe surfaces: implications for neuropathy screening. Neurology 2002;59:611–3.
[77] Boulton AJM, Arezzo JC, Malik RA, et al. Diabetic somatic neuropathies. Diabetes Care 2004;27:1458–86.
[78] Vinik AI. Advances in diabetes for the millennium: new treatments for diabetic neuropathies. Med Gen Med 2004;6:13–9.
[79] Vinik AI, Mehrabyan A. Diabetic neuropathies. Med Clin North Am 2004;88:947–99.
[80] Vinik AI, Mehrabyan A, Colen L, et al. Focal entrapment neuropathies in diabetes. Diabetes Care 2004;27:1783–8.
[81] Gulliford MC, Latinovic R, Charlton J, et al. Increased incidence of carpal tunnel syndrome up to 10 years before diagnosis of diabetes. Diabetes Care 2006;29:1929–30.
[82] Jakobsen J. Peripheral nerves in early experimental diabetes: expansion of the endoneurial space as a cause of increased water content. Diabetologia 1978;14:113–8.
[83] Jakobsen J, Sidenius P. Decreased axonal transport of structural proteins in streptozotocin diabetic rats. J Clin Invest 1980;66:282–6.
[84] Tomlinson DR, Mayer JH. Defects of axonal transport in diabetes mellitus—a possible contribution to the aetiology of diabetic neuropathy. J Auton Pharmacol 1984;4:59–72.
[85] Medori R, Jemich H, Antilio-Gambetti L, et al. Experimental diabetic neuropathy: similar changes of slow axonal transport and axonal size in different animal models. J Neurosci 1988;8:1814–21.
[86] Lundborg G, Rydevik B. Effects of stretching the tibial nerve of the rabbit, a preliminary study of the intraneural circulation and the barrier function of the perineurium. J Bone Joint Surg [Br] 1973;55:390–401.
[87] Rydevik B, Lundborg G. Effects of graded compression on intraneural blood flow. J Hand Surg [Am] 1981;6:3–12.
[88] Mackinnon SE, Dellon AL, Hudson AR, et al. Chronic nerve compression—an experimental model in the rat. Ann Plast Surg 1984;13:112–20.
[89] Dellon AL, Mackinnon SE, Seiler WA. Susceptibility of the diabetic nerve to chronic compression. Ann Plast Surg 1988;20:117–9.
[90] Dellon ES, Dellon AL. Functional assessment of neurologic impairment: track analysis in diabetic and compression neuropathies. Plast Reconstr Surg 1991;88:686–94.
[91] Dellon ES, Dellon AL, Seiler WA IV. The effect of tarsal tunnel decompression in the streptozotocin-induced diabetic rat. Microsurgery 1994;15:265–8.
[92] Kale B, Yuksel F, Celikoz B, et al. Effect of various nerve decompression procedures on the functions of distal limbs in streptozotocin-induced diabetic rats: further optimism in diabetic neuropathy. Plast Reconstr Surg 2003;111:2265–72.
[93] Demir Y, Sari A, Siemionow M. Impact of early decompression on development of superimposed neuropathy in diabetic rats. Presented at the American Association for Surgery of the Hand annual meeting. Puerto Rico, January 1, 2005.
[94] Lam SJS. Tarsal-tunnel syndrome. J Bone Joint Surg [Br] 1967;49:87–92.
[95] Edwards WG, Lincoln R, Bassett FH, et al. Tarsal tunnel syndrome. JAMA 1969;207:716–20.
[96] Linscheid R, Burton R, Fredericks E. Tarsal tunnel syndrome. South Med J 1970;63:1313–20.
[97] Mann RA. Tarsal tunnel syndrome. Orthop Clin North Am 1974;5:109–15.
[98] Stern DS, Joyce MT. Tarsal tunnel syndrome: a review of 15 surgical procedures. J Foot Surg 1989;28:290–4.
[99] Byank RP, Curtis MJ. Diagnosing tarsal tunnel syndrome. Complications in Orthopedics 1992;7:202–202.
[100] Sammarco GJ, Chalk DE, Feibel JH. Tarsal tunnel syndrome and additional nerve lesions in the same limb. Foot Ankle 1993;14:71–7.
[101] Pfeiffer WH, Cracchiolo A. Clinical results after tarsal tunnel decompression. J Bone Joint Surg [Am] 1994;76:1222–30.

[102] Mahan KT, Rock JJ, Hillstrom HJ. Tarsal tunnel syndrome: a retrospective study. J Am Podiatr Med Assoc 1996;86:81–91.
[103] Turan I, Rivero-Melian C, Guntner P, et al. Tarsal tunnel syndrome: outcome of surgery in longstanding cases. Clin Orthop Relat Res 1997;343:151–6.
[104] Baba H, Wada M, Annen S, et al. The tarsal tunnel syndrome: evaluation of surgical results using multivariate analysis. Int Orthop 1997;21:67–71.
[105] Bailie DS, Kelitian AS. The tarsal tunnel syndrome: surgical technique and functional outcome. Foot Ankle Int 1998;19:65–71.
[106] Kohno M, Takahashi H, Segawa H, et al. Neurovascular decompression for idiopathic tarsal tunnel syndrome: technical note. J Neurol Neurosurg Psychiatr 2000;69:87–90.
[107] Gondring WH, Shields B, Wenger S. An outcomes analysis of surgical treatment of tarsal tunnel syndrome. Foot Ankle Int 2003;24:545–9.
[108] Mullick T, Dellon AL. Results of decompression of four medial ankle tunnels in the treatment of tarsal tunnels syndrome. J Reconstr Microsurg, 2007; in press.
[109] Dyck JP, Litchey WJ, Lehman KA, et al. Diabetic polyneuropathy in controlled clinical trials: consensus report of the Peripheral Nerve Society. Ann Neurol 1995;38:478–82.
[110] Young MJU, Breddy JL, Veves A, et al. The prediction of diabetic neuropathic foot ulceration using vibration perception thresholds: a prospective study. Diabetes Care 1994;17: 557–60.
[111] Kumar S, Fernando DJS, Veves A, et al. Semmes-Weinstein monofilaments: a simple, effective and inexpensive screening device for identifying diabetic patients at risk of foot ulceration. Diabetes Res Clin Pract 1995;13:63–7.
[112] Armstrong DG, Lavery LA, Vela SA, et al. Choosing a practical screening instrument to identify patients at risk for diabetic foot ulceration. Arch Intern Med 1998;158:289–92.
[113] Barrett EJ. ADA presidential address: the sheep, the ostrich, the ant, diabetes, and the tragedy of the common. Diabetes Care 2004;27:3005–8.
[114] Hossain P, Kawar B, Nahas ME. Obesity and diabetes in the developing world—a growing challenge. N Engl J Med 2007;356:213–5.
[115] Cornblath DE, Dellon AL, Mackinnon SE. Electrodiagnostic evaluation of peripheral nerve in type I diabetic primate. Muscle Nerve 1989;12:233–5.
[116] Carroll RE, Hurst LC. The relationship of thoracic outlet syndrome and carpal tunnel syndrome. Clin Orthop Relat Res 1982;164:149–53.
[117] Kimura J. Electrodiagnosis in diseases of nerve and muscle. Philadelphia: FA Davis; 1983.
[118] Gilliatt RW, Thomas PK. Changes in nerve conduction with ulnar lesions at the elbow. J Neurol Neurosurg Psychiatry 1960;23:312–20.
[119] Gilliatt RW, Wilson RG. Peripheral nerve conduction in diabetic neuropathy. J Neurol Neurosurg Psychiatry 1962;25:11–6.
[120] AAEM Quality Assurance Committee. Literature review of the usefulness of nerve conduction studies and electromyography for the evaluation of patients with carpal tunnel syndrome. Muscle Nerve 1993;16:1392–414.
[121] Dyck PJ. Correspondence related to the article by Chaudhry, et al. Neurology 2007;68:796.
[122] Lavery LA, Higgins KR, Lanctot DR, et al. Preventing diabetic foot ulcer recurrence in high-risk patients: use of temperature monitoring as a self-assessment tool. Diabetes Care 2007;30:14–20.
[123] Lavery LA, Armstrong DG, Wunderlich RP, et al. Risk factors for foot infections in individuals with diabetes. Diabetes Care 2006;29:1288–93.
[124] Maloney CT Jr, Dellon AL, Heller C Jr, et al. Prognostic ability of a good outcome to carpal tunnel release for decompression surgery in the lower extremity. Clin Podiatr Med Surg 2006;23:559–68.

ELSEVIER
SAUNDERS

Clin Podiatr Med Surg
24 (2007) 449–467

CLINICS IN PODIATRIC MEDICINE AND SURGERY

Vascular Assessment and Reconstruction of the Ischemic Diabetic Limb

Ryan T. Hagino, MD, FACS

Division of Vascular and Endovascular Surgery, University of Texas Health Science Center at San Antonio, 7703 Floyd Curl Drive, San Antonio, TX 78229, USA

Atherosclerosis obliterans complicates the medical and surgical treatment of the diabetic foot. The systemic and local manifestations of the disease have profound effects on wound healing, symptom control, and, ultimately, foot salvage and patient longevity. The medical and surgical treatment of diabetic foot disorders can be drastically effected by the presence or absence of occlusive disease secondary to atherosclerosis and the absolute and relative ischemia induced by such involvement. Before treatment of any lesion involving a diabetic foot, the clinician should consider the degree of involvement of the limb with atherosclerosis and the effects of such treatment and should anticipate the problems and probabilities of success before any incision is actually made on the affected foot. This article discusses the epidemiology, anatomic features, clinical presentation, and treatment of the dysvascular diabetic foot. In addition, an attempt is made to present a rational diagnostic and therapeutic strategy to avoid the common pitfalls associated with the treatment of diabetic foot lesions in limbs affected with atherosclerosis and to maximize the success of any intervention.

Atherosclerosis and peripheral artery disease

Atherosclerosis is a progressive systemic disease that can involve any artery within the body. The common perception is that atherosclerosis represents a continuum of disease initiated through an abnormal response to endothelial injury. The loss of the functionally and physically important barrier of the intima of an artery leads to the increased susceptibility of the endothelium to oxidative injury, lipid accumulation, and inflammatory cell adherence, accumulation, and activation, ultimately leading to

E-mail address: haginor@uthscsa.edu

0891-8422/07/$ - see front matter
doi:10.1016/j.cpm.2007.03.001

a proliferative, progressive accumulation of cellular and noncellular material within the media of an artery. This results in the development of occlusive lesions and thrombotic events [1].

Manifestations of atherosclerosis are largely related to the end organs involved and the degree of ischemia induced by the occlusive disease involving their respective feeding vessels. Typically, the territories affected by atherosclerosis are divided into three regions: (1) the coronary circulation, (2) the cerebrovascular circulation, and (3) the peripheral circulation. By definition, peripheral arterial disease (PAD) involves occlusive or aneurysmal disease involving the arteries outside of the heart and intracranial vessels [2]. Although several medical conditions can affect the peripheral arterial circulation, the most common etiology, by far, is atherosclerosis. Approximately 12 million Americans are affected by symptomatic PAD [3]. For every patient diagnosed with PAD in an office, there are likely three to four patients afflicted by the disease that are not diagnosed, representing a significant proportion of the population [4,5].

Beyond the local effects of such lesions on the end organs supplied by the diseased arteries, the systemic manifestations are germane and profound. Depending on the sensitivity of the diagnostic testing, the prevalence of concomitant coronary artery disease and cerebrovascular disease is 14% to 90% and 25% to 72%, respectively, among patients diagnosed with PAD [6]. In fact, the diagnosis of intermittent claudication, a local manifestation of PAD, is a more profound marker for cardiovascular death than it is for limb loss [7,8]. Patients with known symptomatic coronary disease diagnosed with PAD have been shown to have an increased risk of recurrent myocardial infarction, stroke, and vascular death when compared with patients without PAD [2]. In addition, 25% of patients with PAD who underwent routine coronary angiography before PAD treatment were found to have significant surgically correctable coronary artery disease involving three coronary vessels [9]. Clearly, PAD represents one manifestation of atherosclerosis that has profound implications on long-term survival as well as limb salvage.

Diabetes and atherosclerosis

Epidemiology and pathophysiology

The association between diabetes and atherosclerosis is significant. The prevalence of PAD in the United States among diabetic persons has been estimated to be 9.5% [10]. Matched for age, this is twice the prevalence found among non-diabetic persons. When examining cardiovascular risk factors, the presence of diabetes is associated with a threefold to fourfold greater risk of PAD than in non-diabetic patients; this association is second only to active smoking as a risk factor for PAD [2,7,8]. The American Diabetes Association [3] has gone as far as recommending PAD noninvasive arterial testing with ankle-brachial indices (ABIs) for all patients with diabetes who are 50 years of age or older, for those younger than 50 years if they have other atherosclerotic risk factors, and for subjects who have sustained diabetes for more than 10 years.

Patients who have diabetes have profound abnormalities in arterial physiology and biology that may explain the significant association between the two diagnoses. Patients with diabetes have been shown to have abnormal endothelial-mediated contraction and relaxation through nitric oxide–dependent mechanisms [11]. Nitric oxide is produced by the endothelial cell and is a critical marker for vascular health [12]. Its profound role in endothelial vascular reactivity, platelet and monocyte adherence and activation, and smooth muscle migration and transformation are well known, and dysfunction has been suggested as a precursor for occlusive atherosclerotic plaque development [13]. In addition, diabetes-associated insulin resistance and hyperglycemia have been shown to affect non-endothelial–dependent abnormalities in oxidative metabolism and platelet function, coagulation, and thrombosis [3,11].

Anatomic involvement

An unfortunate nomenclature has developed to describe arteries in diabetic patients affected by atherosclerosis. The blood vessel lesions are typically divided into two groups—large vessel disease and small vessel disease. The implications of such a grouping are profound and have led to the misplaced perception that "small vessel disease" in the foot obviates revascularization as an option for the ischemic diabetic foot. It should be reinforced that "microvascular disease" refers to the important, but separate, obliterative effects at the arteriolar level seen in the retina (diabetic retinopathy), the renal parenchyma (diabetic nephropathy), and, to some degree, the peripheral nervous system (diabetic ischemic neuropathy). The microvascular arteriolar lesion is distinct from atherosclerosis and represents a process involving the basement membrane of the microvasculature on the arteriolar level in these specific end organs. Although this accumulation of matrix within the basement membranes of the nutrient cutaneous vessels within the foot is evident on biopsy in diabetic patients, it is rarely an obliterative process, and the lumen of these vessels is usually preserved [14,15]. Some evidence suggests that this microvascular process leads to abnormalities in nutrient delivery and even hypoxia to the tissues supplied by these nutrient vessels, but the process is not atherosclerosis [15,16]. A recent study noted that the only standard cardiovascular risk factor that contributes to the progression of small vessel PAD in the foot is the presence of diabetes [17]. The risk factors for small vessel PAD are distinct from those contributing to large vessel atherosclerosis [16,17].

Although PAD in diabetic patients tends to be more prevalent and malignant, the peripheral atherosclerosis involving the large vessels of the

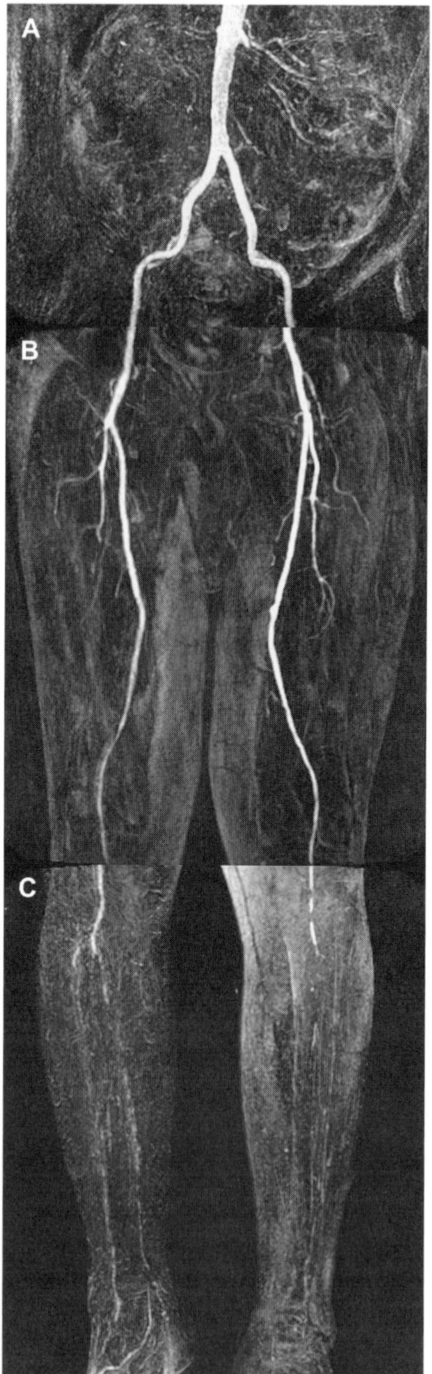
A
B
C

dysvascular diabetic limb is histologically no different from that affecting non-diabetic patients; however, the distribution of the lesions is significantly different. PAD in the non-diabetic patient is typically seen in the more proximal vessels of the lower extremity, specifically, in the aortoiliac and femoral-popliteal system. The distribution of atherosclerotic PAD in the diabetic patient will often be isolated to the infrapopliteal tibial and pedal segments with a relative sparing of the proximal vessels (Fig. 1) [18,19]. An exception to proximal vessel involvement is seen in the predilection for atherosclerotic involvement of the internal iliac arteries and the deep femoral arteries in diabetic patients [19]. Such involvement may influence the ischemic reserve of a diabetic limb because these vessels represent important collateral pathways to the main axial arteries of the limb. Infrapopliteal artery involvement has been show to be more frequent than pedal involvement, but there remains a strong association between the two levels [20].

Some researchers have suggested that involvement with atherosclerosis of the named vessels of the foot often spares the dorsal vessels, whereas others have suggested that the plantar vessels are more often spared [18,21]. The author's group has not able to demonstrate any predilection for sparing of a dorsal versus plantar system in atherosclerotic affected dysvascular diabetic feet [20]. This observation does not mean that the pedal circulation always offers some suitable vessel for revascularization in the foot (Fig. 2). The "microvascular disease" represents microangiopathy seen in the eyes, kidneys, and nerves of diabetic patients and should not be confused with "small vessel" involvement in the foot. The effects of this real phenomenon on patient care and prognosis are discussed further in the section on noninvasive testing.

A separate pathologic entity distinct from atherosclerosis that is often seen in the limbs of diabetic patients is the typical semilunar medial calcinosis of the tibial vessels. This calcification can be seen on plain radiographs in many patients [22]; however, it does not lead to luminal encroachment. The effects of medial calcinosis are largely related to changes in external vessel compressibility and are seen on diagnostic imaging and physiologic testing. Nevertheless, recent investigations suggest that cardiovascular event-free survival in patients with an abnormally elevated ABI (>1.40) may be significantly worse than in patients with normal indices regardless of the presence or absence of diabetes [23].

Fig. 1. Contrast-enhanced MRA demonstrating the typical pattern of occlusive disease in the diabetic patient, notable for internal iliac artery involvement with sparing of the aorta, common, and external iliac arteries (*A*). Relatively disease-free common femoral and superficial femoral arteries, with disease noted in the deep femoral arteries (*B*). (*C*) Severe infrapopliteal disease.

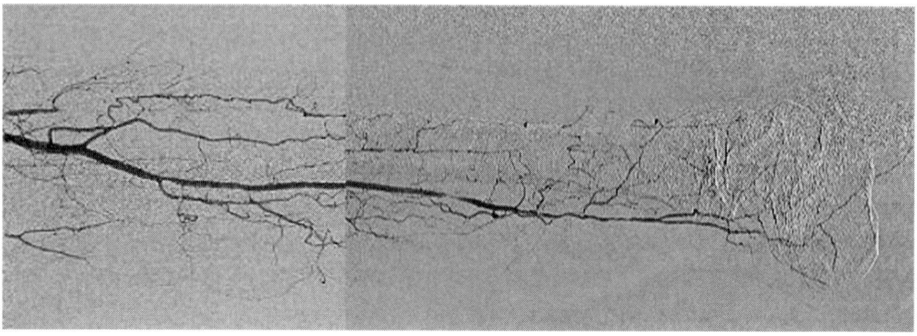

Fig. 2. Selective digital subtraction conventional contrast angiography demonstrating severe tibial artery occlusive disease extending into the pedal circulation.

Clinical manifestations of peripheral arterial disease

The clinical presentation of PAD is variable. The complaints and symptoms associated with PAD represent a continuum ranging from asymptomatic resting arterial insufficiency to profound limb-threatening ischemia. The Fontaine and Rutherford classification systems for chronic lower extremity ischemia have been well described in other publications [2,7]. In brief, the continuum of presentation is as follows: 1—asymptomatic resting ischemia, 2—intermittent claudication, 3—ischemic rest pain, 4—ischemic ulceration, and 5—gangrene. A large subset of "asymptomatic patients" may not complain of classic intermittent claudication but may have other less definable complaints [24].

The asymptomatic patient manifests no overt symptoms of ischemia but has an abnormal examination with or without evidence of ischemia on noninvasive testing. The prognosis for such a diagnosis regarding the involved extremity is good. The likelihood of progression of local disease may be high, but the development of worsening symptoms or limb loss is rare in non-diabetic patients [8]. In stark contrast, the systemic implications of even asymptomatic PAD in a limb are profound. The systemic manifestations of atherosclerosis in these patients lead to an increased long-term risk of cardiac-related events and cardiac death [6,25]. The emphasis of treatment in these patients should be on systemic risk factor modification and anti-platelet therapy as a means of preventing cardiac-related morbidity, rather than on improving the perfusion of an affected limb.

Intermittent claudication is a relatively benign condition from a limb health standpoint. This fairly common condition affects 3% to 6% of patients over the age of 60 years [7]. Typically, the symptoms are described as a cramping, muscular discomfort involving the calf muscles initiated by a reproducible distance of walking that is relieved by a brief period of rest (typically 5 to 10 minutes). The affected muscle group is usually immediately distal to the level of occlusive disease; however, this is not a uniform finding. More than an occasional patient suffering from iliac occlusive disease will present with calf claudication rather than an expected involvement of the hip, buttock, or thigh.

In the patient who has calf claudication, the condition is secondary to the inability of a compromised artery (iliac or superficial femoral artery) above the gastrocnemius muscle group to deliver the increased blood flow required to meet the increased metabolic demands of the muscle associated with exercise. The muscle group is rendered ischemic, leading to the development of symptoms. The symptoms resolve with resting of the muscle group and the subsequent decrease in metabolic demands associated with rest. Hip, thigh, and buttock claudication usually result from proximally located occlusive disease involving the aortoiliac system. The constellation of symptoms related to aortoiliac occlusive disease may include a more frequent complaint of muscular weakness and tiredness, rather than the cramping discomfort usually attributed to vasculogenic claudication in the calf. In addition, males with severe bilateral aortoiliac occlusive disease may manifest vasculogenic impotence because of involvement of the pelvic arterial circulation and the more proximal aorta or common iliac arteries. Likewise, involvement of the buttocks in the ischemic syndrome is an indication of similar pelvic or more proximal arterial involvement. In the absence of hip or buttock complaints, external iliac artery involvement may elicit symptoms of claudication only in the thigh muscle groups.

The diagnosis of foot claudication bears special attention. It is an uncommon finding in which the affected foot suffers from walking-induced cramping, midfoot aching, or pain that is often accompanied by a feeling of numbness. Foot claudication is seen with diffuse infrapopliteal and tibial artery involvement. It is a frequent complaint in patients suffering from Buerger's disease; however, as an independent symptom, the diagnosis of foot claudication is often treated with some skepticism, because it is very uncommon to find a patient with a limb with enough disease present to cause foot claudication who does not suffer from rest pain or tissue loss as the dominant presenting complaint.

The natural history of a particular limb with claudication is good, with only about 5% of limbs progressing to amputation or requiring revascularization for limb salvage over a 5-year period [7]. As noted previously for the asymptomatic limb, intermittent claudication is a marker for overall cardiac morbidity and mortality and should be treated as a risk equivalent for coronary artery atherosclerosis [6]. Although the discomfort associated with claudication can be treated with risk factor modification, exercise therapy, and, in select patients, revascularization, the bulk of counseling and treatment should be directed at reducing the risk of concomitant cardiac death.

The symptoms of ischemic rest pain, ischemic ulceration, and gangrene are distinct from the prior two categories. These clinical syndromes fall into the category of critical ischemia or limb-threatening ischemia. Although they are part of a continuum of complaints seen with arterial insufficiency, distinguishing between claudication and critical ischemia is paramount.

Critical ischemia is usually related to atherosclerotic occlusive disease involving multiple levels within a limb. Although other etiologies such as autoimmune vasculitidies, thromboangiitis obliterans (Buerger's disease), or atheroembolism can lead to similar ischemic damage in a particular foot, these entities are much more infrequent. Critical ischemia due to atherosclerosis carries a grave prognosis for the life and limb of the patient, with each condition (rest pain, ulceration, gangrene) associated with increasing risk. The natural history of patients who have symptoms of chronic critical limb ischemia with ankle pressures less than 40 mm Hg is dismal when they are treated conservatively. Almost 95% of these subjects will require a major amputation or die within 1 year of diagnosis [26].

The typical patient with ischemic rest pain complains of intermittent or continuous forefoot pain unrelated to activity. The pain is often described as an "aching" discomfort deep within the foot that is difficult to relieve with any measures including non-steroidal analgesics or narcotics. The stereotypic description of nocturnal pain occurring while recumbent that requires dangling the foot over the side of a bed, or sleeping in a reclining chair with the affected foot dependent, is surprisingly consistent. As would be expected, the advent of tissue loss or gangrene represents the absolute limits of the foot's ability to compensate for resting arterial insufficiency, with the foot literally dying while still attached to the patient. Intervention in the form of revascularization is imperative if the limb is to be saved.

As is true for most manifestations of atherosclerotic PAD, the systemic consequences for critical lower extremity ischemia are profound. Twenty percent of patients will be dead within 12 months of diagnosis, and 32% will be dead within 2 years [26,27]. The most frequent cause of demise in these patients (as would be expected) is a cardiovascular complication, such as acute coronary syndrome, stroke, or catastrophic peripheral vascular events. In fact, these end-game manifestations of lower extremity PAD are reminiscent of metastatic cancer in terms of the dismal prognosis associated with the diagnosis. Although somewhat nihilistic, the treatment of limb-threatening ischemia should be directed at palliation and maintaining functionality, because any intervention targeted at revascularization will not prolong life per se. The main goal should be directed at maintaining ambulatory status through limb preservation techniques and freedom from pain.

The presentation of PAD in diabetic patients demands special considerations. The manifestation of chronic ischemia may be much more subtle in diabetic patients when compared with non-diabetic patients. The typical symptoms of intermittent claudication may be absent in diabetic patients for several reasons. First, as mentioned earlier, the atherosclerotic burden in the limbs of diabetic patients often spares the proximal vessels; therefore, as the most often affected muscle group in claudicants during walking, the gastrocnemius gets its primary blood supply from the superficial femoral and popliteal arteries and does not suffer from exercise-induced ischemia. No obstructive lesion is present above the muscle group. Second, the peripheral diabetic neuropathy present in many patients may alter existing sensory feedback and pain perception in the limb [28]. What may be called "pain" by non-diabetic persons is perceived as fatigue or tiredness in patients sustaining diabetes. Third, the combinations of impaired protective sensation, impaired immune response, and impaired healing provide a fertile ground for unrecognized trauma and progressive invasive infection. The subsequent increased metabolic demands of an infected foot can outstrip the compromised baseline arterial blood supply, leading to a failure of supply compared with demand. The result is a rapidly deteriorating foot secondary to a relative ischemic state brought on by the infection or trauma.

Physical examination findings among diabetic patients with PAD can be unreliable [3]. The traditional approach of "look, listen, and feel" is germane to the vascular examination. Although the presence of a gangrenous toe is quite obvious, other findings may be subtle. The functional sympathectomy associated with diabetic neuropathy may make the usual autoregulatory response of the cutaneous capillary beds to chronic ischemia less pronounced. Dependent rubor, which is associated with the pooling of blood within the maximally dilated subcutaneous areas of an ischemic foot, may not be present. The classic bland, painful, irregular appearing ulceration associated with ischemia continues to be a common finding in diabetic feet. The neuro-ischemic ulcer may be less apparent because the peripheral neuropathy of diabetes makes the lesion painless [8]. The more usual presentation seems to be a diabetic foot infection requiring rapid debridement and drainage, followed by wound breakdown and progressive involvement of the surrounding tissues with gangrene. It is well known that diabetics with PAD tend to present later and with more profound ischemic complications when compared with their non-diabetic counterparts [3,8,19]. These late presenting ischemic manifestations of PAD present a greater challenge to successful limb salvage.

The absence of or a diminished pulse at a given location suggests an occlusion or stenosis in the artery located proximal to the palpated area. An absent femoral pulse would suggest an aortoiliac lesion. An absent pedal pulse associated with a palpable, more proximal popliteal pulse suggests cural and pedal artery lesions. The latter finding represents a common scenario for a diabetic patient with PAD. Similarly, a bruit heard on auscultation of the femoral artery would suggest occlusive disease at or above the femoral level. The assumption that an absent pedal pulse is diagnostic of a proximal lesion is based on another assumption that the patient actually had the pedal artery present from birth. Pulse examination variability is actually relatively common. Certain hospital-based and community-based studies have noted that the dorsalis pedis artery is absent in 8.1% of patients and the posterior tibial artery in 2.0% [3].

Noninvasive physiologic arterial assessment

Few would question the utility of the Doppler-derived ABI as a diagnostic tool in non-diabetic patients with PAD. The test remains a cheap, reproducible, and portable screening modality. The interobserver and intraobserver variability are low, and the sensitivity and specificity are high (95% and 100%, respectively) for detecting the presence of angiographically confirmed arterial occlusive disease [8]. In addition, its proportionate decrease is a useful measure for quantifying the severity of ischemia. The utility of this study is not only its ability to diagnose the presence of disease but also its ability to quantify the severity of ischemia as well as serially follow the progression of ischemia over time. In its simplest manifestation, the calculation of an ABI requires only a manual blood pressure cuff and a continuous-wave Doppler probe. The Doppler-derived upper extremity systolic brachial arterial cuff pressure is measured in both upper extremities. This measurement is followed by a similar cuff systolic occlusion pressure measurement taken in both feet with the Doppler probe placed over the inframalleolar posterior tibial and dorsalis pedis arteries. The cuff must be placed with its lowest margin just above the ankle in the tendinous portion of the leg. The highest recorded pedal pressure (regardless of the vessel) in a limb is then divided by the highest upper extremity pressure. The resulting ratio is referred to as the ABI. In the absence of an available continuous-wave Doppler probe, Beckman and colleagues [29] have shown that a fairly accurate correlation is noted with systolic pressures derived from automated oscillometric blood pressure cuff readings taken in the arms when compared with those obtained at the ankle level.

Thresholds for the diagnosis of symptomatic and asymptomatic arterial insufficiency at rest have been described [2]. In normal limbs, the ankle pressures are typically equal to or a little higher than those derived at the brachial level. The difference is probably due to the augmentation of the systolic pressure that occurs with reflection of the pressure wave as it is propagated distally. A "normal" ABI is between 0.91 and 1.30. In general, PAD is present if the ABI is less than 0.90. A decreasing ABI is associated with more severe arterial insufficiency. Mild obstruction is defined as an ABI between 0.70 and 0.90, moderate obstruction as an ABI between 0.40 and 0.69, and severe obstruction as an ABI less than 0.40 [2,3].

As alluded to earlier, an ABI greater than 1.30 should be considered fallacious and is due to poorly compressible tibial vessels often seen in patients with medial calcinosis. In these circumstances, the additional measurement of a toe pressure or toe-brachial index (TBI) may provide additionally useful information. The toe pressure is usually obtained with an automated small inflatable cuff and a plethysmographic tracing. The digital vessels are often spared of significant medial calcinosis, and their evaluation may prove valuable in the presence of noncompressible arteries at the ankle [30]. The toe pressure is usually 10 mm Hg less than the ankle pressure, with a generally accepted normal value being greater than 70 mm Hg [7,8]. The TBI is a calculated value similar to the ABI except that the denominator of the ratio is the toe pressure. A normal TBI is expected to be equal to or greater than 0.70. The TBI has been shown to have a similar variability and reproducibility as the ABI [17]. The American Diabetes Association [3] has recommended the combination of ABI and TBI measurements whenever noninvasive arterial testing is performed in diabetic patients.

In general, the ABI can be obtained in an office with relative ease; however, additional noninvasive physiologic tests usually require referral to a vascular laboratory. In this facility, more sophisticated testing can be performed. These tests are designed to provide quantitative assessment of the severity of disease, to localize the sight of disease, and to follow disease progression through serial examinations [2]. The recent AHA/ACC Practice Guidelines for the diagnosis and treatment of PAD reinforce the need for referral to accredited and validated vascular laboratories. These laboratories adhere to strict quality control measures and are subjected to significant scrutiny through an intersocietal and interdisciplinary peer review process [2]. Some of the additional tests available through an accredited vascular laboratory may include segmental pressure measurements, pulse volume recording, directional Doppler waveform analysis, and duplex ultrasound. Less frequently, transcutaneous oxygen testing and laser Doppler oximetry may be available. A detailed summary of the aforementioned tests is beyond the scope of this article. Each particular test has unique benefits and drawbacks, especially in diabetic patients.

The author and his colleagues reviewed their experience with 101 diabetic patients undergoing treatment for symptomatic lower extremity PAD [31]. The results of noninvasive multimodality testing with ABI, TBI, pulse-volume recording, segmental pressure measurements, and segmental Doppler waveform analysis were examined to specifically assess the accuracy in predicting the level of significant (>50% stenosis) infrainguinal arterial disease, as well as the effects of multimodality testing compared with single modality testing on accurate diagnosis. Blinded comparisons of tests with contrast angiograms were performed, and associations between noninvasive diagnoses and angiographically confirmed disease were evaluated for significance. In total, 15% of limbs had uninterpretable ABIs (noncompressible), and 15% could not undergo TBI assessment because of lack of toes or extensive tissue loss involving the toes. Segmental pressures were only accurate in half of the patients due to noncompressible vessels and an inability to tolerate the test. These results have been seen by other investigators [32]. The best predictive combination of testing included pulse-volume recording and Doppler waveform analysis. This combination resulted in a sensitivity of 78% and a specificity of 80% with an associated positive predictive value of 84% in predicting angiographically significant disease. As a result, we have abandoned the use of segmental pressures among our diabetic patients with PAD, relying on Doppler waveform analysis and pulse-volume recording for noninvasive screening.

Imaging techniques

Generally, in a patient who has PAD, a good history will lead the clinician to the suspected diagnosis. The associated physical examination will likely confirm the diagnosis and possibly isolate the proximal extent of occlusive disease. The addition of noninvasive physiologic vascular testing provides a quantitative assessment of the degree of resting or exercise-induced ischemia in an affected limb and, to some degree, provides anatomic localization. These quantitative assessments are important in determining the severity of a given condition and the need for intervention. Although these tests provide a safe and inexpensive means of diagnosis, they arguably may not provide enough anatomic detail to satisfy accurate planning of a particular revascularization procedure.

When revascularization of a dysvascular limb is planned, additional imaging is usually necessary to delineate the location of treatment and to define the best modality of treatment for a particular lesion. Usually, imaging tests are reserved for patients in whom the decision to intervene has already been made because these tests carry more risks than physiologic testing methods.

More expensive imaging modalities such as MR digital subtraction angiography (MRA) and multidetector CT angiography (CTA) have proven roles in the evaluation of vascular anatomy before intervention. These imaging techniques provide spatial anatomic detail of vascular anatomy in relationship to surrounding structures, information regarding lesion severity, length, morphology, and composition, and, in the case of MRI, a possible window into physiologic and metabolic activity of a given plaque [33].

MRA has been shown to provide excellent accuracy when compared with the gold standard of contrast digital subtraction angiography in visualizing atherosclerotic occlusive disease [34]. Because imaging uses a magnetic coil, ionizing radiation is avoided. Earlier imaging with time-of-flight acquisition allowed examination of arteries without the use of iodinated contrast and the attendant risks of nephrotoxicity; however, the mainstay of MRA has become contrast-enhanced imaging, typically using gadolinium chelate as a contrast agent. The imaging quality has improved significantly. Currently, contrast-enhanced MRA is somewhat limited by prolonged image acquisition times and the need for significant post-processing with source images. Acquisition times are improving drastically with the new 3.0 T MRI coils, which should improve image quality and the rapidity of scanning. Although MRA represents an excellent method of imaging the aortoiliac and femoral-popliteal systems, imaging of the infrapopliteal segments (the segments most often involved in diabetic patients with PAD) is more difficult. At this level, deep venous enhancement or "venous contamination" can seriously degrade the images and make interpretation difficult (Fig. 3) [34]. The goal of accurate imaging of these vessels is obtained through limiting the venous enhancement. Unfortunately, the highest risk groups for venous contamination are patients with cellulitis and diabetes [34]. Although MRA has become the default imaging study in patients with chronic renal insufficiency in whom the larger doses of nephrotoxic iodinated contrast required for traditional angiography and CTA would induce renal failure, the use of gadolinium has been associated with acute renal failure, possibly related to acute tubular necrosis [35].

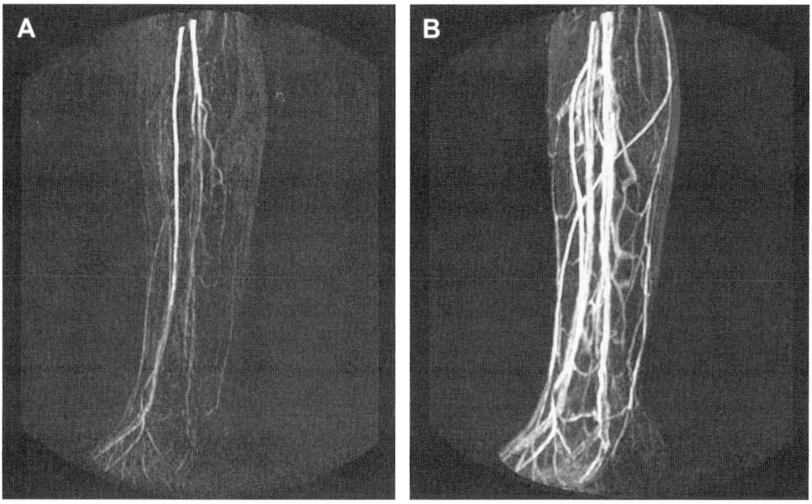

Fig. 3. Contrast-enhanced MRA demonstrating infrapopliteal arteries without venous contamination (*A*) and with venous contamination (*B*) and the associated degradation of the image.

Recently, enthusiasm has been building for the use of CTA in lower extremity arterial imaging. CTA has the benefits of low image acquisition time and ready availability and remains cheaper than conventional angiography. The overall accuracy in diagnosing angiographically significant disease is more than 95%, with sensitivities and specificities of more than 95% and 96%, respectively [36]. Volume rendering and curve planar reconstructions provide images that are nothing less than spectacular to look at; however, as is true for any imaging modality, there are limitations. Although direct arterial access is not required, the test requires the use of potentially nephrotoxic intravenous contrast in doses approaching those used in conventional angiography. The sensitivity and specificity of CTA are greater for the detection of arterial occlusions versus stenoses, and CTA has greater accuracy and less interobserver variability for proximal lesions compared with infrapopliteal lesions [37]. These more distal lesions are often found in diabetic patients with PAD. Willmann and colleagues [36] reported 96% sensitivity, 95% specificity, and 96% accuracy in diagnosing significant infrapopliteal occlusive disease with CTA. Another limitation is seen when imaging calcified vessels (prevalent among patients with diabetes), which may preclude an accurate assessment of the luminal diameter in affected segments.

The final imaging modality, conventional digital subtraction angiography, has long been considered the gold standard for imaging the arteries of a dysvascular limb. Although diagnostic conventional angiography is readily available, improved imaging with MRA and CTA has led to the decline of conventional angiography as a primary diagnostic modality. This diminution is largely the result of its limitations. It is expensive and invasive and provides little information beyond the two-dimensional image of a contrast-filled lumen of an artery. Its utility in imaging diabetic patients sustaining PAD arises from the limitations of newer imaging techniques, specifically, the ability to see the infrapopliteal, calcified segments of diseased tibial and pedal arteries. This visualization often requires superselective cannulation of the distal superficial femoral or popliteal vessels with direct injection at the popliteal level to achieve maximal contrast delivery. This selective imaging proves invaluable in planning for crural and pedal level bypasses.

Revascularization techniques

In general, the decision to attempt revascularization in a critically ischemic limb is based on several factors: (1) Can the patient tolerate an attempt at revascularization? (2) Is the affected foot salvageable? (3) Is the patient ambulatory? (4) What is the patient's current living status? Regarding the first question, the usual confounding comorbid medical conditions that may prohibit an attempt at revascularization are related to complicated cardiac issues. One should expect coronary artery disease in this population [6,25], and most procedures, whether performed percutaneously or through open surgery, can be carried out with acceptable risk and outcomes [38,39]. Assessment of perioperative cardiac risk would entire a separate article and is not discussed herein; however, a few conditions do make any intervention exceptionally dangerous, that is, uncontrolled congestive heart failure, severe aortic stenosis, and acute coronary syndrome. These conditions would make the risk of any intervention exceptionally high, and procedures should be avoided.

The second question is also very pertinent. There is an undefined limit to the amount of tissue loss present in a given foot and the utility of attempting revascularization. Despite the use of vacuum-assisted wound devices, free tissue transfer strategies, and skin grafting, a serious assessment of foot functionality should be made before revascularization. The patient needs to understand the residual disability associated with such heroic measures. The expectations regarding functionality of a viable but mangled foot should not be glossed over. In addition, there must be an informed decision made by the patient that such salvage techniques are associated with considerable pain, hospitalization, additional surgeries, and prolonged recovery. When presented with the reality of the situation, a significant minority of patients may opt for primary amputation rather than aggressive revascularization and reconstructive efforts [24,40]. Likewise, as alluded to in the third and fourth questions, if the patient was nonambulatory before the current crisis, or if the patient was living in an assisted living setting or nursing home, there should be no reasonable expectation that the patient will begin ambulating and live independently despite successful limb salvage [41].

The timing of intervention in diabetic patients with tissue loss or active infection requires special consideration. If an aggressive posture toward limb salvage is to be adopted, delay in revascularization is associated with significant morbidity. Sheahan and colleagues [42] studied a large cohort of 670 patients who underwent 920 minor amputations, defined as interphalangeal, ray, or transmetatarsal, performed on 747 dysvascular limbs. All limbs underwent surgical revascularization. Sixty-five percent of these procedures were performed before (<30 days) amputation, 9.8% after (<30 days) amputation, and the rest at the time of amputation. Conversion to a major amputation occurred in 2.9%. Patients who had bypass subsequent to amputation had twice the risk of limb loss when compared with those who underwent concomitant or early revascularization. It is commonly agreed among vascular surgeons that any form of minor amputation in a dysvascular limb should be performed simultaneously or after the limb has been revascularized. To accomplish this mandate, revascularization procedures in patients with tissue loss requiring some form of minor amputation for ulceration, gangrene, or infection are, by necessity, urgent or emergent procedures.

Once the decision to proceed with revascularization is made, the next critical decision should be what methods to adopt. The broad categories are generally considered catheter-based, percutaneous methods (ie, endovascular techniques), open surgical techniques, or a combination of both (ie, hybrid techniques). The method adopted for treatment is usually based on a combination of systemic risk and local anatomic considerations [43–45].

Endovascular interventions may include conventional balloon angioplasty, "cutting balloon" angioplasty, unconventional balloon angioplasty (so-called "cryoplasty"), intraluminal stenting, plaque excision (mechanical atherectomy), or laser atherectomy, among others. The multitude of treatment options makes independent evaluation of each modality difficult; however, in general, shorter focal lesions usually respond well to endovascular interventions regardless of the particular method used. Because most diabetic patients with critical limb ischemia are afflicted with varying degrees of infrapopliteal occlusive disease, the utility of various forms of endovascular therapy in these patients requires further examination. Technical successes are often excellent, with clinical success occurring with less frequency; however, most would agree that failed angioplasty (or other endovascular intervention) does not preclude surgical bypass. Because endovascular procedures generally have a more favorable risk profile when compared with bypass, it would not be unreasonable to proceed with an attempt at endovascular intervention for anatomically favorable disease before surgical revascularization [8,46–49]. That being said, attempted percutaneous revascularization for longer, less favorable lesions in which failure is more frequent may simply delay revascularization. Unfortunately, not enough research has been devoted to the rapidity of clinical response associated with endovascular therapy for critical ischemia. An important question remains: Do clinical failures of endovascular treatment result in an unacceptable delay before surgical revascularization and a higher risk for limb loss?

Surgical infrainguinal revascularization has been well studied. Several generalities are clear: (1) the complexity of the procedures is increasing, and the patients are getting sicker [50]; (2) autogenous conduits are preferable for all procedures involving infrapopliteal vessels; (3) any artery can serve as a bypass inflow vessel provided the vessels proximal to the anastomotic site are relatively disease free [8]; (4) the distal target of revascularization should be the least diseased vessel that establishes the best continuous runoff to the foot [8]; and (5) pedal artery targets are acceptable [7,15,39]. In patients with diabetes, the bypass graft patency is comparable with that achieved in non-diabetic patients. Although it is generally accepted that limb salvage rates are higher than graft patency rates among patients with critical ischemia, this is less evident among diabetic patients; primary graft failure is associated with substantial limb loss in this population [51].

Although the outcomes of a particular revascularization procedure are generally measured through the patency of a given bypass or intervention and limb salvage rates, the limitations of these survival metrics are seen in their inability to match up with patient satisfaction and well being [44]. Perhaps our traditional measurements of success are becoming more useful for research purposes than as clinically relevant measures of success [24,40,44]. The complex effects of anatomic features of the disease, the clinical presentation, the baseline functional status of the patient, comorbid medical conditions, and various technical considerations may require the use of algorithms guiding therapy in an objective standardized manner to maximize overall success [43,45]. Successful revascularization must always be coupled with successful application of multidisciplinary parallel treatment of local and systemic effects of infection, the systemic manifestations of diabetes, and good foot care [52].

Summary

PAD in diabetic patients is common. Patients with diabetes tend to present with more severe manifestations of the disease and require a more complicated diagnostic and therapeutic strategy for revascularization. Although techniques are rapidly evolving, revascularization remains only one component in the treatment of patients with diabetes and PAD. Because overall cardiovascular morbidity and mortality are high among patients with PAD, treatment to control the systemic atherosclerotic disease cannot be overemphasized. In addition, improvement in arterial perfusion is important, but wound care and pressure point unloading remain vital if more limbs are to be saved. As new treatment paradigms evolve, the assessment of outcomes needs to become more clinically relevant. Traditional measures of success may prove unreliable in measuring patient satisfaction and the perception of well being. Newer patient-oriented (rather than limb-oriented) measures of success will need to be developed and expanded.

References

[1] Berliner JA, Navab M, Fogelman AM, et al. Atherosclerosis: basic mechanisms. Oxidation, inflammation, and genetics. Circulation 1995;91(9):2488–96.

[2] Hirsch AT, Haskal ZJ, Hertzer NR, et al. ACC/AHA 2005 Practice Guidelines for the management of patients with peripheral arterial disease (lower extremity, renal, mesenteric, and abdominal aortic): a collaborative report from the American Association for Vascular Surgery/Society for Vascular Surgery, Society for Cardiovascular Angiography and Interventions, Society for Vascular Medicine and Biology, Society of Interventional Radiology, and the ACC/AHA Task Force on Practice Guidelines (Writing Committee to Develop Guidelines for the Management of Patients With Peripheral Arterial Disease). Endorsed by the American Association of Cardiovascular and Pulmonary Rehabilitation; National Heart, Lung, and Blood Institute; Society for Vascular Nursing; TransAtlantic Inter-Society Consensus; and Vascular Disease Foundation. Circulation 2006;113(11):e463–654.

[3] American Diabetes Association. Peripheral arterial disease in people with diabetes [see comment]. Diabetes Care 2003;26(12):3333–41.

[4] Fowkes FG, Housley E, Cawood EH, et al. Edinburgh Artery Study: prevalence of asymptomatic and symptomatic peripheral arterial disease in the general population. Int J Epidemiol 1991;20(2):384–92.

[5] Hirsch AT, Criqui MH, Treat-Jacobson D, et al. Peripheral arterial disease detection, awareness, and treatment in primary care [see comment]. JAMA 2001;286(11):1317–24.

[6] Golomb BA, Dang TT, Criqui MH. Peripheral arterial disease: morbidity and mortality implications. Circulation 2006;114(7):688–99.

[7] Dormandy JA, Rutherford RB. Management of peripheral arterial disease (PAD). TASC Working Group. TransAtlantic Inter-Society Consensus (TASC). J Vasc Surg 2000;31(1 Pt 2):S1–296.

[8] Norgren L, Hiatt WR, Dormandy JA, et al. Inter-society consensus for the management of peripheral arterial disease (TASC II). J Vasc Surg 2007;45(1 Suppl):S5–67.

[9] Hertzer NR. Clinical experience with preoperative coronary angiography. J Vasc Surg 1985; 2(3):510–4.

[10] Gregg EW, Sorlie P, Paulose-Ram R, et al. Prevalence of lower-extremity disease in the US adult population $\geq$40 years of age with and without diabetes: 1999–2000 National Health and Nutrition Examination Survey. Diabetes Care 2004;27(7):1591–7.

[11] Creager MA, Luscher TF, Cosentino F, et al. Diabetes and vascular disease: pathophysiology, clinical consequences, and medical therapy. Part I. Circulation 2003;108(12): 1527–32.

[12] Landmesser U, Hornig B, Drexler H. Endothelial function: a critical determinant in atherosclerosis? Circulation 2004;109(21 Suppl 1):II27–33.

[13] Kim JA, Montagnani M, Koh KK, et al. Reciprocal relationships between insulin resistance and endothelial dysfunction: molecular and pathophysiological mechanisms. Circulation 2006;113(15):1888–904.

[14] LoGerfo FW, Coffman JD. Current concepts: vascular and microvascular disease of the foot in diabetes. Implications for foot care. N Engl J Med 1984;311(25):1615–9.

[15] Akbari CM, LoGerfo FW. Diabetes and peripheral vascular disease. J Vasc Surg 1999;30(2): 373–84.

[16] Criqui MH, Browner D, Fronek A, et al. Peripheral arterial disease in large vessels is epidemiologically distinct from small vessel disease: an analysis of risk factors. Am J Epidemiol 1989;129(6):1110–9.

[17] Aboyans V, Criqui MH, Denenberg JO, et al. Risk factors for progression of peripheral arterial disease in large and small vessels. Circulation 2006;113(22):2623–9.

[18] Karacagil S, Almgren B, Lorelius LE, et al. Angiographic runoff patterns in patients undergoing lower limb revascularization. Acta Chir Scand 1989;155(1):19–24.

[19] Jude EB, Oyibo SO, Chalmers N, et al. Peripheral arterial disease in diabetic and nondiabetic patients: a comparison of severity and outcome. Diabetes Care 2001;24(8): 1433–7.

[20] Toursarkissian B, D'Ayala M, Stefanidis D, et al. Angiographic scoring of vascular occlusive disease in the diabetic foot: relevance to bypass graft patency and limb salvage. J Vasc Surg 2002;35(3):494–500.

[21] Berceli SA, Chan AK, Pomposelli FB Jr, et al. Efficacy of dorsal pedal artery bypass in limb salvage for ischemic heel ulcers. J Vasc Surg 1999;30(3):499–508.

[22] Emanuele MA, Buchanan BJ, Abraira C. Elevated leg systolic pressures and arterial calcification in diabetic occlusive vascular disease. Diabetes Care 1981;4(2):289–92.

[23] Resnick HE, Lindsay RS, McDermott MM, et al. Relationship of high and low ankle brachial index to all-cause and cardiovascular disease mortality: the Strong Heart Study [see comment]. Circulation 2004;109(6):733–9.

[24] Nehler MR, McDermott MM, Treat-Jacobson D, et al. Functional outcomes and quality of life in peripheral arterial disease: current status. Vasc Med 2003;8(2):115–26.

[25] Criqui MH, Langer RD, Fronek A, et al. Mortality over a period of 10 years in patients with peripheral arterial disease. N Engl J Med 1992;326(6):381–6.

[26] Wolfe JH, Wyatt MG. Critical and subcritical ischaemia. Eur J Vasc Endovasc Surg 1997; 13(6):578–82.

[27] Anonymous. Long-term mortality and its predictors in patients with critical leg ischaemia: the ICAI Group (Gruppo di Studio dell'Ischemia Cronica Critica degli Arti Inferiori) [the Study Group of Criticial Chronic Ischemia of the Lower Extremities]. Eur J Vasc Endovasc Surg 1997;14(2):91–5.

[28] Dolan NC, Liu K, Criqui MH, et al. Peripheral artery disease, diabetes, and reduced lower extremity functioning. Diabetes Care 2002;25(1):113–20.

[29] Beckman JA, Higgins CO, Gerhard-Herman M. Automated oscillometric determination of the ankle-brachial index provides accuracy necessary for office practice. Hypertension 2006; 47(1):35–8.

[30] Young MJ, Adams JE, Anderson GF, et al. Medial arterial calcification in the feet of diabetic patients and matched non-diabetic control subjects [see comment]. Diabetologia 1993;36(7): 615–21.

[31] Toursarkissian B, Mejia A, Smilanich RP, et al. Noninvasive localization of infrainguinal arterial occlusive disease in diabetics. Ann Vasc Surg 2001;15(1):73–8.

[32] Moneta GL, Yeager RA, Lee RW, et al. Noninvasive localization of arterial occlusive disease: a comparison of segmental Doppler pressures and arterial duplex mapping. J Vasc Surg 1993;17(3):578–82.

[33] Castillo M. From the vulnerable plaque to the vulnerable patient: imaging and clinical implications [comment]. Acad Radiol 2006;13(10):1177–9.

[34] Leiner T. Magnetic resonance angiography of abdominal and lower extremity vasculature. Top Magn Reson Imaging 2005;16(1):21–66.

[35] Akgun H, Gonlusen G, Cartwright J Jr, et al. Are gadolinium-based contrast media nephrotoxic? A renal biopsy study. Arch Pathol Lab Med 2006;130(9):1354–7.

[36] Willmann JK, Baumert B, Schertler T, et al. Aortoiliac and lower extremity arteries assessed with 16-detector row CT angiography: prospective comparison with digital subtraction angiography. Radiology 2005;236(3):1083–93.

[37] Fleischmann D, Hallett RL, Rubin GD. CT angiography of peripheral arterial disease J Vasc Interv Radiol 2006;17(1):3–26.

[38] Calle-Pascual AL, Duran A, Diaz A, et al. Comparison of peripheral arterial reconstruction in diabetic and non-diabetic patients: a prospective clinic-based study. Diabetes Res Clin Pract 2001;53(2):129–36.

[39] Akbari CM, Pomposelli FB Jr, Gibbons GW, et al. Lower extremity revascularization in diabetes: late observations. Arch Surg 2000;135(4):452–6.

[40] Goshima KR, Mills JL Sr., Hughes JD. A new look at outcomes after infrainguinal bypass surgery: traditional reporting standards systematically underestimate the expenditure of effort required to attain limb salvage. J Vasc Surg 2004;39(2):330–5.

[41] Abou-Zamzam AM Jr, Lee RW, Moneta GL, et al. Functional outcome after infrainguinal bypass for limb salvage. J Vasc Surg 1997;25(2):287–95 [discussion: 95–7].

[42] Sheahan MG, Hamdan AD, Veraldi JR, et al. Lower extremity minor amputations: the roles of diabetes mellitus and timing of revascularization. J Vasc Surg 2005;42(3):476–80.

[43] Taylor SM, Kalbaugh CA, Gray BH, et al. The LEGS score: a proposed grading system to direct treatment of chronic lower extremity ischemia. Ann Surg 2003;237(6):812–8 [discussion: 8–9].

[44] Taylor SM, Kalbaugh CA, Blackhurst DW, et al. Determinants of functional outcome after revascularization for critical limb ischemia: an analysis of 1000 consecutive vascular interventions. J Vasc Surg 2006;44(4):747–55 [discussion: 55–6].

[45] Kalbaugh CA, Taylor SM, Cull DL, et al. Invasive treatment of chronic limb ischemia according to the Lower Extremity Grading System (LEGS) score: a 6-month report. J Vasc Surg 2004;39(6):1268–76.

[46] Kalbaugh CA, Taylor SM, Blackhurst DW, et al. One-year prospective quality-of-life outcomes in patients treated with angioplasty for symptomatic peripheral arterial disease. J Vasc Surg 2006;44(2):296–302 [discussion: 3].

[47] Faglia E, Dalla Paola L, Clerici G, et al. Peripheral angioplasty as the first-choice revascularization procedure in diabetic patients with critical limb ischemia: prospective study of 993 consecutive patients hospitalized and followed between 1999 and 2003. Eur J Vasc Endovasc Surg 2005;29(6):620–7.

[48] Faglia E, Mantero M, Caminiti M, et al. Extensive use of peripheral angioplasty, particularly infrapopliteal, in the treatment of ischaemic diabetic foot ulcers: clinical results of a multicentric study of 221 consecutive diabetic subjects. J Intern Med 2002;252(3):225–32.

[49] Hanna GP, Fujise K, Kjellgren O, et al. Infrapopliteal transcatheter interventions for limb salvage in diabetic patients: importance of aggressive interventional approach and role of transcutaneous oximetry. J Am Coll Cardiol 1997;30(3):664–9.

[50] Conte MS, Belkin M, Upchurch GR, et al. Impact of increasing comorbidity on infrainguinal reconstruction: a 20-year perspective. Ann Surg 2001;233(3):445–52.

[51] Toursarkissian B, Shireman PK, Schoolfield J, et al. Outcomes following distal bypass graft occlusion in diabetics. Ann Vasc Surg 2003;17(6):670–5.

[52] Anonymous. Consensus Development Conference on Diabetic Foot Wound Care: 7-8 April 1999, Boston, Massachusetts. American Diabetes Association [see comment]. Diabetes Care 1999;22(8).1354–60.

ELSEVIER
SAUNDERS

Clin Podiatr Med Surg
24 (2007) 469–482

CLINICS IN
PODIATRIC
MEDICINE AND
SURGERY

Surgical Management of Diabetic Foot Infections and Osteomyelitis

Robert G. Frykberg, DPM, MPH[a,*],
Brian Wittmayer, DPM[a],
Thomas Zgonis, DPM, FACFAS[b]

[a] *Carl T. Hayden Veterans Affairs Medical Center, 650 East Indian School Road, Phoenix, AZ 85012, USA*

[b] *Department of Orthopaedics, Podiatry Division, The University of Texas Health Science Center at San Antonio, 7703 Floyd Curl Drive, MSC 7776, San Antonio, TX 78229, USA*

With diabetes at almost epidemic proportions worldwide, complications directly related to the disease will become more prevalent [1–3]. Foot ulceration is a frequent complication of diabetes, and is estimated to affect approximately 15% of patients during the course of their lifetimes [4–6]. Ulceration is often complicated by infection, contributing to 20% of diabetes-related hospital admissions, as well as being a major factor in nontraumatic lower extremity amputation (LEA) [7,8]. Diabetes-related amputation accounts for more than 60% of nontraumatic LEAs in the United States; the estimated 3- and 5-year survival rates following surgery are only 50% and 40%, respectively [2,9]. Studies have also demonstrated the substantial economic impact of diabetic foot infection and subsequent LEAs [5,10–12]. Infection in the diabetic foot is often complicated by other comorbidities, including neuropathy, peripheral vascular disease, immunopathy, and renal disease. Accordingly, a multidisciplinary team approach to foot infections is deemed essential to maximize outcomes and decrease patient morbidity [13].

Risk factors and identification of diabetic foot infections

Foot ulceration is the most common single precursor to LEAs among persons who have diabetes. Significant risk factors for ulceration include peripheral vascular disease (PVD), neuropathy, structural deformity, trauma,

* Corresponding author.
E-mail address: robert.frykberg@med.va.gov (R.G. Frykberg).

0891-8422/07/$ - see front matter. Published by Elsevier Inc.
doi:10.1016/j.cpm.2007.04.001

and limited joint mobility [13–15]. Often it is a cumulative effect of these risk factors that leads to ulceration. Similarly, these same risks factors are also significant for the development of foot infection. A recent prospective study of over 1600 diabetic patients followed for more than 2 years found that 9.1% of this cohort developed a foot infection [12]. Almost exclusively, these infections were associated with open wounds or penetrating injuries. The associated risk for hospitalization and amputation were 56 and 154 times greater, respectively, than in those patients who did not develop a foot infection.

One often overlooked risk factor for infection in the diabetic patient is immunopathy, with its attendant increased susceptibility to infection. It has been found that leukocyte phagocytosis and chemotaxis are greatly impaired in those patients who have poorly controlled diabetes [16–18]. It is also well-documented that infection potentiates uncontrolled hyperglycemia. Thus in the diabetic patient, infection adversely affects diabetes control, and uncontrolled diabetes adversely affects the host's immunologic response [7].

Ulceration, whether neuropathic or neuroischemic, is the most common precursor to diabetic foot infection. Neuropathy in the presence of trauma, structural deformity, or limited joint mobility allows for development of ulceration that may go unrecognized, thereby delaying treatment. The open wound allows for entry of bacteria, which proliferate in the immunocompromised diabetic host. In those patients who have PVD, the infection can rapidly progress to limb- or life-threatening infection (Fig. 1A–C).

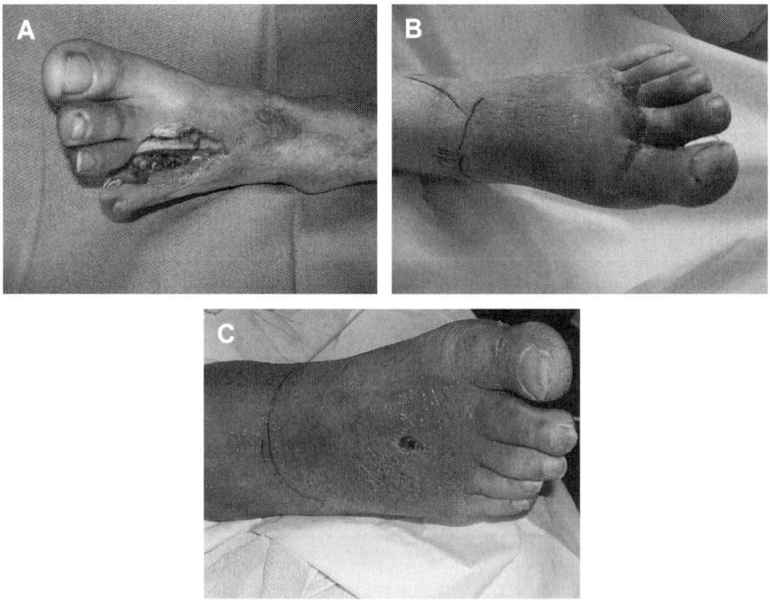

Fig. 1. (*A–C*) Three different clinical presentations of severely ischemic diabetic foot infections.

Unfortunately, such presentations increase the need for emergent amputation. Initial evaluation should focus on thorough clinical examination, with supplemental laboratory and imaging studies, to determine the severity of infection. Common clinical findings of infection include gangrene, purulent drainage, malodor, erythema, warmth, induration, lymphangitis, and soft tissue emphysema. Pain and tenderness in the foot of a patient previously known to be insensate should also raise suspicion of an underlying infection. Recalcitrant hyperglycemia and complaints of fever, malaise, and chills that are referred to as "the diabetic foot flu" are also indicators of possible deep infection [13,19].

Classification: limb-threatening versus non–limb-threatening infections

Several schemes have been developed to classify the severity of diabetic foot infections [7,20–22]. To be clinically useful, a classification system should not only communicate severity, but should also help to guide treatment and lead to a predictable outcome. Although not as thorough as that one recently adopted by the Infectious Disease Society of America in 2004 [22], a well-accepted scheme classifies infection as non–limb-threatening versus limb-threatening [20,23]. This system is simplistic, but provides the essentials in determining severity and subsequent treatment.

Non–limb-threatening infections generally involve superficial ulcerations without significant ischemia, bone or joint involvement, or systemic toxicity. There is associated cellulitis extending more than 2 cm around the wound [23]. Patients who have non–limb-threatening infections are usually medically stable, and can be treated in the outpatient setting. Treatment should focus on local wound care, debridement, proper offloading, and culture-directed oral and topical antibiotic therapy. Aerobic gram-positive cocci are the organisms of primary concern, and appropriate empirical antibiotic coverage for these pathogens is necessary. First-generation cephalosporins, penicillinase-resistant penicillins, clindamycin, or doxycycline are frequently prescribed as initial therapy. Antimicrobial therapies include

Cephalosporin (cephalexin, cefadroxil, cefdinir)
Penicillins (dicloxacillin, amoxicillin/clavulanate)
Clindamycin
Doxycycline
Trimethoprim/sulfamethoxazole
Fluoroquinolones (levofloxacin, moxifloxacin)
Linezolid

Antimicrobial therapy is then tailored according to cultures and sensitivities as well as clinical progress. Plain film radiography initially ruling out any acute soft tissue emphysema or underlying osteomyelitis is also warranted. If there is uncertainty as to the arterial perfusion status, noninvasive vascular testing should also be pursued. As necessary, comorbid conditions such as uncontrolled diabetes, hypertension, or renal disease should be brought to the attention of the appropriate provider. The patient should then be reassessed within 48 to 72 hours to evaluate the response to therapy. If there is no improvement or if the infection has progressed, hospital admission for intravenous antibiotics and possible surgical intervention should be considered [13,22,24].

Moderate to severe infections with 2 cm or more of periwound cellulitis, abscess formation, lymphangitis, gangrene, osteomyelitis, or critical limb ischemia are classified as limb-threatening [19,23]. These deep infections generally require hospitalization for intravenous antibiotics, with a likelihood of surgical intervention. Classic systemic signs of infection including fevers, chills, malaise, and leukocytosis may also be present; however, one must not rely solely on these signs and symptoms, given that up to 50% of diabetic patients do not elicit a typical systemic response because of diabetes-related immune suppression [23,25]. Broad-spectrum antimicrobial therapy is considered adjunctive to surgical intervention for deep infections (Box 1) [22,26]. Usually administered parenterally, empirical therapy should be targeted to gram positive cocci, gram-negative rods, and anaerobes, with close

Box 1. Empirical antimicrobial therapy for limb-threatening infections[a]

Cefazolin
Ceftriaxone
Ceftazidime
Cefepime
Aztreonam
Oxacillin, nafcillin
Ampicillin/sulbactam
Piperacillin/tazobactam
Ertapenem
Imipenem
Clindamycin
Metronidazole
Tigecycline
Vancomycin
Daptomycin
Linezolid
Trimethoprim/sulfamethoxazole
Fluoroquinolones (ciprofloxacin, levofloxacin, moxifloxacin)

[a]Most agents are administered intravenously. Combination therapy is often warranted depending upon allergy profile and presence of resistant organisms.

attention being paid to resistant organisms. As with non–limb-threatening infections, radiographs should be obtained to evaluate for presence of osteomyelitis, foreign bodies, or gas in the soft tissues. Consultation with internal medicine, endocrinology, nephrology, cardiology, vascular surgery, and infectious disease are often warranted to better manage comorbid disease states. A multidisciplinary approach has been shown to significantly improve outcomes in the presence of complicated infection [27].

Early surgical management of diabetic foot infections

Surgery performed on the infected diabetic foot frequently involves incision and drainage or amputation. A new scheme has recently been proposed for classifying surgery in the diabetic foot into four classes [28,29]:

- Class I: elective. Reconstructive procedures on patients who do not have loss of protective sensation (LOPS)
- Class II: prophylactic. Reconstructive procedures performed to reduce the risk of ulceration or reulceration in patients who have LOPS and do not have a wound present
- Class III: curative. Procedures performed to assist in healing of open wounds
- Class IV: emergent. Procedures performed to arrest or limit progression of infection

Historically, elective surgery in the diabetic foot has been looked upon as somewhat ill-advised; however, recent reports indicate that elective and prophylactic procedures do provide significant benefit in properly selected patients [29–32].

In the presence of infection, most surgery in the diabetic foot falls into the categories of emergent or curative, and generally involves a limb-threatening infection. When this is the case, early surgical intervention is essential, whether it involves simple debridement of soft tissues, drainage of a deep abscess, or even an open amputation.

In emergent cases where the infection is potentially life-threatening, immediate surgery foregoing formal consultation from other specialties (ie, medicine, vascular surgery, nephrology, and so on) may be indicated. Simple incision and drainage may be performed in the clinic setting or at the bedside in the insensate patient who is medically stable. Not all patients are insensate, and this must be addressed with proper anesthesia including local, regional, general, or in combination.

A retrospective study of 112 patients by Tan and colleagues [33] determined that early aggressive surgical intervention and appropriate antibiotic therapy significantly improved outcomes. There were two groups of interest: Group I included patients who received intravenous antibiotics and no surgical intervention during the first 3 days of hospitalization; Group II consisted of patients who received intravenous antibiotics along with surgical intervention within the first 3 days of admission. Group II was further divided into an "A" group, who received surgical debridement, and a "B" group, who received localized amputation below the ankle level. Statistically significant findings included a higher incidence of above-ankle amputation in Group I compared with those who received early surgical intervention (92.3% versus 20%) for the treatment of deep infection. Furthermore, the surgical group also had a reduced length of hospital stay by at least 6 days [33]. The necessity for surgical management of deep diabetic foot infections was also corroborated by Eneroth and colleagues [26], who found that surgical intervention was necessary in 86% of patients. In this study, approximately one third of such infections were treated with minor amputation, whereas 8% required a major amputation before healing.

Thorough debridement of all grossly necrotic and infected tissue should be the main goals of the initial surgery. An understanding of foot anatomy and function is imperative [34]. Initial skin incisions and dissection should take into consideration future surgical plans. Care must be taken to preserve viable tissues and prevent unwanted damage to neighboring structures that may be needed to achieve a functional outcome with a curative procedure [35].

Upon initial drainage, reliable aerobic, anaerobic, and fungal cultures should be obtained. If bone is resected, it too should be sent for culture as well as histology to determine the presence of any underlying osteomyelitis. Once the infection is under control and the patient is medically stable, additional assessments should be undertaken, with special attention paid to underlying vascular disease or osteomyelitis. If pedal pulses are nonpalpable or clinical signs of ischemia are present, noninvasive vascular studies should be performed. Such studies include ankle brachial indices (ABI), pulse volume recordings, or transcutaneous oxygen pressures (TCPO2) [36–38]. These studies are beneficial in ascertaining the need for vascular surgery consultation with subsequent angiogram and possible revascularization. Noninvasive tests also assist in preoperative planning by determining adequacy of tissue perfusion (and probability for healing) at various sites on the foot. If there is suspicion of underlying osteomyelitis and plain film radiographs do not demonstrate any early osseous changes, further imaging with radionucleotide bone or leukocyte scans, CT, or MRI is warranted [39–41].

Management of osteomyelitis in the diabetic foot

It is estimated that approximately 20% of diabetic patients who present with foot infections have evidence of osteomyelitis [42]. The presence of bone infection is an additional variable that complicates treatment in diabetic foot infections, in terms of the duration of required antimicrobial therapy as well as the likelihood for surgery. The diagnosis of osteomyelitis is not always straightforward, especially when plain radiographs are ostensibly normal, or in the presence of underlying osteoarthropathy. There are multiple clinical findings that may raise suspicion for osteomyelitis, but only some have been shown to be of any predictive value. In one study, ulcerations with an area of more than 2 cm^2, a depth of more than 3 mm, or with exposed bone were more likely to have underlying osteomyelitis [43]. Grayson and colleagues [44] have reported that infected foot ulcerations in which bone can be probed at the ulcer base have a high positive predictive value for osteomyelitis. The validity of the "probe-to-bone" test has recently been challenged by Lavery and colleagues [42], who found in their series that although a positive test had an 87% sensitivity, the predictive value of this test for osteomyelitis was only 57%. In a predominantly outpatient population in which the prevalence of osteomyelitis was only 12%, they found that a negative test could reliably exclude the diagnosis, with a negative predictive value of 91%. In this regard, it seems as though the prevalence of osteomyelitis in the population under study (mild or severe infection) plays a critical role in the validity of this simple test. Notwithstanding, bone biopsy in concert with bone culture is often considered the gold standard, having sensitivity and specificity of 95% and 99%, respectively [45]. Sampling error is not uncommon when obtaining bone biopsies, and false negatives may occur.

Much of present day diagnosis relies on the use of multiple imaging studies, including nuclear bone and leukocyte scans, MRI, and CT. Plain film radiographic findings include focal osteopenia and cortical erosions. Limitations to plain films include a delay of 10 to 20 days before acute changes are seen, as well as nonspecific findings that may be present with other osseous pathology, most notably Charcot neuroarthropathy. This lack of specificity in the presence of neuropathic bone disease also affects the accuracy of nuclear scans and MRI [46]. CT has similar drawbacks as plain films, but may be of benefit in cases where cortical bone involvement is suspected, because of the high cortical resolution in CT scans.

Once the diagnosis has been made, a treatment regimen must be initiated. Treatment for osteomyelitis has generally been described as medical (conservative) or surgical. Medical treatment usually consists of "limited" or no debridement, with a 6 to 8 week course of intravenous or oral antibiotics. Often therapy consists of initial intravenous (IV) therapy followed by a course of oral therapy [22]. There is no substantial scientific evidence that lays forth a protocol of medical therapy that gives a consistent, predictable result. There are studies that attempt to demonstrate that osteomyelitis may be treated solely by medical means [47,48]. As with many studies investigating osteomyelitis, diagnosis was mainly based on clinical findings and bone biopsy was lacking in most cases. The question therefore remains as to whether osteomyelitis is indeed present in these studies, or whether skin and soft tissue infection alone are being treated [48–50].

There is no doubt that medical therapy plays an important part in treating osteomyelitis, but when medical therapy alone fails, surgical therapy is needed [22]. The authors' contention is that osteomyelitis is a "surgical disease," and when it is diagnosed, surgical intervention should be part of primary treatment. There is literature supporting the fact that surgical treatment of osteomyelitis improves morbidity and mortality, but once again, the method of diagnosis comes into question, as it does in most studies evaluating treatment of this disease [13,50,51].

A 1996 study by Ha Van and colleagues [52] compared two cohorts of diabetic patients who had ulceration and underlying osteomyelitis. One group received only medical therapy consisting of antibiotics, wound care, and proper offloading. The second group received the same medical therapy along with "conservative" surgical treatment, defined as limited resection of a phalanx or metatarsal bone. The primary end point was duration of time until the wound was completely healed. Of the medical therapy group, 57% healed in a mean of 462 days, versus 78% healing within an average of 181 days in the conservative surgery group. Duration of antibiotic use was also significantly reduced in the conservative surgery group—111 days versus 246 days on average. The number of secondary surgical procedures (revascularization or amputation) after failing initial treatment was also significantly higher in the medical treatment group versus the conservative surgery group (14 patients versus 3 patients) [52].

At this time there is no conclusive evidence to suggest whether medical therapy alone is sufficient to treat osteomyelitis and when surgical intervention is absolutely indicated [50]. A consensus of the present day literature will support the benefits of a combined approach of antibiotic therapy with aggressive surgical debridement of infected bone [13,22,51]. The surgical approach to osteomyelitis should be aimed at resecting as much infected bone as possible, with focus on preserving foot function. Wide excision of necrotic and infected bone with 5 mm or greater of clearance has been shown to reduce the risk for recurrence in cases of chronic osteomyelitis when compared with groups in which marginal resection (<5 mm of clearance) or intralesional debridement was obtained [53]. If diffuse bone destruction is evident, primary partial foot amputation versus limited resection should be considered. Box 2 lists the common types of procedures used to manage these potentially limb-threatening bone infections.

Following bone resection or debridement, appropriate culture-guided antibiotic therapy should be instituted for 2 to 6 weeks, depending on the extent of bone infection [22]. When there is no acute soft tissue infection or purulent drainage, and if there is adequate soft tissue coverage, primary closure may be performed. If soft tissue infection remains, delayed primary closure can be performed when the infection clears, or the wound may be allowed to close by secondary intention. Negative pressure wound therapy (V.A.C., KCI, San Antonio, Texas) is frequently used in this setting, and has been found to expedite healing of such open wounds [54]. An adjunct to surgical resection of bone is placement of antibiotic-impregnated polymethylmethacrylate beads or absorbable calcium sulfate pellets. Randomized control trials in humans are not readily available, but several studies do

Box 2. Commonly used procedures within each surgical category

Class I: elective
Bunionectomy
Hammertoe repair
Ingrown toenail removal
Metatarsal osteotomy

Class II: prophylactic
Bunionectomy
Sesamoidectomy
Hammertoe
Metatarsal osteotomy
Charcot exostectomy
Achilles tendon lengthening

Class III: curative
Metatarsal head resection, pan-metatarsal head resection
Keller arthroplasty
Metatarsal-phalangeal or interphalangeal joint resection
Plantar midfoot exostectomy
Partial foot amputation: digital, ray, transmetatarsal amputation (TMA), Chopart, Syme
Partial calcanectomy

Class IV: emergent
Incision and drainage
Guillotine amputation at appropriate level
Staged partial foot amputations
Major (above ankle) amputation

show evidence that antibiotic-impregnated beads can be effective in eradicating osteomyelitis [55,56].

Amputation considerations in the diabetic foot

Amputation in the diabetic foot can generally be classified as an emergent or curative procedure [28]. In the presence of life-threatening infection such as necrotizing fascitis or gas gangrene emergent, open amputation is warranted. Profound peripheral vascular disease should not be an immediate indication for amputation. If infection can be controlled with debridement or limited amputation, the definitive level of amputation should be determined following revascularization. Recent advances in distal revascularization procedures have allowed for more distal limb-sparing amputations [25,36,37]. This is significant, given the impact on energy expenditure and quality of life with more proximal level amputations [57]. As a general rule, amputation should be performed as far distal as possible, although there are exceptions. Digital amputations have shown to be of little functional deficit. Patients such as paraplegics and quadriplegics or those who are otherwise nonambulatory are exceptions, in that level of amputation should focus around prevention of future contractures and decubitus ulceration.

Clinical practice guidelines set forth by the American College of Foot and Ankle Surgeons [13] give the following goals in selection of amputation level

- Creation of a distal stump that can be easily accommodated with footgear, orthotic device, or prosthesis
- Creation of a distal stump that is durable and resistant to pressure breakdown
- Creation of a distal stump that will not cause muscle or other dynamic imbalances
- Healing by primary intention if at all possible

Ignoring the aforementioned goals may lead to a poorly functional limb and a more proximal amputation in the future. As mentioned previously, factors that impact wound healing are also of importance in selecting a viable amputation level. Poor perfusion and extensive bone or soft tissue loss are of key importance. The importance of noninvasive vascular studies (ABI, toe pressures, TcPO2, and so forth) has previously been discussed, and is invaluable in assessing patients who have suspected vascular disease. In the presence of abnormal or marginal noninvasive studies, vascular surgery consultation is needed to evaluate for revascularization before definitive amputation. Revascularization procedures should be avoided in the presence of uncomplicated claudication pain, nonambulatory patients who essentially have nonfunctional limbs, and patients who have significant comorbidities who are at high risk for severe postoperative complications.

The amount of infected osseous and soft tissue as well as necrosis are crucial in determining a functional amputation level. Soft tissue deficits that are encountered can often be overcome by use of adjunctive wound care modalities such as vacuum assisted closure (VAC) devices or hyperbaric oxygen therapy. Plastic surgery techniques using skin flaps and grafts have also been of benefit in obtaining soft tissue coverage. Necrotic and infected bone generally needs to be resected, and therefore primary amputation needs to be considered. In determining the final amputation level, the surgeon must weigh several factors: removal of necrotic tissue (including bone) while also minimizing the residual functional deficit, available flaps for closure, biomechanical alterations and risk for transfer lesions, and finally, tissue perfusion [13,58]. For example, multiple ray amputations are frequently required to arrest infection in the forefoot. Although such

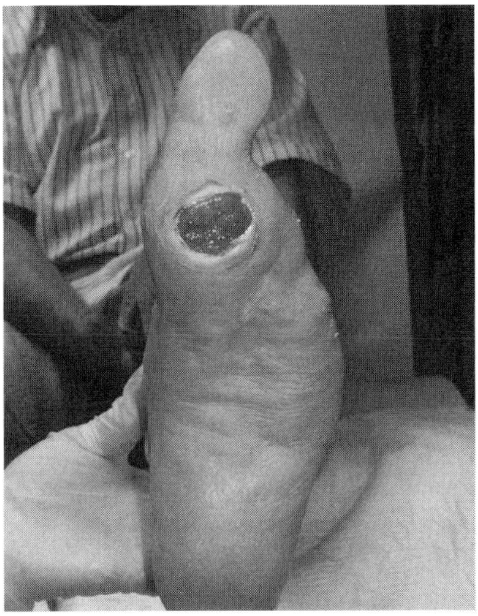

Fig. 2. Residual deformity with plantar ulceration after lesser ray amputations. This problem should be anticipated and avoided by appropriate preoperative planning.

procedures can ultimately heal, excessive pressures transferred to the remaining metatarsals subject the foot to recurrent ulcerations (Fig. 2). In this situation it is therefore advisable to perform a transmetatarsal amputation that can still provide an adequate weight bearing surface without the disadvantages of leaving two or three rays to bear the load [58,59].

The dynamic consequences of performing an amputation must always be considered. More proximal amputations lead to loss of numerous muscle and tendon attachments. This leads to muscle imbalances, which may in turn cause future functional deficits. Often these imbalances or deficits can be overcome with proper prosthetic and orthotic accommodation. There are other situations where an adjunct curative procedure is needed, such as a tendo-Achilles lengthening [60,61]. This is frequently necessary with a transmetatarsal or Chopart's amputation secondary to a loss of dorsiflexory power and dynamic contracture of the triceps surae. In all cases after foot surgery and amputation in these high-risk individuals, attention must be paid to protective footwear to aid in the prevention of subsequent ulceration and infection [13].

Summary

Foot infections are a major complication of diabetes and subsequent amputation. Special attention must be directed to proper identification and treatment. The podiatric physician is often the "gatekeeper" of a multidisciplinary team. Efficient use of ancillary services has been shown to significantly improve outcomes. For limb-threatening infections often complicated by osteomyelitis, a combined approach with prompt surgical intervention and appropriate antibiotic therapy is generally the accepted treatment. Without proper identification and treatment, these infections often lead to amputation. When faced with amputation, the goals should focus on a functional level of amputation, with strategies directed at prevention of ulceration of the amputated side as well as the contralateral limb.

References

[1] Wild S, Roglic G, Green A, et al. Global prevalence of diabetes: estimates for the year 2000 and projections for 2030. Diabetes Care 2004;27(5):1047–53.

[2] Centers for Disease Control and Prevention National diabetes fact sheet: general information and national estimates on diabetes in the United States, 2005. Atlanta (GA): U.S. Department of Health and Human Services, Centers for Disease Control and Prevention; 2005.

[3] Boulton AJ, Vileikyte L, Ragnarson-Tennvall G, et al. The global burden of diabetic foot disease. Lancet 2005;366(9498):1719–24.

[4] Reiber GE. Epidemiology of foot ulcers and amputations in the diabetic foot. In: Bowker JH, Pfeifer MA, editors. The diabetic foot. St. Louis (MO): Mosby; 2001. p. 13–32.

[5] Reiber GE, Boyko E, Smith DG. Lower extremity foot ulcers and amputations in diabetes. In: Harris MI, Cowie C, Stern MP, editors. Diabetes in America. 2nd edition; 1995, NIH Publication No. 95-1468.

[6] Frykberg RG, Habershaw G, Chrzan JS. Epidemiology of the diabetic foot: ulcerations and amputations. In: Veves A, editor. Contemporary endocrinology: clinical management of diabetic neuropathy. Totowa (NJ): Humana Press; 1998. p. 273–90.

[7] Gibbons GW, Eliopoulos G. Infection of the diabetic foot. In: Kozak GP, Campbell D, Frykberg RG, et al, editors. Management of diabetic foot problems. 2nd edition. Philadelphia: WB Saunders; 1995. p. 121–9.

[8] Reiber GE, Lipsky BA, Gibbons GW. The burden of diabetic foot ulcers. Am J Surg 1998; 176(2A Suppl):5S–10S.

[9] American Diabetes Association. Diabetes 1996 vital statistics. Alexandria (VA): American Diabetes Association; 1996.

[10] Tennvall GR, Apelqvist J, Eneroth M. Costs of deep foot infections in patients with diabetes mellitus. Pharmacoeconomics 2000;18(3):225–38.

[11] American Diabetes Association. Economic costs of diabetes in the U.S. in 2002. Diabetes Care 2003;26(3):917–32.

[12] Lavery LA, Armstrong DG, Wunderlich RP, et al. Risk factors for foot infections in individuals with diabetes. Diabetes Care 2006;29(6):1288–93.

[13] Frykberg RG, Zgonis T, Armstrong DG, et al. Diabetic foot disorders: a clinical practice guideline [revision]. J Foot Ankle Surg 2006;45(5 Suppl):S1–66.

[14] Boulton AJ, Kirsner RS, Vileikyte L. Clinical practice. Neuropathic diabetic foot ulcers. N Engl J Med 2004;351(1):48–55.

[15] Boyko EJ, Ahroni JH, Stensel V, et al. A prospective study of risk factors for diabetic foot ulcer. The Seattle Diabetic Foot Study. Diabetes Care 1999;22(7):1036–42.

[16] Bagdade JD, Root RK, Bulger RJ. Impaired leukocyte function in patients with poorly controlled diabetes. Diabetes 1974;23:9–17.

[17] Nolan CM, Beaty HN, Bagdade JD. Further characterization of the impaired bactericidal function of granulocytes in patients with poorly controlled diabetes. Diabetes 1978;27(9): 889–94.

[18] Delamaire M, Maugendre D, Moreno M, et al. Impaired leucocyte functions in diabetic patients. Diabet Med 1997;14(1):29–34.

[19] Frykberg RG. An evidence-based approach to diabetic foot infections. Am J Surg 2003; 186(5A):44S–54S [discussion: 61S–4S].
[20] Karchmer AW, Gibbons GW. Foot infections in diabetes: evaluation and management. Curr Clin Top Infect Dis 1994;14:1–22.
[21] Lipsky BA. A report from the international consensus on diagnosing and treating the infected diabetic foot. Diabetes Metab Res Rev 2004;20(Suppl 1):S68–77.
[22] Lipsky BA, Berendt AR, Deery HG, et al. Diagnosis and treatment of diabetic foot infections. Clin Infect Dis 2004;39(7):885–910.
[23] American Diabetes Association. Consensus development conference on diabetic foot wound care: 7-8. Boston: American Diabetes Association; Diabetes Care 1999;22(8):1354–1360.
[24] Armstrong DG, Lipsky BA. Diabetic foot infections: stepwise medical and surgical management. Int Wound J 2004;1(2):123–32.
[25] Caputo GM, Cavanagh PR, Ulbrecht JS, et al. Assessment and management of foot disease in patients with diabetes. N Engl J Med 1994;331(13):854–60.
[26] Eneroth M, Apelqvist J, Stenstrom A. Clinical characteristics and outcome in 223 diabetic patients with deep foot infections. Foot Ankle Int 1997;18(11):716–22.
[27] Sumpio BE, Aruny J, Blume PA. The multidisciplinary approach to limb salvage. Acta Chir Belg 2004;104(6):647–53.
[28] Armstrong DG, Frykberg RG. Classifying diabetic foot surgery: toward a rational definition. Diabet Med 2003;20(4):329–31.
[29] Armstrong DG, Lavery LA, Frykberg RG, et al. Validation of a diabetic foot surgery classification. Int Wound J 2006;3(3):240–6.
[30] Frykberg R, Giurini J, Habershaw G, et al. Prophylactic surgery in the diabetic foot. In: Kominsky SJ, editor. Medical and surgical management of the diabetic foot. St. Louis (MO): Mosby; 1993. p. 399–439.
[31] Armstrong DG, Lavery LA, Vazquez JR, et al. Clinical efficacy of the first metatarsophalangeal joint arthroplasty as a curative procedure for hallux interphalangeal joint wounds in persons with diabetes. Diabetes Care 2003;26:3284–7.
[32] Berner A, Sage R, Niemela J. Keller procedure for the treatment of resistant plantar ulceration of the hallux. J Foot Ankle Surg 2005;44(2):133–6.
[33] Tan JS, Friedman NM, Hazelton-Miller C, et al. Can aggressive treatment of diabetic foot infections reduce the need for above-ankle amputation? Clin Infect Dis 1996;23(2):286–91.
[34] Gibbons GW, Habershaw GM. Diabetic foot infections. Anatomy and surgery. Infect Dis Clin North Am 1995;9(1):131–42.
[35] van Baal JG. Surgical treatment of the infected diabetic foot. Clin Infect Dis 2004;39(Suppl 2):S123–8.
[36] Akbari CM, Macsata R, Smith BM, et al. Overview of the diabetic foot. Semin Vasc Surg 2003;16(1):3–11.
[37] Sumpio BE, Lee T, Blume PA. Vascular evaluation and arterial reconstruction of the diabetic foot. Clin Podiatr Med Surg 2003;20(4):689–708.
[38] Kalani M, Brismar K, Fagrell B, et al. Transcutaneous oxygen tension and toe blood pressure as predictors for outcome of diabetic foot ulcers. Diabetes Care 1999;22(1):147–51.
[39] Alazraki N, Dalinka MK, Berquist TH, et al. Imaging diagnosis of osteomyelitis in patients with diabetes mellitus. American College of Radiology. ACR appropriateness criteria. Radiology 2000;215(Suppl):303–10.
[40] Ledermann HP, Morrison WB, Schweitzer ME. MR image analysis of pedal osteomyelitis: distribution, patterns of spread, and frequency of associated ulceration and septic arthritis. Radiology 2002;223(3):747–55.
[41] Johnson JE, Kennedy EJ, Shereff MJ, et al. Prospective study of bone, indium-111-labeled white blood cell, and gallium-67 scanning for the evaluation of osteomyelitis in the diabetic foot. Foot Ankle Int 1996;17(1):10–6.
[42] Lavery LA, Armstrong DG, Peters EJ, et al. Probe-to-bone test for diagnosing diabetic foot osteomyelitis; reliable or relic? Diabetes Care 2007;30(2):270–4.

[43] Newman LG, Waller J, Palestro CJ, et al. Unsuspected osteomyelitis in diabetic foot ulcers. Diagnosis and monitoring by leukocyte scanning with indium in 111 oxyquinoline. JAMA 1991;266(9):1246–51.
[44] Grayson ML, Gibbons GW, Balogh K, et al. Probing to bone in infected pedal ulcers. A clinical sign of underlying osteomyelitis in diabetic patients. JAMA 1995;273(9):721–3.
[45] Mushlin AI, Littenberg B. Diagnosing pedal osteomyelitis: testing choices and their consequences. J Gen Intern Med 1994;9(1):1–7.
[46] Palestro CJ, Mehta HH, Patel M, et al. Marrow versus infection in the Charcot joint: indium-111 leukocyte and technetium-99m sulfur colloid scintigraphy. J Nucl Med 1998;39(2):346–50.
[47] Bamberger DM, Daus GP, Gerding DN. Osteomyelitis in the feet of diabetic patients. Long-term results, prognostic factors, and the role of antimicrobial and surgical therapy. Am J Med 1987;83(4):653–60.
[48] Venkatesan P, Lawn S, Macfarlane RM, et al. Conservative management of osteomyelitis in the feet of diabetic patients. Diabet Med 1997;14(6):487–90.
[49] Pittet D, Wyssa B, Herter-Clavel C, et al. Outcome of diabetic foot infections treated conservatively: a retrospective cohort study with long-term follow-up. Arch Intern Med 1999;159(8):851–6.
[50] Jeffcoate WJ, Lipsky BA. Controversies in diagnosing and managing osteomyelitis of the foot in diabetes. Clin Infect Dis 2004;39(Suppl 2):S115–22.
[51] Lipsky BA. Osteomyelitis of the foot in diabetic patients. Clin Infect Dis 1997;25(6):1318–26.
[52] Ha Van G, Siney H, Danan JP, et al. Treatment of osteomyelitis in the diabetic foot: contribution of conservative surgery. Diabetes Care 1996;19:1257–60.
[53] Simpson AH, Deakin M, Latham JM. Chronic osteomyelitis. The effect of the extent of surgical resection on infection-free survival. J Bone Joint Surg Br 2001;83(3):403–7.
[54] Armstrong DG, Lavery LA. Negative pressure wound therapy after partial diabetic foot amputation: a multicentre, randomised controlled trial. Lancet 2005;366(9498):1704–10.
[55] Armstrong DG, Findlow AH, Oyibo SO, et al. The use of absorbable antibiotic-impregnated calcium sulphate pellets in the management of diabetic foot infections. Diabet Med 2001;18(11):942–3.
[56] Roeder B, Van Gils CC, Maling S. Antibiotic beads in the treatment of diabetic pedal osteomyelitis. J Foot Ankle Surg 2000;39(2):124–30.
[57] Waters RL, Perry J, Antonelle D, et al. Energy cost of walking of amputees: the influence of level of amputation. J Bone Joint Surg Am 1976;58:42–6.
[58] Attinger C, Venturi M, Kim K, et al. Maximizing length and optimizing biomechanics in foot amputations by avoiding cookbook recipes for amputation. Semin Vasc Surg 2003;16(1):44–66.
[59] Sanders LJ, Dunlap G. Transmetatarsal amputation. A successful approach to limb salvage. J Am Podiatr Med Assoc 1992;82(3):129–35.
[60] Mueller MJ, Sinacore DR, Hastings MK, et al. Effect of achilles tendon lengthening on neuropathic plantar ulcers. A randomized clinical trial. J Bone Joint Surg Am 2003;85(8):1436–45.
[61] Nishimoto GS, Attinger CE, Cooper PS. Lengthening the Achilles tendon for the treatment of diabetic plantar forefoot ulceration. Surg Clin North Am 2003;83(3):707–26.

ELSEVIER
SAUNDERS

Clin Podiatr Med Surg
24 (2007) 483–503

CLINICS IN PODIATRIC MEDICINE AND SURGERY

Nonoperative Treatment of Neuro-Osteoarthropathy of the Foot: Do We Need New Criteria?

Ernst Chantelau, MD, PhD[a,*],
Renate Kimmerle, MD, PhD[b],
Ludger W. Poll, MD, PhD[c]

[a]*Diabetes Foot Clinic, Department of Endocrinology, Diabetes and Rheumatology, Heinrich-Heine-University Düsseldorf, PO Box 10 10 07, D-40001 Düsseldorf, Germany*
[b]*Practice of Endocrinology and Diabetes, Aachener Strasse 196, D-40223 Düsseldorf, Germany*
[c]*Practice of Radiology and Nuclear Medicine, Beekstrasse 41, 47051 Duisburg, Germany*

Neuro-osteoarthropathy is defined as an acute or subacute condition that may affect patients with pain insensitivity from diabetic polyneuropathy, leprosy, or other disorders such as hereditary neuropathy [1–5]. It is characterized by painless osteoarticular damage of load-bearing parts of the skeleton, such as the feet, which is accompanied by soft tissue edema.

The trigger is common (so-called "minor environmental") trauma, the consequences of which are uncommon. The damage is usually extensive because of persistent load bearing due to the absence of the pain-guided, normal aversion reaction. Pain insensitivity is the primary risk factor for neuro-osteoarthropathy of the foot, including the Charcot foot. Secondary risk factors are osteoporosis and load-bearing intensity [6]. The pathogenesis of neuro-osteoarthropathy has been a matter of controversy since the days of Charcot and Virchow [3,7]. Charcot believed a neurogenic, endogenous bone dystrophy to be the cause of osteoarticular destruction (neurotrophic theory), whereas Virchow and colleagues assumed unperceived traumatization as the primum movens (neurotraumatic theory) [3,7]. Neither of the opponents could prove their theory due to imperfect diagnostic techniques 125 years ago.

* Corresponding author.
E-mail address: lobnig@med.uni-duesseldorf.de (E. Chantelau).

doi:10.1016/j.cpm.2007.03.006
podiatric.theclinics.com

At that time, syphilis was a frequent underlying condition of neuro-osteoarthropathy, whereas, currently, it is pain insensitivity from diabetic polyneuropathy. Accordingly, it was speculated that in diabetic subjects osteoarticular damage would result from a specific diabetic osteopathy; however, diminished bone quality predisposing to (pathologic) insufficiency fractures could not be demonstrated in diabetic polyneuropathy [8]. Qualitative bone histology was unremarkable in two studies on amputation specimens from diabetic patients with pain insensitivity and gangrene [9,10]. Bone-healing properties were found to be normal after correcting the insulin deficit (or the hyperglycemia, respectively) in experiments with diabetic animals (Table 1) [11–13].

The Charcot foot

The Charcot foot is the most extensive manifestation of neuro-osteoarthropathy of the foot, with osteoarticular destructions of the Lisfranc joint or other weight-bearing bones and joints. As such, the Charcot foot marks the end stage of neuro-osteoarthropathy of the foot. Its manifestations affect the feet in approximately 0.5% to 1% of the current diabetic population. A Charcot foot is defined "on plain radiographs as massive destruction, dissolution or disruption of foot or ankle bony architecture" [4]. The acute destruction process is followed by a chronic quiescent stage, the long-term prognosis of which is poor due to the high risk of skin ulceration over bony deformities and subsequent infection and amputation [4,14,15]. Radiographic studies showed that bones and joints eventually would fracture and dissolve (Charcot foot stage I: bone dissolution), repair (stage II: bone coalescence), and remodel (stage III), ending invariably in a severely deformed foot skeleton with joint ankylosis and bone deformities. The orthopedic

Table 1
Bone healing or bone quality, respectively, in relation to diabetic control (experimental studies)

Parameter	Study: Macey, et al 1989 [11]	Follak, et al 2004 [12]	Thrailkill, et al 2005 [13]
Animal species	Rats	Rats	Mice
Control animals			
Blood glucose, mg/d	110	90	190
Bone quality/healing	Normal	Normal	Normal
Diabetic animals untreated			
Blood glucose, mg/dL	560	360	480
Bone quality/healing	Impaired	Impaired	Impaired
Diabetic animals + insulin			
Blood glucose, mg/dL	260	170	260
Bone quality/healing	Normal	Normal	Normal

surgeon Sidney N. Eichenholtz believed long before the inception of MRI that "the appearance of the roentgenological features were sufficient to establish the diagnosis" [16] of a Charcot foot, and he consequently described the three radiographic stages mentioned previously. Unfortunately, this description has been taken as representative of the entire fatal evolution of the condition, which is a misconception.

Today we know from MRI that the "roentgenological features" of osteoarticular destructions in pain-insensitive feet, and of the Charcot foot in particular, are triggered by "silent" (fatigue) injury [17–20]. Persistent weight bearing over weeks and months causes the skeletal breakdown [6]. The first clinical symptom, which is a relatively painless inflammatory foot and ankle edema, is the physiologic consequence of nonfracture bone or joint injury (eg, fatigue trauma, bone contusion). This injury may not appear on plain radiographs but is seen on MR images as bone marrow edema. The foot edema increases heavily with nonfracture bone injuries progressing to complete fractures (Charcot foot stage I), regresses with bone coalescence (stage II), and fully resolves after completion of stage III (bone remodeling), like any fracture edema does [21–23]. At variance to the edema of deep vein thrombosis, with which it is often confused because of comparable painlessness, a foot edema from bone stress injury increases during weight bearing and subsides upon rest.

Persons who have pain insensitivity do not develop a Charcot foot unless they sustain an overuse injury. Less than 10% of all patients with diabetic polyneuropathy ever sustain neuro-osteoarthropathy. Persons without pain insensitivity do not develop a Charcot foot, even if they sustain a bone injury, because they tolerate overusing an injured foot (eg, with a "march-fracture") [18,24,25] for only 2 to 8 days [26] in contrast to persons with pain-insensitive feet, who may tolerate persistent weight bearing on an injured foot for 2 to 10 months [17,20] before seeking medical help.

Neuro-osteoarthropathy can be treated, and many methods and techniques have been advocated in the literature. Established treatment procedures, including immediate immobilization and off-loading in a total contact cast (TCC), will heal acute nonfracture (and fracture) bone injuries in feet with impaired sensitivity [20,27–29] in the same manner as they heal such injuries in feet with normal sensitivity [24,25,30–32].

Osteoarticular destruction including the devastating Charcot foot can be aborted if painless nonfracture skeletal injuries from common trauma (eg, foot sprain, fatigue stress) in pain-insensitive feet are treated as urgently and as stringently as if they were painful. "Not all hyposensitive feet with a fracture or dislocation are automatically Charcot feet.... If a skeletal injury is promptly diagnosed and carefully and adequately treated, the lesions may heal as any bony, ligamentous, or capsular lesion in a foot with normal sensation" [3]. The evolution of neuro-osteoarthropathy is schematically shown in Fig. 1.

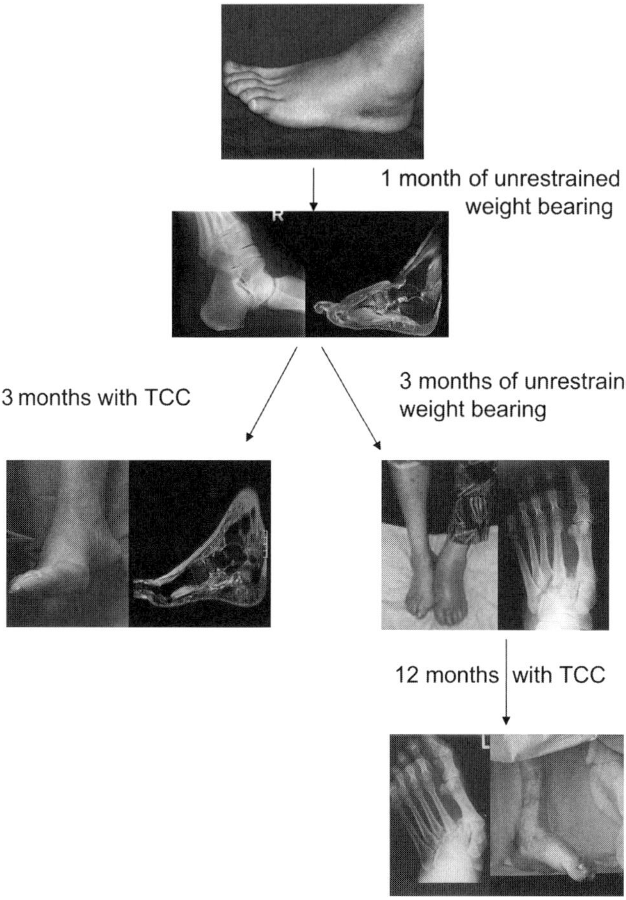

Fig. 1. Schematic presentation of the evolution of neuro-osteoarthropathy. Upper panel: hyperflexion injury of the left foot, with painless inflammatory edema (painful only during load bearing) in a patient with diabetic polyneuropathy. Radiograph and MR image (T1-weighted, fat-suppressed, with contrast media) 1 month later show unremarkable skeletal structure on radiograph and bone marrow edema (bright appearance) of the Lisfranc joint on MRI, indicative of stress injury. Left hand side, middle: clinical picture and MR image of injury (as above) after 3 months of treatment with TCC show regression of the bone and soft tissue edema, indicative of healing (cure). Right hand side, middle: clinical picture and plain radiograph of a Lisfranc joint dislocation fracture in a patient with diabetic polyneuropathy after 3 months of unrestrained weight bearing show soft tissue edema and bone dissolution (Charcot foot stage I). Right hand side, bottom: clinical picture and plain radiograph of Lisfranc joint fracture (as above) after 12 months of treatment with TCC show bone remodeling, joint ankylosis, and skeletal deformity, indicative of faulty healing (Charcot foot stage III).

Nonoperative treatment of acute neuro-osteoarthropathy of the foot: off-loading and immobilization

The mainstay of nonoperative treatment of acute neuro-osteoarthropathy is immobilization and off-loading of the injured foot, as is true for stress injuries in sports' traumatology [24,25,31,32]. The rationale for this approach, its putative mechanism of action, and its criteria and effectiveness are outlined in the following sections.

Rationale for off-loading and immobilization

Immobilization and off-loading is an established treatment of minor and major mechanical skeletal injuries. From observations that skeletal injuries can trigger neuro-osteoarthropathy of the foot, it has been concluded that common fracture treatment might be an option for treating this condition [7,33,34]. Evidence of complete fractures contributing to neuro-osteoarthropathy stems from case reports [35–40]. Likewise, cases of iatrogenic bone or joint injury (eg, from deliberate foot surgery) have been reported documenting the postoperative development of a Charcot foot [41–44]. Evidence of nonfracture injuries contributing to neuro-osteoarthropathy stems from imaging studies early after the onset of first symptoms (ie, after the onset of foot swelling).

In a case report [18] and two case series [17,29], it was shown that the absence of radiographic pathology was associated with the presence of bone or joint pathology on MRI in acutely swollen pain-insensitive feet. A case report [45] and two case series have shown that, with persistent weight bearing, these imaging abnormalities progress to radiographically visible bone/joint pathology and deformities in pain-insensitive feet [6,17]. Evidence of stress injury perception is barely obtainable from the history in patients with pain insensitivity [2,5]. Nevertheless, Slowman-Kovacs and colleagues [46] have reported three patients with pain-insensitive feet in whom minor trauma triggered osteoarthropathy. Armstrong and colleagues [41] reported that 26% of 55 patients with Charcot foot were able to recall a foot trauma as the preceding event (including 4% with recent foot surgery), and Onvlee [3] noted a patient-reported foot trauma in 14% of 64 patients who had Charcot feet. Larsen and Holstein [47] found a recent history of overuse fractures in 5 cases (10%), or a history of mobilization after prolonged periods of restricted weight bearing in 28 (60%) of 47 cases of Charcot foot as trigger events. Thompson and colleagues [38] reported a history of acute fracture in 9 (82%) of 11 cases with Charcot foot. In neither of the case reports or series was objective confirmation of the patient-reported positive or negative trauma history presented, such as by concurrent MRI. This imaging would have been necessary considering the imprecision of trauma perception and the low reliability of self-reporting due to pain insensitivity of the feet.

Putative mechanism of action of off-loading and immobilization

Putting at rest a foot with acute neuro-osteoarthropathy invariably decreases swelling and inflammation [7,33,34]. Such observations have encouraged the use of immobilization and off-loading (eg, by application of a cast) for treating this condition. Immobilization and off-loading mitigate fatigue processes and tear-and-wear that inevitably occur in a damaged foot skeleton during everyday unprotected ambulation (comprising approximately 5000 strides per day in patients with diabetic polyneuropathy [48]). Onvlee [3] in his review has noted that most authorities advise a (partially weight-bearing) walking cast rather than a non–weight-bearing cast for the treatment of acute Charcot foot, consistent with contemporary understanding of bone healing. Partial weight bearing is generally indicated as a therapeutic means to support osteochondral healing [49]; however, the exact strain environment of a partially loaded foot remains unknown [49]. Interfragmentary movements impair fracture healing [50]; therefore, rigid rather than soft or semi-rigid immobilization is advisable for bone healing [51]. The authors prefer the treatment scheme outlined by Onvlee [3] using the rigid bivalved fiberglass TCC, which is assumed to support bone healing by reducing peak contact stresses, decreasing shear forces and interfragmentary movements, and providing redistribution of loads necessary to accommodate abnormal skeletal anatomy [4]. McGill and colleagues [34] have shown that application of a walking TCC reduces the inflammatory activity in an acute Charcot foot within 6 months.

Criteria for immobilizing and off-loading injured pain-insensitive feet

Previously, only the acute fracture state of neuro-osteoarthropathy that could be visualized by plain radiographs (Charcot foot stages I and II) was taken as a criterion to off-load and immobilize a swollen pain-insensitive foot [4,14,15,17,41,47]. Currently, acute nonfracture bone injuries (ie, bone bruise and bone marrow edema) that can be visualized by MRI (rather than plain radiographs) must be taken as criterion to off-load and immobilize a swollen pain-insensitive foot, because persistent weight bearing in this condition will cause neuro-osteoarthropathy with complete fractures and Charcot foot [6]. Clinical tests to diagnose foot injuries (eg, the Ottawa [52] and Bernese [53] ankle rules) require an undisturbed, subjective pain perception as a prerequisite. Such tests apply only to subjects with normal pain sensitivity and must not be used in patients with pain insensitivity. We (Chantelau, Kimmerle, and Poll) and others [20,28] have recommended the use of MRI rather than plain radiographic examination for patients experiencing painless swelling in the foot or leg. The authors agree with Thompson's [38] suggestions that, even when there is no fracture identified, the patient should be given crutches or a cast at the initial treatment.

Evidence for the effectiveness of immobilization and off-loading therapy

Several case series and one comparative study of immobilization and off-loading of fracture injuries in patients with polyneuropathy have been reported, most of which were retrospective studies. Controlled clinical trials are not available. Thompson and colleagues [38] emphasized that, "with adequate external immobilization and protection from continued stress, the fractures heal." Kristiansen [37] observed that foot deformities occurred in three patients with fracture injuries despite being taped or using a walking cast for 6 to 8 weeks; one of the patients required amputation. Boninger and Leonard [54] reported on six patients with acute Charcot changes using a molded total-contact, ankle-foot orthosis for 7 to 45 months until healing of the foot. Subsequently, custom shoes were required by three of their patients, while three other patients needed prolonged use of the TCC because of residual inflammatory activity.

Larsen and Holstein [47] reported on the outcome of 47 feet with Charcot fractures subjected to restricted weight bearing using crutches (n = 39), a plaster cast (n = 3), or no treatment (n = 5). Full weight bearing was accomplished within 5 to 6 months. The outcome was fair at best: 17 feet healed with minor deformity, and 28 feet healed with major deformity. There was one amputation and one death. Fourteen feet developed pressure ulcers, and 6 feet developed fracture relapses. Many patients (80%) required hand-made shoes, 14% were managed with molded insoles and conventional shoes, and 6% remained confined to a wheelchair [47]. Fabrin and colleagues [15] reported on 115 diabetic patients with acute (stage I-II) Charcot foot who were treated by weight-bearing restriction using crutches and "therapeutic footwear" (no TCC). Most feet healed with major deformities (70% required bespoke shoes or boots); 30% of patients had multiple fracture relapses; the incidence of foot ulcers was 7%; and two patients died before the fractures healed [15]. Saltzmann and colleagues [4] reported on 59 patients with acute (stage I) Charcot foot and 56 with Charcot foot of other stages, with and without concomitant foot ulcers. All of the patients wore a TCC for a median of 12 months, and approximately 25% of all limbs required the TCC for more than 18 months. Saltzmann and coworkers observed a 2.7% annual rate of amputation in their cohort (during a median follow-up of 3.8 years), mostly in patients with active ulcers ($P = .016$ versus patients without open foot or ankle ulcers). They cautioned that, in their cohort, the use of TCC in ulcerated Charcot feet was associated with greater levels of ulcer recurrence and maintained that "additional study of the use of orthotics to treat Charcot deformities is needed"[4]. Armstrong and colleagues [41] and Sinacore [55] reported on patient series with acute (stage I) Charcot fractures in whom treatment by TCC achieved healing of the acute osteoarticular destructions, albeit, with devastating deformities (Table 2).

The one comparison study of immobilization and off-loading versus persistent weight bearing in fracture injuries was provided by Clohisi and Thompson [56], who retrospectively assessed a series of patients with kidney transplantation and acute Charcot fractures of the foot. A group of seven patients was treated with a "non–weight-bearing protective device," while another group of 11 patients was not (persistent weight-bearing group).

Table 2
Summary of some studies on nonoperative treatment of neuro-osteoarthropathy

Reference	Number of patients	Bone injury	Mode (duration) of intervention	Outcome: major deformities (%)		
				Forefoot	Midfoot	Hindfoot
[41]	55	Fractures	TCC (4.5 mo)	3	82	15
[55]	30	Fractures	TCC (3 mo)	20	69	11
[15]	115	Fractures	Crutches (4–6 mo)	19	74	7
[17]	13	Fractures	TCC (4.5 mo)	8	92	0
[62]	9	Fractures	TCC (5.8 wk)	NA	NA	NA
[64]	21	Fractures	Pamidronate[a]	NA	NA	NA
[66]	11	Fractures	Alendronate (6 mo)	NA	NA	NA
[67]	16	Fractures	Calcitonin (6 mo)	NA	NA	NA
[17]	11	BME	TCC (3 mo)	0	8	0
[29]	12	BME	TCC (6 mo)	0	0	0
[20]	11	BME	TCC (4 mo)	0	0	0

Abbreviations: BME, bone marrow edema on MRI; NA, not analyzed; TCC, total contact cast.

[a] One single intravenous infusion of 90 mg of pamidronate; follow-up period, 12 months.

During follow-up of a median of 5 years, in the persistent weight-bearing group there were three amputations and four patients with inability to walk, whereas no amputation and walking inability was observed in the group that had been treated with the non–weight-bearing protective device [56]. A comparison of nonoperative versus operative treatment of Charcot fractures was, unfortunately, avoided by Simon and colleagues [57], who chose to retrospectively evaluate 14 operated cases out of a series of 43 cases. The remaining 29 cases with Charcot fractures were treated nonoperatively with off-loading among other methods but were not evaluated.

Off-loading and immobilization of nonfracture bone injuries was assessed by two case series and a retrospective comparative study. Edmonds and colleagues [29] reported on "12 diabetic patients with Charcot osteoarthropathy presenting with a hot swollen foot, hot isotope bone scan and normal radiograph." MRI showed bone marrow edema alone in six patients and bone marrow edema in association with subchondral fracture or subchondral cystic changes in the remaining six patients. Off-loading with a TCC resulted in resolution of the bone marrow edema; fractures healed in three patients; and cysts remained unchanged. "On follow-up of all patients, radiographs showed no subluxation and there was no clinical deformity" [29]. Chantelau and colleagues [20] reported prospectively on 11 consecutive diabetic patients with insensitive feet and stress bone injuries who were treated with a TCC shortly after the onset of first symptoms and who were cured without major deformities after an average of 16 weeks of off-loading and immobilization (Tables 3 and 4).

A retrospective comparison of immobilization and off-loading in fracture versus nonfracture injuries [17] has shown that treatment by a TCC prevents

Table 3
Demographic and clinical characteristics of 11 patients with insulin-treated diabetes mellitus and silent stress bone injures, prospectively treated with TCC

Patient number	Gender, female/male	Age, years	Diabetes type	Duration of diabetes, years	Risk factors for foot stress injury	Trauma history
1	Male	49	I	25	Obesity	Walking
2	Female	64	I	51	Hypoglycemic attacks	Sprain
3	Female	56	II	19	Unknown	Unknown
4	Male	57	II	6	Obesity/osteoporosis	Walking
5	Female	65	II	29	Unknown	Sprain
6	Female	54	I	35	Unknown	Sprain
7	Male	48	I	27	Unknown	Unknown
8	Male	70	II	10	Obesity	Unknown
9	Male	70	II	40	Unknown	Unknown
10	Male	65	II	20	Osteoporosis	Repeat blunt trauma
11	Female	62	I	20	Unknown	Sprain

Charcot deformities and fractures only if applied to nonfracture injuries (see Table 2). Likewise, the results of arthrodesis treatment were excellent in terms of restoration of foot shape and function when the operation was done at a very early stage of Charcot fractures [57].

Table 4
Treatment details of diabetic patients with polyneuropathy and silent stress bone injuries as described in Table 3

Patient number	Grade of bone injury[a]	Duration of symptoms before treatment, weeks	Duration of TCC treatment, weeks	Outcome	Follow-up, months	Number of relapses
1	III	4	6	Cured	24	0
2	IV	1	10	Cured	15	0
3	III–IV	8	8	Cured	12	1
4	III	4	20	Osteoarthrosis	17	0
5	III–IV	12	8	Cured	17	1
6	III–IV	2	8	Osteoarthrosis	12	0
7	III	2	20	Cured	6	0
8	III	4	28	Cured	14	0
9	III	1	8	Cured	4	0
10	III	12	52	Osteoarthrosis	26	3
11	III	12	18	Cured	13	0

[a] The bone injuries were diagnosed by MRI and were graded according to Kiuru and colleagues [25] as follows: grade I, endosteal marrow edema; grade II, periosteal edema and endosteal marrow edema; grade III, muscle edema, periosteal edema, and endosteal marrow edema; grade IV, fracture line; grade V, callus in cortical bone.

How to ensure immobilization and off-loading of a pain-insensitive injured foot

At variance to the previous recommendations, some foot and ankle experts claim that "immobilization has been the mainstay of treatment for all ankle sprains, but functional treatment (including elastic bandage, soft cast, tape, or orthoses and coordination training with a physical therapist) has been shown to have greater benefit in terms of improving symptoms and functional outcomes in short-term, intermediate-term and long-term follow-up" [58]. A flexible bandage is probably not protective enough for ankle sprains in pain-insensitive patients. One of the three patients reported on by Kristiansen [37] developed severe foot deformity while being treated with a tape only. Tape treatment is contraindicated in fractures. Moreover, tape treatment of foot injuries requires a functioning pain sensation. The aversion reaction against offending forces is lost in patients with pain insensitivity. Even patients with normal pain sensitivity are unable to fully accomplish pain-guided restrictions, such as partial restricted weight bearing following fracture healing [59].

Treatment results have been suboptimal when immobilization and off-loading has been delayed or insufficient in patients with acute neuro-osteoarthropathy. Larsen and Holstein [47] withheld TCC treatment from their patients with neuro-osteoarthropathy after they had experienced gangrene caused by a nonremovable, circular, and ill-fitting cast. Their treatment results were fair at best. The judgment by Fabrin and colleagues [15] that "the TCC is considered by some to be the 'gold standard' of treatment of the acute Charcot foot, but crutches and therapeutic protective shoes (possibly after a few days of using a wheelchair) are adequate in most cases" seems to be unfounded after comparing their results (obtained with crutches and shoes) with those of other researchers obtained with a TCC. The superiority of a TCC for treating bone injuries in pain-insensitive feet has been demonstrated repeatedly; however, caution is necessary because of the inability of patients to indicate ill-fitting of the cast and the potential of cast-induced ulcerations and amputations [4,15,47].

The TCC is the treatment of choice at the authors' institution. Patients with a foot injury, preferably before a complete fracture has occurred, should be subjected to bed rest for a few days to immediately and completely off-load and elevate the affected foot. A compression stocking is applied to support edema reduction and to prevent vein thrombosis. Subsequently, the limb is casted with the foot in the neutral position. A bivalved rigid walking cast is applied made of fiberglass, padded with cotton-covered rubber foam, and furnished with a rocker-bottom walking sole. The TCC is placed in an attempt to evenly distribute forces across the plantar surface of the foot while immobilizing foot and ankle joints in a neutral position. It allows restrained ambulation while immobilizing and off-loading the injured foot. The fitting of the cast is checked regularly, and potentially dangerous pressure points are removed as recommended by Saltzmann and colleagues [4]. Patients are advised to use the TCC all day long, together with crutches, and to take it off only during sleep at night. TCC treatment is applied until healing of the injury, defined as the absence of clinical signs of inflammation (ie, absence of edema, erythema, and hyperthermia of the affected foot) during ambulation, together with resolution of bone marrow edema on follow-up MRI (or bone remodeling on plain radiographs). After healing, a gradual return to weight-bearing activity is advised during 4 to 8 weeks, replacing the TCC by appropriate footwear for increasing periods of time.

Potential adverse effects of the TCC may be related to insufficient casting. The authors have observed a case of malalignment and a pressure ulcer due to a poorly fitted TCC [17]. We have never seen gangrene from a TCC, as reported by Larsen and Holstein [47], probably because we have always used bivalved removable casts rather than nonremovable circular casts. Heparin may not be necessary, because compression stockings for prophylaxis of deep vein thrombosis after foot and ankle trauma have been regarded as sufficient by most orthopedic surgeons [60]. Moreover, the removable bivalved TCC is taken off during bed rest, allowing unloaded limb movements, at least for several hours of sleep at night (Fig. 2).

How can the response to immobilization and off-loading therapy be monitored?

Previous investigators have observed the response of fracture injuries to immobilization and off-loading by monitoring the hyperthermia of the foot

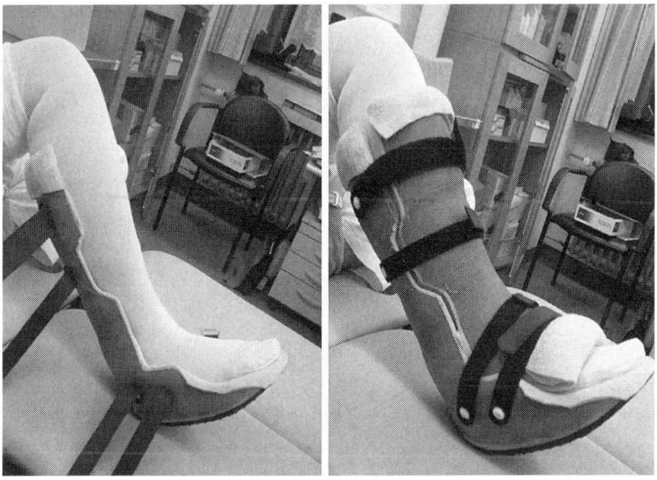

Fig. 2. Bivalved TCC, open/closed. Foot in a neutral position. Leg covered with compression stocking. Rubber-foam padding. Rocker sole.

decreasing and the edema resolving [15,34,41,47], and by observing bone coalescence and bone consolidation/remodeling on repeated plain radiographs [4,41]; however, tailoring treatment duration according to the normalization of foot temperature, the resolution of foot edema, or bone remineralization on plain radiographs is associated with a considerable rate of fracture relapse [15,41]. A more refined method of follow-up that should be applied, particularly in cases of nonfracture injuries, would be based on repeated MRI. The authors have found during the return to weight-bearing activity that follow-up MRI sometimes discloses residual bone marrow edema that is not accompanied by relevant clinical symptoms.

Accordingly, we argue that the duration of immobilization and off-loading should be determined in relation to MRI improvement [61] and should probably be longer than might be suggested by clinical and radiographic improvement. Likewise, the return to weight bearing and the monitoring of the re-activation procedure should be based on the more sensitive MRI findings rather than on crude temperature or plain radiographic findings as has been tradition.

Apparently, the duration of off-loading and immobilization varies with the physician's treatment objectives, the patient's compliance with the TCC, and the extent of bone injury. Pinzur and colleagues [62] reported that 5.8 weeks of TCC treatment relieved acute stage I Charcot symptoms, whereas Chantelau [17] and Armstrong and colleagues [41] reported an average of 4.5 months of TCC treatment healed acute Charcot fractures. Moreover, Armstrong and colleagues [41] reported an average of 6 months of immobilization before the patients wore permanent footwear. Saltzmann and colleagues [4] reported on average 12 months of cast treatment, whereas Bates and colleagues [63] reported 20 months of TCC treatment to heal Charcot fractures. The average duration of cast treatment to heal nonfracture injuries has ranged from 3 to 6 months (see Table 2).

Nonoperative treatment of acute neuro-osteoarthropathy of the foot: medical treatment

Two drug classes, bisphosphonates and calcitonin, have been tried on the acute Charcot foot in small, short-term studies. Bisphosphonates are widely used for the treatment of osteoporosis and osteogenesis imperfecta. The exact mechanism of the drug class in halting bone loss by preventing osteoclastic resorption is not completely understood. Pamidronate was administered in a randomized controlled trial to 21 patients [64] and in a nonrandomized trial to 11 patients [65]. All patients showed a significant decrease in foot temperature and bone turnover markers. Effects on foot deformities were not reported. Comparable results were obtained in 11 patients during treatment with alendronate over 6 months [66]. Calcitonin was given to 16 patients over 6 months with some effect on foot temperature and bone turnover markers but, like bisphosphonates, without any clinical benefit [67]. Potential side effects of calcitonin (flush, nausea, tachycardia) and of bisphosphonates (jaw osteonecrosis) have to be considered. A summary of reports on nonoperative treatment of acute neuro-osteoarthropathy of the foot is presented in Table 2.

Nonoperative treatment of healed, quiescent neuro-osteoarthropathy of the foot: footwear

Footwear is required to protect any foot from injury during walking, including the pain-insensitive foot with healed bone or joint injury or joint dysfunction.

In cases of uneventfully healed bone or joint injury without skeletal deformities, "normal" footwear used previously may be used again. However, painful stress injuries of the talus if insufficiently off-loaded and immobilized may heal with complications (eg, subchondral degeneration) in 50% of cases [68]. After healing of a painful sports trauma, subjects may sustain repeated injuries of the same type and location without proper prevention [69]. Likewise, 3 of 11 neuropathic patients with healed "silent" stress injuries had one to three relapses in the same foot within 12 to 26 months of follow-up (see Table 4). The persistence of undetected residual morphologic or functional damage (eg, osteoarthrosis, subchondral cysts, tendon weakness, joint instability) after healing of even minor neuro-osteoarthropathy must be assumed, a locus minoris resistentiae, which requires future protection; therefore, after healing of a silent foot injury, the use of particular protective footwear is preferable to prevent relapses.

In patients with minor deformity after healed neuro-osteoarthropathy (eg, little or no depression of the longitudinal arch), industrially fabricated "diabetic" shoes with a stiff walking sole and a rocker bottom [70,71] may be sufficient. These shoes, when furnished with custom-molded, full-contact, rigid insoles to provide arch support [72], will adequately minimize load bearing and mobility of the tarsometatarsal and tarsophalangeal joints during walking. They also shorten stride length (Fig. 3).

In cases of severe deformities, custom-made shoes are necessary requiring individualized lasts, which can be made traditionally by the use of plaster of Paris or by using contemporary computerized scanning (Fig. 4). Both techniques do not guarantee the necessary peak-pressure relief during walking, because the ground-reaction forces exerted by a moving foot with Charcot deformity are difficult to predict, especially inside a shoe. Moreover, the shape of the foot varies unpredictably with weight bearing [73]. Hence, the making of suitable bespoke footwear for the healed Charcot foot remains confined to trial-and-error. The foot and the shoe should be checked frequently after the first use of bespoke shoes to notice and correct dangerous pressure points in the shoe as early as possible before a full-thickness foot ulcer has occurred (Fig. 5).

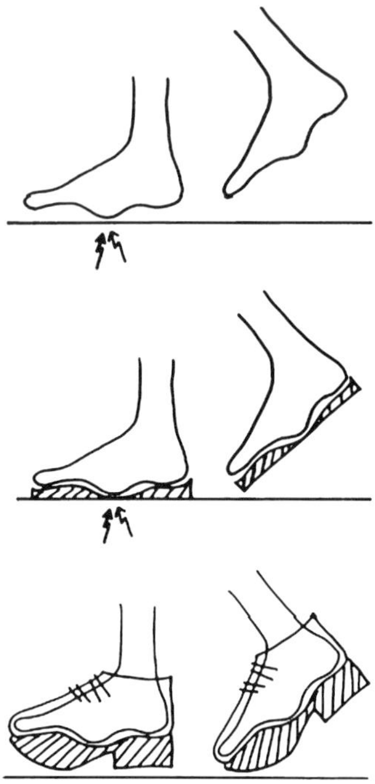

Fig. 3. Construction principle of footwear for a foot with healed osteoarticular destructions from neuro-osteoarthropathy. The immobilized foot is moved by the shoe. Upper part: foot characteristics of stiff joints, bony deformities, and poor skin coverage (arrows indicate peak pressure points). Middle part: customized, full-contact orthosis with rigid construction, load evenly distributed, and no pressure peaks. Requires rocker sole [71] for functioning. Lower part: rocker sole enables forward movement of the rigid shoe with the immobilized foot with rolling-over, no propulsion, no push-off ground reaction forces.

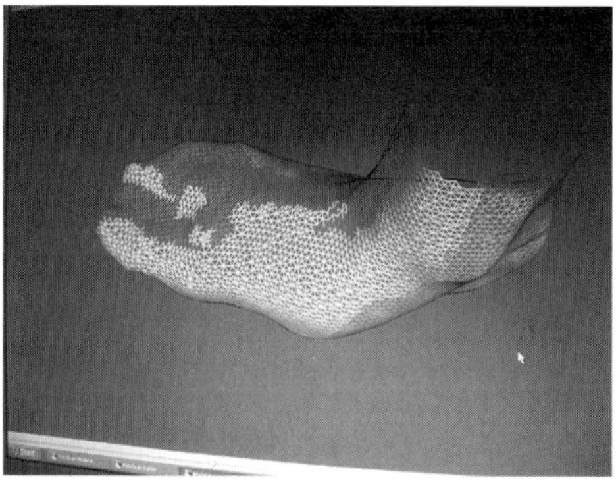

Fig. 4. Computer scan of a healed (stage III) Charcot foot, the basis for making individual customized lasts.

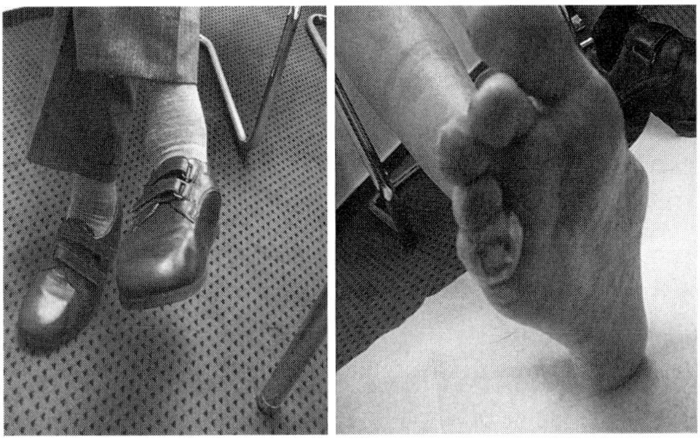

Fig. 5. Pressure ulcer that has developed 1 week after the first use of an ill-fitted, hand-made rocker shoe in a patient with a healed (stage III) Charcot foot.

In the series by Armstrong and colleagues [41], 4 to 10 weeks passed from the cessation of TCC treatment until the first use of custom footwear, referred to as "prescription footwear," "accommodative footwear," "permanent footwear," or "custom molded footwear," produced and fitted by a "pedorthic shoe specialist." Technical details of the footwear were not given. Eight of 55 patients had a Charcot relapse, and four patients had an ulcer at a toe (n = 2) or metatarsal head (n = 2) within 10 months of using this footwear [41].

Potential adverse effects from rocker bottom shoes relate to instability during standing and walking and stair climbing. At the time of writing this article, no studies were available on the clinical effectiveness and safety of footwear for the pain-insensitive foot with healed neuro-osteoarthropathy.

Discussion

> "Disease is very old, and nothing about it has changed. It is we who change, as we learn to recognise what was formerly imperceptible."
>
> —Jean Martin Charcot

The inception of MRI [19,66,74–76] has taught us to recognize what was formerly (on plain radiographs) imperceptible—the traumatic nature of neuro-osteoarthropathy. There are only two necessary component causes for neuro-osteoarthropathy (including the Charcot foot) to develop, similar to the component causes of neuropathic foot ulcers [77]: (1) a foot skeletal injury, and (2) ongoing traumatization from persistent weight bearing. The primary risk factor for neuro-osteoarthropathy is pain insensitivity, which increases the likelihood of continued traumatization. Secondary risk factors are impact force intensity (eg, from obesity and weight-bearing physical activity [6]) and bone weakness (eg, from osteoporosis/osteopathy of any cause), which lower the fracture threshold. Increased local blood flow, which previously was assumed to be a risk factor [8,57], is likely to be the consequence rather than the cause of Charcot foot [8].

Foot and ankle experts and other professionals need to adopt new criteria to treat neuro-osteoarthropathy and Charcot foot in particular. What we have learned thus far includes the following theories, thoughts, and suggestions:

Pain, which is a cardinal, albeit, unspecific symptom of stress bone injuries, may not be displayed as a cardinal symptom in subjects with pain insensitivity. In these patients, relatively painless foot edema, which is unspecific, becomes the presenting sign of a skeletal injury in a medical consultation. This sign must be accepted like the concept of painless silent myocardial infarction in diabetic patients with polyneuropathy. The first examination in a patient presenting with a painless swollen foot must be the examination of pain sensitivity to elucidate the significance of the reported painlessness.

Well-established clinical techniques to assess the severity of foot injuries, such as the Ottawa or Bernese ankle rules [52,53], must not be applied to subjects with pain insensitivity. The confirmation of a suspected foot bone injury in pain-insensitive patients requires the application of appropriate techniques such as MRI rather than plain radiographs or clinical examination techniques [58].

Not only examination techniques but also established traumatology therapies need to be modified to suit pain-insensitive patients. Off-loading and immobilization are the mainstays of treatment in cases of foot injury from fatigue or common (environmental) trauma. So-called "functional treatment" with tapes and soft bandages has never been studied in pain-insensitive patients. Their benefits have not been demonstrated unequivocally in controlled clinical trials [78–82]; therefore, functional treatment should probably not be applied in common injuries in pain-insensitive feet.

Early diagnosis is important to avoid unnecessary pointless or even harmful treatment [17,83]. A swollen foot in a pain-insensitive patient is an emergency. Early treatment avoids complications. The overall aim of musculoskeletal treatment is to prevent severe articular destruction and avoid the need for amputation [2,5]. This goal can be accomplished if treatment is started in the state of nonfracture injuries [17,20,29]. Previous suggestions by Thompson and colleagues [38], who maintained "the presence of painless swelling in the lower extremity of…at-risk patients…should be considered an early sign of impending pathological fracture, joint disruption, or both," and of Greider [2], who emphasized that "signs of…swelling, local warmth…must be investigated and treated immediately" in patients with insensitivity to pain, are important parameters of the patient's treatment.

At-risk patients should be screened and educated to avoid strenuous exercise and falls and to seek early advice in the event of any foot abnormality, such as an abnormal shape, temperature, color, or function, and with any common (environmental) foot trauma.

The role of drugs to heal neuro-osteoarthropathy of the foot, including the Charcot foot, remains unproven.

Summary

Neuro-osteoarthropathy originates from a bone or joint injury followed by the persistence of strain in pain insensitivity. It is characterized by painless osteoarticular damage of load-bearing parts of the skeleton such as the feet. The worst manifestation of neuro-osteoarthropathy is the Charcot foot with its devastating osteoarticular destructions and irreversible deformities. New diagnostic tools like MRI have revealed that mechanical stress is causative of the condition. Consequently, neuro-osteoarthropathy must no longer be regarded as an incurable disease. New diagnostic and treatment criteria are needed. Any painless, MRI-proven nonfracture injury should be subjected to off-loading and immobilization until healing, because this strategy has shown to be highly effective in preventing neuro-osteoarthropathy including the Charcot foot. Whether drug treatment has a role in terms of prevention or healing of osteoarticular destructions remains to be demonstrated.

Acknowledgment

The comments by Dr. G.J.Onvlee, an orthopedic surgeon formerly at the University of Leiden (The Netherlands), on an earlier version of this article are gratefully acknowledged.

References

[1] Brand PW. Insensitive feet: a practical handbook on foot problems in leprosy. London: The Leprosy Mission; 1977.

[2] Greider TD. Orthopedic aspects of congenital insensitivity to pain. Clin Orthop Relat Res 1983;172:177–85.

[3] Onvlee GJ. The Charcot foot: a critical review and an observational study of a group of 60 patients [thesis]. Medical Faculty, University of Leiden/The Netherlands;1998.

[4] Saltzmann CL, Hagy ML, Zimmerman B, et al. How effective is non-operative initial treatment of patients with diabetes and Charcot arthropathy of the feet? Clin Orthop Relat Res 2005;435:185–90.

[5] Minde JK, Svensson O, Holmberg M, et al. Orthopedic aspects of familial insensitivity to pain due to a novel nerve growth factor beta mutation. Acta Orthop 2006;77:198–202.

[6] Kimmerle R, Chantelau E. Weight-bearing intensity produces Charcot deformity in injured neuropathic feet in diabetes. Exp Clin Endocrinol Diabetes 2007;115:360–64.

[7] Bradshaw TW. Aetiopathogenesis of the Charcot foot: an overview. Practical Diabetes International 1998;15:22–4.
[8] Chantelau E, Onvlee GJ. Charcot foot in diabetes: farewell to the neurotrophic theory. Horm Metab Res 2006;38:361–7.
[9] Craig JG, Amin MB, Wu K, et al. Osteomyelitis of the diabetic foot: MR imaging-pathologic correlation. Radiology 1997;203:849–55.
[10] Chantelau E, Wolf A, Özdemir S, et al. Bone histomorphology may be unremarkable in diabetes mellitus. Med Klin 2007;102:429–33.
[11] Macey LR, Kana SM, Jingushi S, et al. Defects of early fracture-healing in experimental diabetes. J Bone Joint Surg Am 1989;71:722–33.
[12] Follak N, Klöting I, Wolf E, et al. Improving metabolic control reverses the histomorphometric and biomechanical abnormalities of an experimentally induced bone defect in spontaneously diabetic rats. Calcif Tissue Int 2004;74:551–60.
[13] Thrailkill KM, Liu L, Wahl EC, et al. Bone formation is impaired in a model of type 1 diabetes. Diabetes 2005;54:2875–81.
[14] Sinacore DR, Withrington NC. Recognition and management of acute neuropathic (Charcot) arthropathies of the foot and ankle. J Orthop Sports Phys Ther 1999;29:736–46.
[15] Fabrin J, Larsen K, Holstein PE. Long-term follow-up in diabetic Charcot feet with spontaneous onset. Diabetes Care 2000;23:796–800.
[16] Eichenholtz SN. Charcot joints: with a foreword by Philip D. Wilson. Springfield (IL): Charles C. Thomas; 1966. (quoted by Simon, et al [57]).
[17] Chantelau E. The perils of procrastination: effects of early vs. delayed detection and treatment of incipient Charcot fracture. Diabet Med 2005;22:1707–12.
[18] Chantelau E, Richter A, Schmidt-Grigoriadis P, et al. The diabetic Charcot foot: MRI discloses bone stress injury as trigger mechanism of neuroarthropathy. Exp Clin Endocrinol Diabetes 2006;114:118–23.
[19] Chantelau E, Poll L. Evaluation of the diabetic Charcot foot by MR imaging or plain radiography—an observational study. Exp Clin Endocrinol Diabetes 2006;114:428–31.
[20] Chantelau E, Richter A, Ghassem-Zadeh N, et al. "Silent" bone stress injuries in the feet of diabetic patients with polyneuropathy—a report on 12 cases. Arch Orthop Trauma Surg 2007;127:171–7.
[21] Szczesny G, Olszewski WL. The pathomechanism of posttraumatic edema of lower limbs. I. The effect of extravasated blood, bone marrow cells, and bacterial colonization on tissues, lymphatics, and lymph nodes. J Trauma 2002;52:315–22.
[22] Szczesny G, Olszewski WL. The pathomechanism of posttraumatic edema of lower limbs. II. Changes in the lymphatic system. J Trauma 2003;55:350–4.
[23] Veihelmann A, Szczesny G, Refior HJ, et al. Microcirculatory changes in the soft tissues of the mouse lower limb after mechanical trauma [abstract]. J Bone Joint Surg Br 2002; 84(Suppl 1):21.
[24] Lassus J, Tulikoura I, Konttinen Y, et al. Bone stress injuries of the lower extremity. Acta Orthop Scand 2002;73:359–68.
[25] Kiuru MJ, Pihlajamäki HK, Ahovuo JA. Bone stress injuries. Acta Radiol 2004;45:317–26.
[26] Schulte D. Die sogenannte Fussgeschwulst. Arch Klin Chir 1897;55:872–92 [in German].
[27] Edmonds ME, Petrova N, Elias D. The earliest magnetic resonance imaging sign of mid-foot Charcot osteoarthropathy is oedema of the subchondral (subarticular) bone marrow which needs prompt therapeutic offloading [abstract]. Diabet Med 2005;22 (Suppl 2):93.
[28] Edmonds ME, Petrova NL, Edmonds A, et al. Early identification of bone marrow oedema in Charcot foot on MRI allows rapid intervention to prevent deformity [abstract]. Diabetic Med 2006;23(Suppl 2):70.
[29] Edmonds ME, Petrova NL, Edmonds A, et al. What happens to the initial bone marrow oedema in the natural history of Charcot osteoarthropathy [abstract]? Diabetologia 2006; 49(Suppl 1):684.

[30] Eichenholtz SN, Levine DB. Fractures of the tarsal navicular bone. Clin Orthop 1964;34: 142–57.
[31] Perron AD, Brady WJ, Keats TA. Principles of stress fracture management. Postgrad Med 2001;110:115–24.
[32] Perron AD, Brady WJ, Keats TA. Management of common stress fractures: when to apply conservative therapy, when to take an aggressive approach. Postgrad Med 2002; 111:95–106.
[33] Sinha J, Thomas EM, Foster A, et al. Fractures in the neuropathic diabetic foot. The Foot 1994;4:28–30.
[34] McGill M, Molyneaux L, Bolton T, et al. Response of Charcot's arthropathy to contact casting: assessment by quantitative techniques. Diabetologia 2000;43:481–4.
[35] Lister J, Maudsley RH. Charcot joints in diabetic neuropathy. Lancet 1951;ii:1110–3.
[36] Johnson JTH. Neuropathic fractures and joint injuries: pathogenesis and rationale of prevention and treatment. J Bone Joint Surg Am 1967;49:1–30.
[37] Kristiansen B. Ankle and foot fractures in diabetics provoking neuropathic joint changes. Acta Orthop Scand 1980;51:975–9.
[38] Thompson RC, Havel P, Goetz F. Presumed neurotrophic skeletal disease in diabetic kidney transplant recipients. JAMA 1983;249:1317–9.
[39] Williams WW, Stiles PJ. Silent fracture of the ankle joint in juvenile-onset diabetes mellitus. Injury 1991;22:412–4.
[40] Graves M, Tarquinio TA. Diabetic neuroarthropathy (Charcot joints): the importance of recognizing chronic sensory deficits in the treatment of acute foot and ankle fractures in diabetic patients. Orthopedics 2003;26:415–8.
[41] Armstrong DG, Todd WF, Lavery LA, et al. The natural history of acute Charcot's arthropathy in a diabetic foot specialty clinic. Diabet Med 1997;14:357–63.
[42] Medhat MA, Krantz H. Neuropathic ankle joint in Charcot-Marie-Tooth disease after triple arthrodesis of the foot. Orthop Rev 1988;17:873–80.
[43] Pell RF, Myerson MS, Schon LC. Clinical outcome after primary triple arthrodesis. J Bone Joint Surg Am 2000;82:47–57.
[44] Senneville E, Melliez H, Beltrand E, et al. Culture of percutaneous bone biopsy specimens for diagnosis of diabetic foot osteomyelitis: concordance with ulcer swab cultures. Clin Infect Dis 2006;42:57–62.
[45] Classen JN, Rolley RT, Carneiro R, et al. Management of foot conditions of the diabetic patient. Am Surg 1976;42:81–8.
[46] Slowman-Kovacs SD, Braunstein EM, Brandt KD. Rapidly progressive Charcot arthropathy following minor joint trauma in patients with diabetic neuropathy. Arthritis Rheum 1990;33:412–7.
[47] Larsen K, Holstein P. Stress fractures as the cause of Charcot feet. In: Bakker K, Nieuwenhuijzen Kruseman AC, editors. The diabetic foot. Proceedings of the 1st International Symposium on the Diabetic Foot. Excerpta Medica Amsterdam, The Netherlands; 1991. p. 108–16.
[48] Kanade RV, van Deursen RWM, Harding K, et al. Walking performance in people with diabetic polyneuropathy: benefits and threats. Diabetologia 2006;49:1747–54.
[49] Duda GN, Maldonado ZM, Klein P, et al. On the influence of mechanical conditions in osteochondral defect healing. J Biomech 2005;38:843–51.
[50] Augat P, Simon U, Liedert A, et al. Mechanics and mechano-biology of fracture healing in normal and osteoporotic bone. Osteoporos Int 2005;16:S36–43.
[51] Schell H, Epari DR, Kassi JP, et al. The course of bone healing is influenced by the initial shear fixation stability. J Orthop Res 2005;23:1022–8.
[52] Stiell IG, Greenberg GH, McKnight RG, et al. Decision rules for the use of radiography in acute ankle injuries. JAMA 1993;269:1127–32.
[53] Eggli S, Sclabas GM, Eggli S, et al. The Bernese ankle rules: a fast, reliable test after low-energy, supination-type malleolar and midfoot trauma. J Trauma 2005;59:1268–71.

[54] Boninger ML, Leonard JA. Use of bivalved ankle-foot orthosis in neuropathic foot and ankle lesions. J Rehabil Res Dev 1996;33:16–22.
[55] Sinacore DR. Acute Charcot arthropathy in patients with diabetes mellitus: healing times by foot location. J Diabetes Complications 1998;12:287–93.
[56] Clohisi DR, Thompson RC. Fractures associated with neuropathic arthropathy in adults who have juvenile-onset diabetes. J Bone Joint Surg Am 1988;70:1192–200.
[57] Simon SR, Tejwani SG, Wilson DL, et al. Arthrodesis as an early alternative to nonoperative management of Charcot arthropathy of the diabetic foot. J Bone Joint Surg Am 2000;82: 939–50.
[58] Paige NM, Nouvong A. The top 10 things foot and ankle specialists wish every primary care physician knew. Mayo Clin Proc 2006;81:818–22.
[59] Vasarhelyi A, Baumert T, Fritsch C, et al. Partial weight bearing after surgery for fractures of the lower extremity: is it achievable? Gait Posture 2006;23:99–105.
[60] Moriatis Wolf J, DiGiovanni CW. A survey of orthopedic surgeons regarding DVT prophylaxis in foot and ankle trauma surgery. Orthopedics 2004;27:504–8.
[61] Krüger K, Heindel W, Burger C, et al. MR tomographic imaging of uncomplicated secondary fracture healing: distal radius fracture as an example [in German]. Fortschr Röntgenstr 1999;170:262–8.
[62] Pinzur MS, Lio T, Posner M. Treatment of Eichenholtz stage I Charcot foot arthropathy with a weight bearing total contact cast. Foot Ankle Int 2006;27:324–9.
[63] Bates M, Petrova NL, Edmonds ME. How long does it take to progress from cast to shoes in the management of Charcot osteoarthropathy? [abstract]. Diabet Med 2006;23(Suppl 2):27.
[64] Jude EB, Selby PL, Burgess J, et al. Bisphosphonates in the treatment of Charcot neuroarthropathy: a double-blind randomised controlled trial. Diabetologia 2001;44:2032–7.
[65] Anderson JJ, Woelffer KE, Holtzmann JJ, et al. Bisphosphonates for the treatment of Charcot neuroarthropathy. J Foot Ankle Surg 2004;43:285–9.
[66] Pitocco D, Ruotolo V, Caputo S, et al. Six-month treatment with alendronate in acute Charcot neuroarthropathy. Diabetes Care 2005;28:1214–5.
[67] Bem R, Jirkovska A, Fejfarova V, et al. Intranasal calcitonin in the treatment of acute Charcot neuro-osteoarthropathy: a randomized controlled trial. Diabetes Care 2006;29: 1392–4.
[68] Sormaala MJ, Niva MH, Kiuru MJ, et al. Outcomes of stress fractures of the talus. Am J Sports Med 2006;34:1809–14.
[69] Hagglund M, Walden M, Ekstrand J. Previous injury as a risk factor for injury in elite football: a prospective study over two consecutive seasons. Br J Sports Med 2006;40:767–72.
[70] Busch K, Chantelau E. Effectiveness of a new brand of stock 'diabetic' shoes to protect against diabetic foot ulcer relapse: a prospective cohort study. Diabetic Med 2003;20:665–9.
[71] van Schie C, Ulbrecht JS, Becker MB, et al. Design criteria for rocker shoes. Foot Ankle Int 2000;21:833–44 [Erratum in: Foot Ankle Int 2001;22:184–5].
[72] Actis RL, Ventura LB, Smith KE, et al. Numerical simulation of the plantar pressure distribution in the diabetic foot during push-off stance. Med Biol Eng Comput 2006;44: 653–63.
[73] Houston VL, Luo GM, Mason CP, et al. Changes in male foot shape and size with weight bearing. J Am Podiatr Med Assoc 2006;96:330–43.
[74] Moore TE, Yuh WTC, Kathol MH, et al. Abnormalities of the foot in patients with diabetes mellitus: findings on MR imaging. AJR Am J Roentgenol 1991;157:813–6.
[75] Lohmann M, Kivisaari A, Vehmas T, et al. MRI abnormalities of foot and ankle in asymptomatic, physically active individuals. Skeletal Radiol 2001;30:61–6.
[76] Muthukumar T, Butt SH, Cassar-Pullicino VN. Stress fractures and related disorders in foot and ankle: plain films, scintigraphy, CT, and MR imaging. Semin Musculoskelet Radiol 2005;9:210–26.
[77] Pecoraro R, Reiber G, Burgess EM. Pathways to diabetic limb amputation: basis for prevention. Diabetes Care 1990;15:513–21.

[78] Kerkhoffs GM, Rowe BH, Assendelft WJ, et al. Immobilisation and functional treatment for acute lateral ankle ligament injuries in adults. Cochrane Database Syst Rev 2002;3: CD003762.
[79] Kerkhoffs GM, Struijs PA, Raaymakers EL, et al. Functional treatment after surgical repair of acute Achilles tendon rupture: wrap vs walking cast. Arch Orthop Trauma Surg 2002;122: 102–5.
[80] Kerkhoffs GM, Handoll HH, de Bie R, et al. Surgical versus conservative treatment for acute injuries of the lateral ligament complex of the ankle in adults. Cochrane Database Syst Rev 2002;3:CD000380.
[81] Kerkhoffs GM, Struijs PA, Marti RK, et al. Different functional treatment strategies for acute lateral ankle ligament injuries in adults. Cochrane Database Syst Rev 2002;3: CD002938.
[82] Kerkhoffs GMMJ, Struijs PAA, Marti RK, et al. Functional treatments for acute ruptures of the lateral ankle ligament: a systematic review. Acta Orthop Scand 2003;74:69–77.
[83] Petrova NL, Foster AVM, Edmonds ME. Why is there a delay in diagnosis and management of the Charcot foot? [abstract]. Diabet Med 2003;20(Suppl 2):30.

ELSEVIER
SAUNDERS

Clin Podiatr Med Surg
24 (2007) 505–517

CLINICS IN
PODIATRIC
MEDICINE AND
SURGERY

Charcot Foot and Ankle Reconstruction: Current Thinking and Surgical Approaches

Thomas Zgonis, DPM, FACFAS[a,*],
Thomas S. Roukis, DPM, FACFAS[b],
Bradley M. Lamm, DPM, AACFAS[c]

[a]*Department of Orthopaedics, Podiatry Division, University of Texas Health Science Center at San Antonio, 7703 Floyd Curl Drive, MC 7776, San Antonio, TX 78229, USA*
[b]*Department of Surgery, Madigan Army Medical Center, 9040-A Fitzsimmons Avenue, MCHJ-SV, Tacoma, WA 98431, USA*
[c]*Rubin Institute for Advanced Orthopedics, International Center for Limb Lengthening, Sinai Hospital of Baltimore, 2401 West Belvedere Avenue, Baltimore MD 21215, USA*

Diabetic Charcot foot deformity (ie, neuropathic osteoarthropathy) is a progressive, disfiguring, and debilitating condition characterized by joint subluxation and dislocation, fracture, and extensive osseous destruction of the foot architecture due to severe peripheral neuropathy. This progressive disease process is precipitated with repetitive trauma that goes unrecognized because of a loss of sensation (ie, dense peripheral neuropathy) and reactive hyperemia (ie, osteopenia, reduced bone stiffness, reduced bone density). If left untreated, the end result is commonly a deformed foot that is difficult to properly shoe and brace, often with recurrent ulceration and infection that ultimately may lead to an amputation of the lower limb [1–6].

The goal in any treatment regimen involving the diabetic Charcot foot deformity is to create a plantigrade and stable foot free from significant risk for further breakdown or infection [1,4–6]. Conservative and surgical intervention has been discussed for all stages of disease as well as anatomic locations of deformity. Achilles tendon lengthening, plantar ostectomy, osseous débridement, realignment osteotomy, selective or extended arthrodesis, and open reduction with various forms of internal fixation with or without external fixation are surgical reconstructive procedures that have

* Corresponding author.
E-mail address: zgonis@uthscsa.edu (T. Zgonis).

0891-8422/07/$ - see front matter
doi:10.1016/j.cpm.2007.03.004

been described to realign and stabilize the deformed diabetic Charcot foot [1–14]. The actual decision between conservative and surgical intervention depends on an assessment of the risks and benefits of each in terms of the deformity present, the expected recovery course, the ability of the patient to comply, comorbidities, nutritional status, psychosocial issues, family support capabilities, and many others. The "lesser of two evils" is usually present when one has to choose between conservative care using immobilization and strict non–weight bearing (eg, reliance on casting/bracing to maintain reduction, skin breakdown, deep venous thrombosis) or surgical intervention (eg, incision breakdown, infection, hardware failure). Because patients in whom diabetic Charcot foot deformity develops universally have dense peripheral neuropathy with loss of pain as a factor, the worst case scenario must be assumed and the treatment plan made as "patient proof" as possible.

Surgical construction of the deformed diabetic Charcot foot using external fixation has received much attention recently. Although no peer-reviewed, scientifically sound manuscripts have been published, the various forms of external fixation employed and the techniques used have allowed for a sound working knowledge to be developed. Herein, the authors present each of their techniques, including the rationale for constructing the deformed diabetic Charcot foot that has failed, or is inappropriate for, conservative care or lesser involved surgical procedures. The components of each author's technique can be incorporated into the podiatric foot and ankle surgeon's armamentarium.

Acute correction using static or Taylor spatial external ring fixation alone

Multiplane circular external fixation alone minimizes the need for extensive surgical exposure in Charcot foot and ankle reconstruction and may provide a means of reducing deformities while maintaining the reduction during consolidation. It can also provide rigid fixation with open reduction and primary arthrodesis techniques. Acute deformity correction via a single or multiple wedge osteotomies and primary arthrodesis with application of an external circular multiplane fixator or Taylor Spatial Frame (Smith & Nephew, Memphis, Tennessee) for severe deformities is usually recommended for a longer term successful outcome (Fig. 1A–E).

In the presence of an ulcer or osteomyelitis, single or multiple-staged reconstruction procedures including ulcer resection, biopsy, wedge osteotomy, soft tissue coverage via local, muscle, or distant pedicle flaps, and primary arthrodesis through circular external fixation techniques provide better changes for a shoe or brace fitting with a lesser chance of ulcer recurrence and instability.

In the midfoot, a single medial or combined lateral incision may be used to address the tarso-metatarsal instability, and primary arthrodesis is

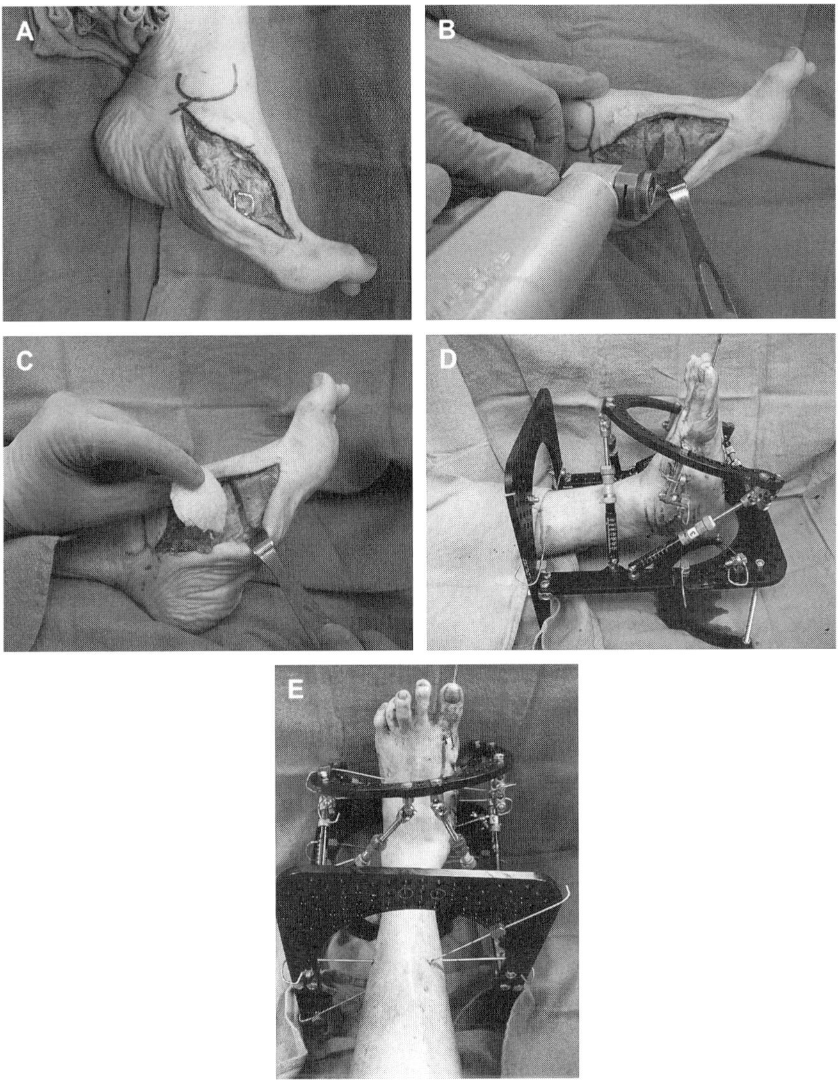

Fig. 1. Previous failure of a Charcot midfoot reconstruction with internal fixation (*A*), followed by an acute correction (*B*) and arthrodesis with the use of an allogenic bone graft (*C*) and a Taylor Spatial Frame (*D* and *E*).

performed with the use of allogenic bone graft material with or without autogenous platelet-rich plasma and bone growth electrical stimulation. In the rearfoot/ankle, the most common primary arthrodesis techniques via multiplane circular fixators include triple, pantalar, and talectomy with tibiocalcaneal or concomitant tibionavicular and calcaneocuboid arthrodesis.

The use of internal fixation including screws, plates, staples, or intramedullary nails is usually not advisable in the diabetic patient with a dense peripheral neuropathy and a significant amount of decreased cortical stiffness and overall bone mineral density. In addition, internal fixation may be a source of a seeded infection and loosening and further surgical reconstruction. Most patients who have foot and ankle Charcot deformities present to the surgeon's office with a concomitant ulceration or soft tissue and bone infection. The use of an external fixation device alone becomes suitable in these surgical reconstruction procedures because it provides a source of rigid fixation and stabilization. In the absence of a concomitant ulcer or infection, a combination of internal and external fixation techniques may be entertained.

Acute correction using static external ring fixation with internal fixation

With the patient positioned on the operating room table in the supine position and a well-padded gel bolster placed under the ipsilateral buttock to control physiologic external rotation of the lower limb, the foot, ankle, lower leg, and thigh are prepared and draped using an aseptic technique. First, the equinus contracture that is nearly universally present in diabetic patients with a Charcot deformity [15–17] is addressed through a percutaneous tendo-Achilles triple hemisection [18,19] or endoscopic gastrocnemius recession, which is the preferred method because the correction is equal but the potential for overlengthening, rupture, and neurologic injury to the sural nerve markedly reduced [20]. The only concern with the endoscopic gastrocnemius recession is the need to use a tourniquet to allow sufficient visualization.

Next, a subtalar arthroeresis is performed to place an oversized subtalar arthroeresis implant within the sinus tarsi (Horizon; Biopro, Port Huron, Michigan). The rationale behind this procedure is that frontal plane deformities are frequently associated with the diabetic Charcot foot deformity that is difficult to control. Placement of an oversized subtalar arthroeresis implant is simple to perform, minimally invasive, allows for correction of significant frontal plane deformities about the hindfoot, is reversible, and stiffens the hindfoot significantly [21], allowing protection of the subsequent midfoot stabilization procedures.

The involved articulations about the medial column are identified under image intensification, and minimally invasive incisions are carried directly to the underlying articulations. A large trephine is used to core out the diseased articulation with care taken to properly expose and fenestrate the subchondral bone plate to expose bleeding, healthy cancellous bone. If any diseased bone is present following this technique, the incision should be extended and any nonviable bone removed. The osseous defect is then packed with a combination of allogenic bone graft material impregnated with either bone marrow aspirate harvested through the lateral wall of the calcaneus or autologous platelet-rich plasma. This combination of products exploits the ability to promote osteoinduction and osteoconduction across large osseous voids in an immunocompromised host and avoids the associated morbidity of autogenous bone graft harvest from the proximal tibia or iliac crest. This packing is followed by manipulation of the midfoot to correct the deformity and then percutaneous placement of a large diameter guidewire from the plantar aspect of the hallux into the first metatarsal head under image intensification that is driven proximally into the talus.

Once proper placement and alignment are verified under image intensification, the incision is extended to allow the first metatarsal head to be properly countersunk and the distal first metatarsal to be tapped. A proper length 8.0-mm cannulated titanium screw (Asnis III; Stryker Orthopaedics, Mahwah, New Jersey) is then driven across the entire medial column until seated below the subchondral bone in the first metatarsal head. Next, a large diameter guidewire is placed in similar fashion through either the second and third or third and fourth metatarsals, across the midfoot, and into the hindfoot. A proper length 6.5-mm cannulated titanium screw (Asnis III) is then driven across the aforementioned regions and seated below the subchondral bone in the respective metatarsal heads [22]. The alignment of the entire foot and location of the hardware is inspected through clinical and image intensification visualization. If satisfactory, the surgical sites are irrigated and closed in a single layer using 2-0 nylon suture and skin staples.

An external ring fixation system with a carbon fiber foot plate, which allows for enhanced visualization of the reconstructed osseous articulations, is then used with a double-stacked foot plate to allow off-loading of the internal fixation construct, permit weight-sharing during the initial healing phase of 6 to 8 weeks [23–27], and allow inspection of the incision sites on a regular basis. An external bone growth stimulator is applied immediately postoperative and continued on a daily basis for 6 months to maximize osseous incorporation [28]. The rationale for this is that plain radiographs are notoriously inconclusive when used to evaluate osseous union, and specialized imaging techniques like CT scans provide limited detail due to the presence of metallic implants. Furthermore, clinical signs of union, such as the resolution of edema, warmness, and stability of the midfoot to manual stress, are imprecise. Surgical correction of a diabetic Charcot foot deformity is difficult; however, surgical revision of a previously failed surgical attempt at reconstruction of a diabetic Charcot deformity is even more challenging. For this reason, the use of multiple forms of technology to enhance osseous incorporation should be employed. The external ring fixation system is removed in the operative room and a weight-sharing cast applied for an additional 3 to 4 weeks. Gradual conversion to a weight-bearing cast, a removable walking boot, and, finally, custom-molded shoe gear and in-shoe orthoses occurs over the ensuing 4 to 6 months.

The following is a summary of the key points when performing acute correction of the diabetic Charcot foot deformity using static external ring fixation with internal fixation (Fig. 2A–F):

The foot must be aligned such that the heel is under the mechanical axis of the lower leg with the metatarsal heads sharing equal weight distribution and aligned perpendicular to the heel.

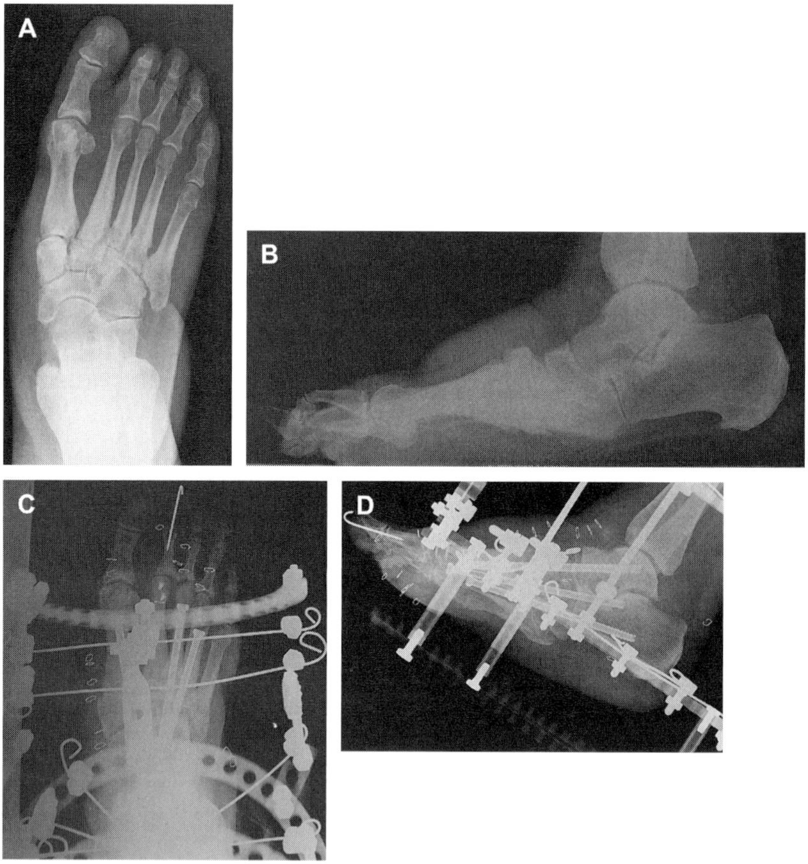

Fig. 2. Chronic diabetic Charcot deformity involving multiplane deformity of the forefoot, midfoot, and hindfoot as evidenced by weight-bearing anteroposterior (*A*) and lateral (*B*) radiographs. Immediate postoperative anteroposterior (*C*) and lateral (*D*) radiographs following "pan-pedal" stabilization. Final postoperative anteroposterior (*E*) and lateral (*F*) weight-bearing radiographs demonstrate osseous union throughout the midfoot complex without migration or loss of alignment throughout remaining midfoot and hindfoot articulations. Note that a distal oblique lesser metatarsal osteotomy (ie, Weil) was performed for the second metatarsophalangeal joint dislocation with some residual dislocation present.

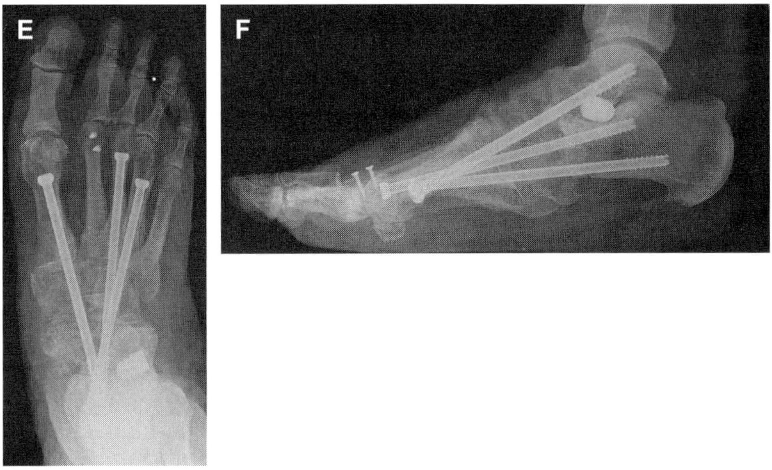

Fig. 2 (*continued*)

The joints adjacent to the involved fracture-dislocation must be stabilized. This "pan-pedal" stabilization is less prone to breakdown than is isolated or regional arthrodesis of only those obviously involved articulations.

The foot must be able to be passively dorsiflexed 5 degrees past neutral (ie, a 90-degree angle between the lateral border of the foot and the length of the fibula) with the foot fully stabilized and aligned as detailed previously.

Minimally invasive techniques that do not involve a great amount of soft tissue dissection are mandatory.

The use of orthobiologics such as platelet-rich plasma, bone marrow aspirate, and osteoinductive/osteoconductive allogenic bone graft material becomes mandatory.

The use of bone growth stimulation becomes mandatory.

The use of supplemental external ring fixation becomes mandatory.

Minimally invasive gradual Charcot foot reconstruction

Gradual correction with external fixation is preferred for large Charcot foot deformity reductions. Correction with external fixation is minimally invasive, allows for gradual accurate anatomic realignment of the dislocated/subluxated Charcot joints without loss of foot length or bone mass, provides for partial weight bearing, and limits neurovascular compromise because the correction occurs slowly during a period of time.

A stable or coalesced foot with Charcot deformity requires an osteotomy for correction of the deformity. For an unstable or an incompletely coalesced

Charcot foot, correction can be obtained through gradual distraction. Despite the radiographic appearance of coalescence, most Charcot deformities can be distracted through the joints to realign the pedal anatomy [29] without osteotomy. The first stage, osseous realignment, is achieved with a Taylor Spatial Frame using the principle of ligamentotaxis. After realignment, the correction is maintained by arthrodesis (the second stage) using percutaneously inserted intramedullary metatarsal [30].

The first stage consists of osseous realignment achieved by performing ligamentotaxis. The Taylor Spatial Frame forefoot 6×6 butt frame construct is applied and provides gradual relocation of the forefoot on the hindfoot. The distal tibia, talus, and calcaneus are fixed with two U-plates joined and first mounted orthogonal to the tibia in the anteroposterior and lateral planes. The U-plate is affixed to the tibia with one lateromedial 1.8-mm wire and two to three other points of fixation (combination of smooth wires or half-pins). For additional stability, a second distal tibial ring can be added to create a distal tibial fixation block. It is essential to fix the hindfoot in a neutral position; an Achilles tendon lengthening typically is required to achieve a neutral hindfoot position. With the hindfoot manually held in a neutral position, the U-plate is fixed to the calcaneus with two crossing 1.8-mm wires. A 1.8-mm medial-lateral talar neck wire also is inserted and fixed to the U-plate. Next, two 1.8-mm stirrup wires are inserted through the osseous segment just proximal and distal to the Charcot joints. Stirrup wires are bent 90 degrees just outside the skin to extend and attach, but are not tensioned to, their respective external fixation rings distant from the point of fixation. These stirrup wires capture osseous segments that are far from an external fixation ring, providing accurate and precise Charcot joint distraction.

A full external fixation ring is then mounted to the forefoot with two 1.8-mm crossing metatarsal wires and the aforementioned distal stirrup wire. Digital pinning often is required whereby the digital wires (1.5 or 1.8 mm) are attached to the forefoot ring. Smooth wires in the foot are preferred in the neuropathic population. The six Taylor Spatial Frame struts are placed and final radiographs obtained (anteroposterior and lateral views of the foot to include the tibia). Orthogonal anteroposterior and lateral view fluoroscopic images are obtained of the reference ring. The images provide the mounting parameters that are needed for computer planning. The choice of which ring (distal or proximal) to use as the reference ring is per the surgeon's preference; typically, a distal reference is chosen for foot deformity correction. Superimposition of the reference ring on the final films is critical for accurate postoperative computer deformity planning (www.spatialframe.com).

One must fully understand the Taylor Spatial Frame planning before attempting this procedure. The surgeon enters the deformity and mounting parameters into an Internet-based software program that produces a daily schedule for the patient to perform adjustments on each of the six struts. The rate and duration of the patient's schedule is controlled by the surgeon's

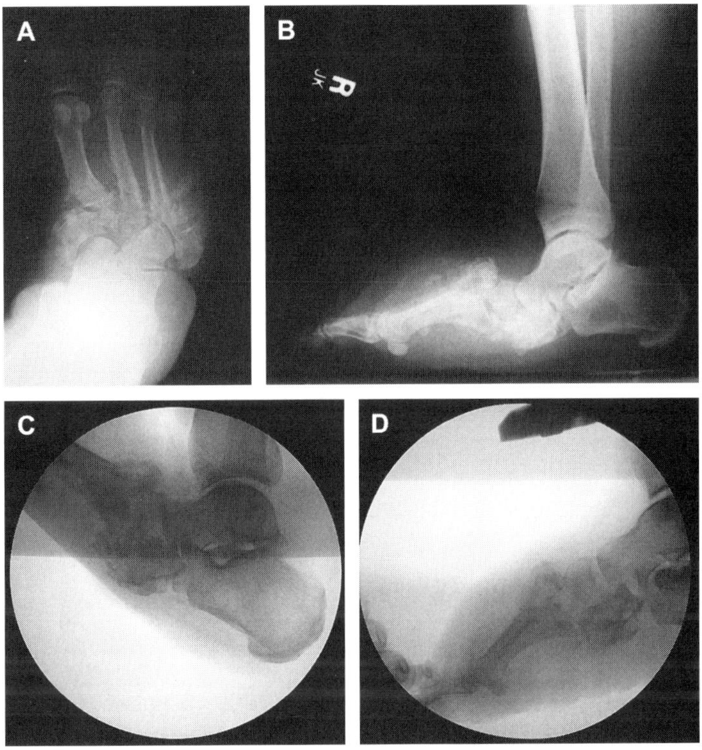

Fig. 3. Anteroposterior view of a midfoot Charcot neuroarthropathy deformity (*A*). Lateral view radiograph shows rockerbottom and equinus deformities. Note the dorsal displacement of the forefoot and the break in Meary's angle (*B*). The lateral view still image, obtained by using video fluoroscopy, confirms the instability of the midfoot Charcot, demonstrating significant forefoot dorsiflexion (*C*) and plantarflexion (*D*). Immediate postoperative anteroposterior radiograph shows midfoot adduction (20 degrees). The stirrup wires (90-degree bent wires that are not tensioned) are placed adjacent to the region of distraction and realignment (midfoot in this case). These stirrup wires ensure focused distraction. Note the Taylor Spatial Frame planning lines and reference points (*E*). Immediate postoperative lateral radiograph shows plantarflexion of the forefoot (10 degrees). The change in forefoot position when compared with the preoperative radiographs is due to the acute manipulation intraoperatively. The stirrup wires (90-degree bent wires that are not tensioned) are placed adjacent to the region of distraction and realignment (midfoot in this case). Note the Taylor Spatial Frame planning lines and reference points (*F*). Clinical photograph shows the Taylor Spatial Frame (forefoot 6×6 butt) applied. Note the delta configuration of the tibial half-pins and the build out (two-hole plate) off the distal foot ring to allow for soft tissue clearance (*G*). A clinical lateral photograph shows the Taylor Spatial Frame (forefoot 6×6 butt) applied. Note the stirrup wires adjacent to the distraction region (*H*). Lateral view radiograph after 1 month of gradual Taylor Spatial Frame correction showing a normal or zero Meary's angle and distraction of the midfoot. The dorsal foot ulcer has healed, and the foot is correctly positioned (*I*). Immediately after removal of the external fixator, a minimally invasive fusion of the midtarsal joint was performed to prevent future Charcot foot collapse. A weight-bearing anteroposterior radiograph shows two percutaneous intramedullary metatarsal screws and a lateral column screw that were inserted for stabilization of the fusion of the midtarsal joint. Note the accurate anatomic reduction (*J*). A postoperative lateral view photograph shows a healed plantigrade foot with intact intramedullary metatarsal screws (*K*).

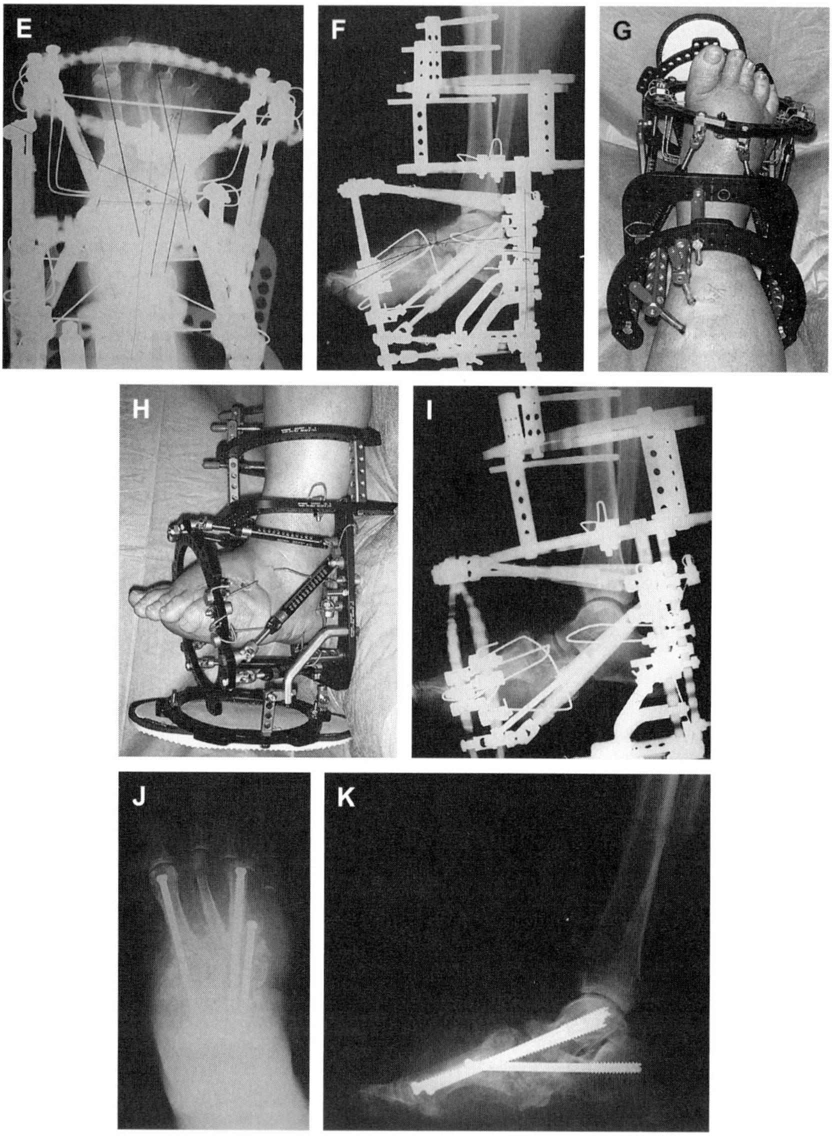

Fig. 3 (*continued*)

data entry. The patient is followed up clinically and radiographically in the office on a weekly or biweekly basis.

Creative frame construction is required because of the small pedal anatomy, which renders it difficult to apply external fixation. When applying the forefoot 6×6 butt frame, it is important to mount the U-plate on the hindfoot and the full ring on the forefoot as posterior and anterior as possible, respectively. The greatest distance between the forefoot and hindfoot ring is critical to accommodate the struts of the Taylor Spatial Frame. Bone segment fixation is important; otherwise, failure of osteotomy separation or incomplete anatomic reduction occurs. Small wire fixation is preferred in the foot because of the size and consistency of the bones. When treating a patient with neuropathy, building extremely stable constructs is of great importance. External fixation for Charcot deformity correction should include a distal tibial ring with a closed foot ring.

After gradual distraction with the Taylor Spatial Frame has realigned the anatomy of the foot, the second stage of correction is performed. In the second stage, the external fixator is removed while simultaneously performing minimally invasive arthrodesis of the affected joints with percutaneous insertion of internal fixation. Gradual distraction for realignment of the dislocated Charcot joints is obtained in approximately 1 to 2 months. Before frame removal, small transverse incisions (2 to 3 cm in length) overlying the appropriate joints are made to perform cartilage removal and joint preparation for arthrodesis. Minimally invasive arthrodesis is easily preformed because the Charcot joints are already distracted. Under fluoroscopic guidance, the guidewires for the large diameter cannulated screws are inserted percutaneously through the plantar skin incision into the metatarsal head by dorsiflexing the hallux. After the lateral and medial column guidewires are inserted to maintain the corrected foot position, the frame is removed and the foot is re-prepared. Typically, three large diameter cannulated intramedullary metatarsal screws are inserted—medial and lateral column partial threaded screws for compression of the arthrodesis site and one central fully threaded screw for additional stabilization. These screws span the entire length of the metatarsals to the calcaneus and talus, provide compression across the minimally invasive arthrodesis site, and stabilize adjacent joints. The intramedullary metatarsal screws cross an unaffected joint, the Lisfranc joint, thereby protecting it from experiencing a future Charcot event. The minimally invasive incisions are then closed, and a well-padded U and L splint is applied. Before hospital discharge (length of hospital stay ranges from 1 to 4 days), the patient's operative splint and dressing are removed and a short leg cast is applied. A non–weight-bearing short leg cast is maintained for 2 to 3 months, and then gradual progression to weight bearing is achieved. The entire treatment is completed in 4 to 5 months (Fig. 3A–K).

Summary

The techniques described herein present some of the current theories and approaches to the surgical management of patients with severe Charcot foot and ankle deformities. These procedures may be performed in large academic and teaching centers with the wide availability of all the services needed to perform major limb salvage surgeries. In addition, surgical experience and availability become necessary in the overall process of Charcot foot and ankle reconstruction.

References

[1] Frykberg RG, editor. The high risk foot in diabetes mellitus. New York: Churchill Livingstone; 1991.
[2] Eichenholtz SN. In Charcot joints. Springfield (IL): Charles C. Thomas; 1966.
[3] Sanders LJ, Frykberg RG. Diabetic neuropathic osteoarthropathy: the Charcot foot. In: Frykberg RG, editor. The high risk foot in diabetes mellitus. New York: Churchill Livingstone; 1991. p. 325–33.
[4] Larsen K, Fabrin J, Holstein PE. Incidence and management of ulcers in diabetic Charcot feet. J Wound Care 2001;10:323–8.
[5] Bowering CK. Diabetic foot ulcers: pathophysiology, assessment, and therapy. Can Fam Physician 2001;47:1007–16.
[6] Brem H, Sheehan P, Boulton AJM. Protocol for treatment of diabetic foot ulcers. Am J Surg 2004;187:1S–10S.
[7] Schon LC, Easley ME, Weinfeld SB. Charcot neuroarthropathy of the foot and ankle. Clin Orthop Relat Res 1998;349:116–31.
[8] Jolly GP, Zgonis T, Polyzois V. External fixation in the management of Charcot neuroarthropathy. Clin Podiatr Med Surg 2003;20(4):741–56.
[9] Wang JC, Le AW, Tsukuda RK. A new technique for Charcot's foot reconstruction. J Am Podiatr Med Assoc 2002;92(8):429–36.
[10] Trepman E, Nihal A, Pinzur MS. Current topics review: Charcot neuroarthropathy of the foot and ankle. Foot Ankle Int 2005;26(1):46–63.
[11] Shibata T, Tada K, Hashizume C. The results of arthrodesis of the ankle for leprotic neuroarthropathy. J Bone Joint Surg [Am] 1990;72(5):749–56.
[12] Brodsky JW, Rouse AM. Exostectomy for symptomatic bony prominences in diabetic Charcot feet. Clin Orthop Relat Res 1993;296:21–6.
[13] Simon SR, Tejwani SG, Wilson DL, et al. Arthrodesis as an early alternative to nonoperative management of Charcot arthropathy of the diabetic foot. J Bone Joint Surg [Am] 2000; 82(7):939–50.
[14] Catanzariti AR, Mendicino R, Haverstock B. Ostectomy for diabetic neuroarthropathy involving the midfoot. J Foot Ankle Surg 2000;39(5):291–300.
[15] Salsich GB, Muller MJ, Sahrmann SA. Passive ankle stiffness in subjects with diabetes and peripheral neuropathy versus age-matched comparison group. Phys Ther 2000;80:352–62.
[16] Lavery LA, Armstrong DG, Boulton AJ. Ankle equinus deformity and its relationship to high plantar pressure in a large population with diabetes mellitus. J Am Podiatr Med Assoc 2002;92:479–82.
[17] Rao SR, Saltzman CL, Wilken J, et al. Increased passive ankle stiffness and reduced dorsiflexion range of motion in individuals with diabetes mellitus. Foot Ankle Int 2006;27:617–22.
[18] Nishimoto GS, Attinger CE, Cooper PS. Lengthening the Achilles tendon for the treatment of diabetic plantar forefoot ulceration. Surg Clin North Am 2003;83(3):707–26.
[19] Haro AA, DiDomenico LA. Frontal plane-guided percutaneous tendo Achilles' lengthening. J Foot Ankle Surg 2007;46(1):55–61.
[20] DiDomenico LA, Adams HB, Garchar D. Endoscopic gastrocnemius recession for the treatment of gastrocnemius equinus. J Am Podiatr Med Assoc 2005;95(4):410–3.
[21] Husain ZS, Fallat LM. Biomechanical analysis of Maxwell-Brancheau arthroeresis implants. J Foot Ankle Surg 2002;41(6):352–8.
[22] Grant WP, Jerlin EA, Pietrzak WS, et al. The utilization of autologous growth factors for the facilitation of fusion in complex neuropathic fractures in the diabetic population. Clin Podiatr Med Surg 2005;22:561–84.

[23] Roukis TS, Zgonis T. Postoperative shoe modifications for weight bearing with the Ilizarov external fixation system. J Foot Ankle Surg 2004;43:433–5.

[24] Zgonis T. Surgical correction of severe Charcot foot and ankle deformities with external fixation devices. Foot and Ankle Quarterly 2006;18(04):149–57.

[25] Zgonis T, Roukis TS, Frykberg RG, et al. Unstable acute and chronic Charcot's deformity: staged skeletal and soft tissue reconstruction. J Wound Care 2006;15(06):276–80.

[26] Zgonis T, Roukis TS, Polyzois V, et al. Surgical management of the unstable diabetic Charcot deformity using the Taylor spatial frame. Operative Techniques in Orthopaedics 2006; 16:10–7.

[27] Roukis TS, Zgonis T. The management of acute Charcot fracture-dislocation with a Taylor's spatial external fixation system. Clin Podiatr Med Surg 2006;23:467–83.

[28] Petrisor B, Lau JT. Electrical bone stimulation: an overview and its use in high risk and Charcot foot and ankle reconstructions. Foot Ankle Clin 2005;10(4):609–20.

[29] Lamm BM, Paley D. Deformity correction planning for hindfoot, ankle, and lower limb. Clin Podiatr Med Surg 2004;21(3):305–26.

[30] Lamm BM, Paley D. Charcot neuroarthropathy of the foot and ankle. In: Rozbruch RS, Ilizarov S, editors. Limb lengthening and reconstruction surgery. New York: Informa Healthcare; 2006. p. 221–31.

ELSEVIER
SAUNDERS

Clin Podiatr Med Surg
24 (2007) 519–528

CLINICS IN
PODIATRIC
MEDICINE AND
SURGERY

Closure of Major Diabetic Foot Wounds and Defects with External Fixation

Ali Oznur, MD[a,*], Thomas Zgonis, DPM, FACFAS[b]

[a]*Department of Orthopaedics and Traumatology, Guven Hospital, Block A: Simsek Sokak No: 29, Ankara, Turkey*

[b]*Department of Orthopaedics/Podiatry Division, University of Texas Health Science Center at San Antonio, 7703 Floyd Curl Drive, MSC 7776, San Antonio, TX 78229, USA*

Twenty percent of all diabetic patients' admissions to the hospital are caused by a foot problem or an ulceration at a certain point of their lifetime. Diabetic foot ulcers and their sequelae, amputations, are a major cause of disability, morbidity, mortality, and significant cost for the diabetic patient. Neuropathy, whether sensory, motor, or autonomic, plays an important role in the pathogenesis of diabetic foot ulcers. Although decreased sensation plays an essential role in ulcer formation, it will not cause an ulceration in the absence of abnormal pressure and deformity. Autonomic neuropathy inhibits skin temperature regulation and prevents normal sweating. Motor neuropathy results in intrinsic muscle atrophy, causing an imbalance in intrinsic and extrinsic muscle control of the toes, leading to clawing of the lesser toes. The combination of deep ulcer and underlying osteomyelitis in patients who have diabetes frequently leads to chronic nonhealing foot ulcers. Plantar ulcers are the result of pressure exerted by weight bearing, whereas dorsal ulcers result from a poor shoe fit or hot pack application. Simple closure of these wounds is difficult because of pre-existing bone deformity, tissue inelasticity, location of defect, and underlying osteomyelitis [1–3].

Inadequately diagnosed or treated osteomyelitis in a diabetic foot ulcer increases the risk for amputation. Thorough preoperative examination is necessary to maximize treatment outcome. Optimal medical control of diabetes and associated comorbidities is essential before complex foot and ankle surgery is undertaken. Diabetic control status with serum glycosylated hemoglobin (Hg A1C) levels as well as nutritional status with serum

* Corresponding author.
E-mail address: alioznur@yahoo.com (A. Oznur).

doi:10.1016/j.cpm.2007.03.013 *podiatric.theclinics.com*

albumin levels greater than 3.5 g/dL are a few of the tests assessing the patient's overall medical status and compliance.

Most diabetic foot infections are caused by a mixture of aerobic and anaerobic pathogens; however, the most common organisms cultured are the aerobic gram-positive cocci, including *Staphylococcus aureus*, coagulase-negative staphylococci, and group B streptococci. Some of the aerobic gram-negative organisms frequently cultured are *Proteus* species, *Eschericia coli*, and other Enterobacteriaceae. Enterococcus and *Corynebacterium* species can also be considered as potential pathogens in foot infection. *Pseudomonas aeruginosa* is found in no more than 10% to 20% of diabetic foot cultures [4,5].

The treatment of diabetic patients who have large ulcers and underlying osteomyelitis is not well-described in the current literature, however. Currently, there are only a few reports describing salvage of the diabetic foot with external fixation in the English literature. Surgeons worldwide have been using external fixators for all types of fracture management, arthrodeses, complex deformities, limb lengthening, and osteotomy stabilization. External fixators are able to perform multiplane corrections, including distraction, compression, angulation, translation, stabilization, and neutralization [6–12].

In addition, procedures such as repeated debridements, dressing changes, skin grafting, and bone grafting can be performed without disturbing the fixation. External fixation can be used to treat defects of practically any size after aggressive resection. External fixation can provide good stability in those patients who have severe osteoporosis caused by infection, disuse, or diabetes mellitus. Application of external fixation is performed rapidly and often under spinal or local anesthetic. External fixation pins and wires are not benign in the setting of bone and soft tissue infection. Safe corridors for pins or wires should be chosen with caution.

Closure of large defects after resection of the necrotic bone with external fixation is a powerful modality that has the ability to save extremities that normally would go onto amputation; however, caution should be taken to avoid creating a useless, permanently painful, or senseless limb. Relative contraindications for this approach include but are not limited to the following conditions: venous stasis disease, complex regional pain syndrome, nonambulatory status of the patient, and noncompliance [13–15].

The surgical technique differs in terms of the anatomical location of the ulcer, soft tissue defect, and osteomyelitis. The goal of this suggested protocol and treatment is a shorter hospital stay, limited antibiotic administration, and the achievement of functionally stable feet when compared with other conventional methods.

Technique for heel ulcers

The surgical approach to chronic ulcers of the calcaneus presents considerable difficulty in the diabetic patients. All necrotic, infected, and fibrotic tissue needs to be excised, with the addition of partial or total calcanectomy that is performed according to the size of the ulcer and the concomitant osteomyelitis. With osteomyelitis of the calcaneus, it is difficult to determine how much bone needs to be resected; however, the amount of the resection is critical for eradication of the infection. A plantar longitudinal incision is used, through which the ulcer is excised as an ellipse. Exposure is obtained by splitting the Achilles tendon and reflecting it sharply off the bone. The large wound is closed primarily or is left open for wound care and dressing, with a delayed primary closure or plastic reconstructive techniques.

A multiplane circular external Illizarov fixator with hinges is applied to decrease the soft tissue defect in equinus position of the ankle. The protocol involves the application of a two-ring construct to the tibia, with two 1.8-mm Kirschner wires per ring attached by way of four threaded rods to a foot ring. Center-of-rotation wire is placed through the ankle axis (tip of medial malleolus to the tip of lateral malleolus). This is a reference wire for positioning the medial and lateral ankle hinges. Universal hinges are placed to intersect the ankle axis wire. The lateral hinge is more distal and posterior than the medial hinge. The foot ring is mounted parallel to the sole of the foot. Fixation of the foot ring is achieved with two metatarsal wires and one talar neck wire. Plantar flexion is decreased gradually during the healing period. The external fixator allows monitoring of wounds and eases daily wound dressing changes. This technique eliminates the use of postoperative cast application and its complications. Another advantage of the external fixator is relieving the bed pressure over the heel. The external fixation device is usually removed after between 6 to 8 weeks. Patients subsequently ambulate in a polypropylene splint with plastizote and foam filler in the region of the heel defect (Fig. 1).

Technique for midfoot ulcers

A medial incision is made from the tip of the medial malleolus to the medial site of the first metatarsal. An elliptical incision circumscribing the ulcer is then made to the depth of the bone. All necrotic bone and soft tissue is excised, and a deep bone culture is taken. Resection of the bony prominence causing the ulceration is then performed to treat the underlying osteomyelitis. Surgical debridement is based on previous MRI findings. Pulsatile lavage is used (at least 6 L of normal saline) for copious irrigation. Resection of the infected midfoot bony architecture allows for a decrease in the size of the overlying ulceration. Distraction for joint preparation can be accomplished by the use of a lamina spreader. The large void after surgical debridement is filled with an antibiotic-impregnated bone cement. Smooth wires or pins may be placed to fix the forefoot to the hindfoot through the bone cement. Repeated extensive debridements are followed by the bone cement removal 3 to 4 weeks after the initial surgery. Midfoot wounds are closed without tension after the bone cement removal and the shortening of the foot. After

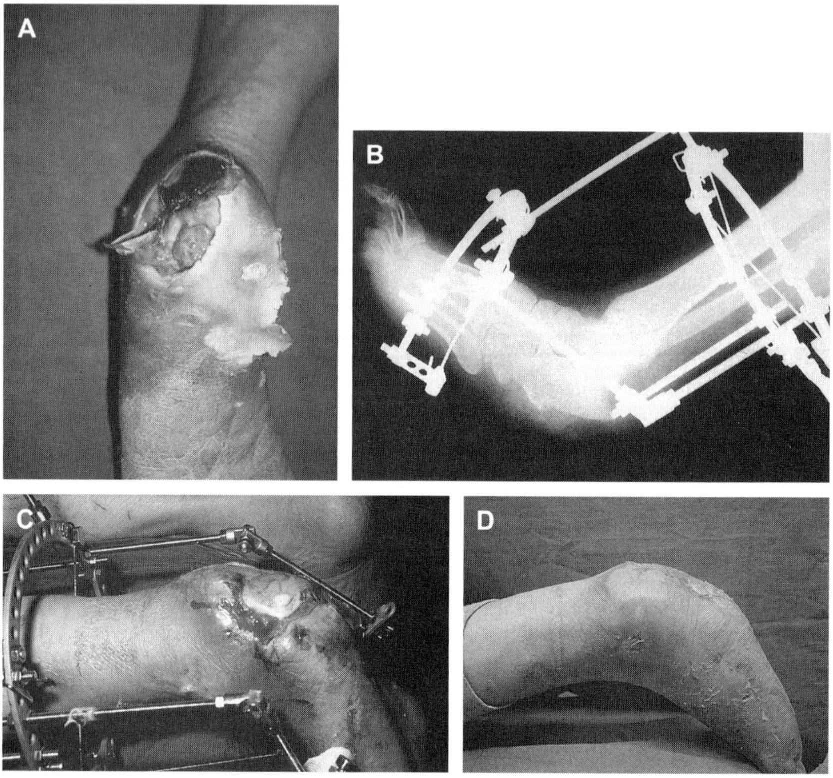

Fig. 1. An initial presentation of an infected calcaneus with a large ulceration (*A*), followed by an aggressive debridement and partial calcanectomy (*B*), an Ilizarov external fixator with hinges to decrease the soft tissue defect in an equinus position (*C*), and removal of the external fixator 6 weeks after the operation with an uneventful recovery (*D*).

the bone cement is removed, an Ilizarov external fixation frame is used with pin placement outside of the infected area, to hold the hindfoot and midfoot under compression and alignment. When all of the ulcerations and previous wounds have healed, the hindfoot is fixed to the forefoot with multiple percutaneous cannulated screws, and the external fixation device is removed. The patients are mobilized in an ankle foot orthosis with custom footplate, lined with pressure-dissipating material. Some of the complications associated with this procedure include but are not limited to the following: persistent infection, soft tissue dehiscence, overcorrection, undercorrection, pseudoarthrosis, and amputation. Pseudoarthrosis may be an acceptable result if the foot is stable and ulcer-free (Fig. 2).

Technique for central rays

Single- or double-ray resections are generally preferable to transmetatarsal amputation. A single amputation of the second, third or fourth ray

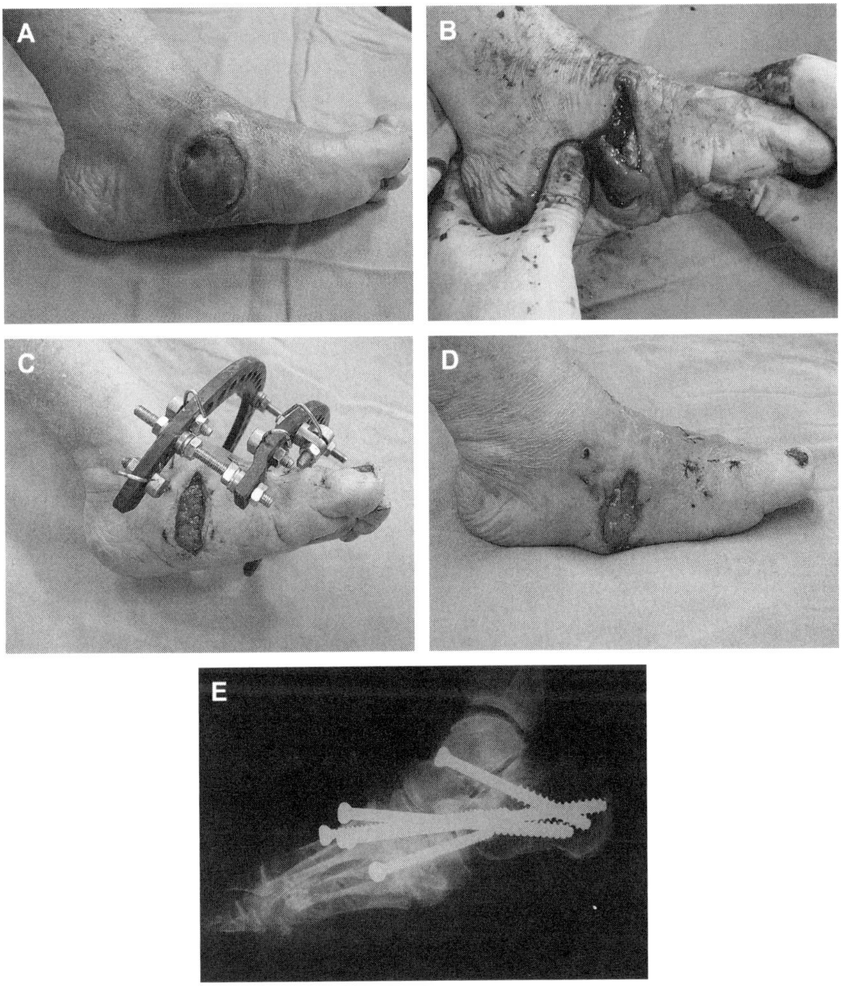

Fig. 2. Initial presentation of a large midfoot ulcer and osteomyelitis of multiple bones (*A*), followed by a large midfoot bony and soft tissue resection (*B*), and external fixation device to allow narrowing of the associated defect (*C*). Eventually, the wounds healed with the application of a split-thickness skin graft (*D*), and the external fixator was removed 7 weeks after the initial surgery followed by percutaneous cannulated screw insertion to further stabilize the foot (*E*).

affects only the width of the forefoot. In cases of an extensive forefoot infection and gangrene, multiple central ray resections may be required. Single-ray resection of the one of the three central rays is technically more difficult than the border ray resections.

The contiguous ulcer site provides a portal of entry for pathogens, which can result in an infection of both soft tissue and bone. Metatarsophalangeal joints are in close proximity to one another, and osteomyelitis can easily result in joint sepsis. The traditional approaches to central metatarsal head ulcerations have involved either limited osseous resection, with or without ablation of the associated toe, or resection of the entire metatarsal ray, with the subsequent development of a "cleft foot" deformity that is prone to transfer ulceration and recurrent wound breakdown resulting from the unstable nature of the forefoot.

To expedite healing and create a stable, plantigrade forefoot after central metatarsal ray resection, "narrowing" of the forefoot through manual apposition of the resultant medial and lateral forefoot segments has been advocated, using widely spaced, heavy gauge sutures, and prolonged non–weight-bearing mobilization to provide stability until soft tissue healing has occurred. The authors describe their technique of using external fixation in closing the diabetic forefoot cleft wounds.

Once the recipient wound has undergone proper extensive irrigation and debridement to remove all necrotic and nonviable tissue and necrotic bone, the appropriate central metatarsal rays are partially resected or excised, with or without concomitant tarsal osteotomy. One of the authors (AO) proposed a modified technique of ray excision [15]. In the classical approach, a "tennis-racquet" incision is made circumferentially around the toe, with a single limb over the dorsum of the involved metatarsal; however, the proximal extension of the incision may jeopardize incisions for more proximal amputations if the ray excision procedure fails. The purpose of this modification is to decrease the dorsal soft tissue dissection to expose the metatarsals. An incision is made over the base of the involved metatarsal that is less than half inches. One hemostat is used to determine the borders of the metatarsal. A small osteotome is introduced and metatarsal is osteotomized. Care is taken not to remove uninvolved the metatarsal. The toe is grasped with a towel clamp and amputated up to healthy skin margin. Then a small gauge is used to dissect soft tissues all around the metatarsal in blind fashion up to the osteotomy level.

The remaining defect in the central foot is then covered with a split-thickness skin graft (STSG) that is usually harvested from the medial arch of the foot, posterior calf, or thigh region of the ipsilateral limb. The harvested STSG is then prepared for soft-tissue wound coverage, by either fenestrating the graft manually with repeated passes of a surgical scalpel (ie, "pie-crusting") or meshing it at a ratio of 1:1.5 or greater using a commercially available mesher.

All necrotic and nonviable tissues including infected and necrotic central rays are removed, and an Ilizarov external fixator frame is applied to compress the remaining metatarsals to decrease the soft tissue defect. When a ray excision is needed, the incision for ray excision is not extended too far proximally. The aim of this modification is to decrease the dorsal soft tissue dissection to expose the involved metatarsal. Another modification is the osteotomy of the base of fifth metatarsal through stab incision. This maneuver is very helpful for closing cleft defects with the tensioning of the olive wires. Medial and lateral olive wires are inserted and fixed to external fixation device. The amount of tensioning of the wires (70–90 kg) depends on the bone quality of the metatarsals, and the soft tissue defect. The midtarsal half ring is attached to the half ring of the hindfoot with threaded rods. External fixation devices may or may not extend to the ankle. The wounds are then closed with interrupted sutures without any tension. Patients are mobilized in a custom-made boot when the pain and swelling has subsided. The described technique is used in patients who need more than one central ray excision for the treatment of osteomyelitis with an associated large soft tissue defect over the dorsum of the foot (Fig. 3).

Discussion

Diabetes mellitus has been estimated to affect 11 million Americans, and of these, approximately 25% will develop foot problems. Furthermore, it

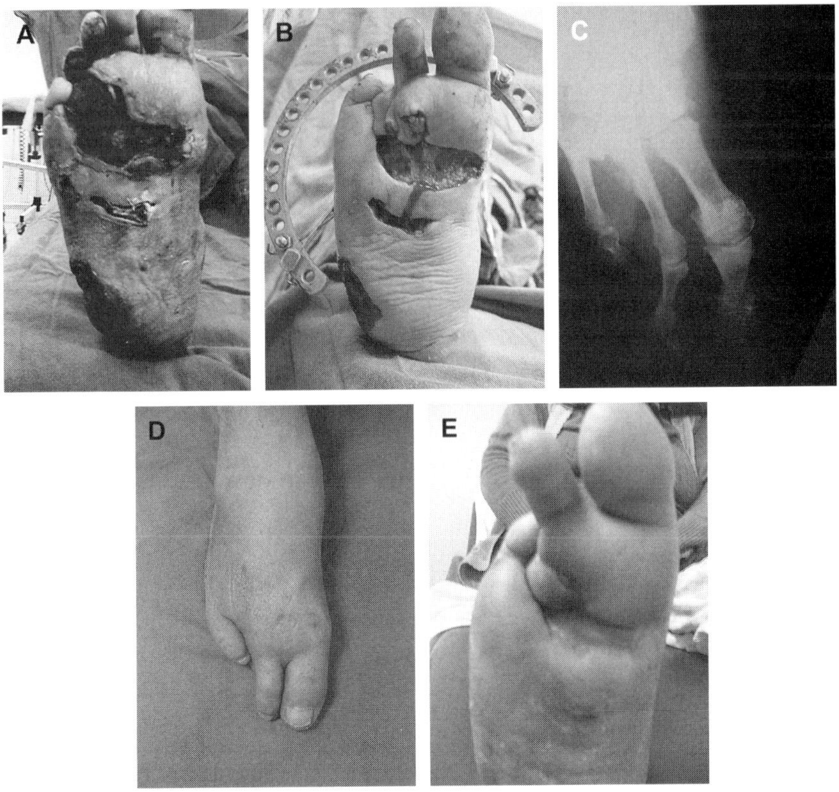

Fig. 3. Initial presentation of a severe midfoot abscess, ischemia, and central ray osteomyelitis (*A*), followed by a resection of the central rays three and four and Ilizarov external fixation (*B*), and final clinical and radiographic presentation after split-thickness skin grafting (*C–E*).

has been shown that at least 15% of hospital admissions are directly related to foot infections. Superficial and deep ulcers can be treated with nonoperative techniques such as daily wound care, immobilization, and serial debridements. Treatment of osteomyelitis in diabetic patients is time-consuming because of vascular insufficiency, peripheral neuropathy, and poor soft tissue coverage. If osteomyelitis or an abscess is present, an incision and drainage should be performed for treatment and obtaining a deep tissue and bone culture [16–19].

A number of surgical techniques can maximize the success of wound healing. The most important is aggressive debridement of all infected tissue and bone, while sparing the healthy tissue for closure. If the wound is grossly infected at the initial debridement, serial surgical debridements is necessary until the wound has responded and started to heal. Leaving large wounds to heal by granulation and secondary intention may take several months or years for a complete closure [20,21].

Antibiotic beads have primarily been used in the treatment of osteomyelitis and compound fractures of the extremities. Antibiotic beads are fabricated by mixing antibiotic powder into polymethylmethacrylate (PMMA) cement pellets. While the PMMA mixture is still soft, small pellets are rolled into shape and placed on a nonabsorbable suture. Too much antibiotic prevents the beads from hardening, and too little antibiotic will limit the effectiveness of the antibiotic beads. The chain of PMMA beads is loosely packed into the wound or bone defect after radical surgical debridement of all infected tissue and bone. A closed compartment is required to obtain high local concentrations of antibiotic. The antibiotic is then released into the wound by diffusion, with local antibiotic levels remaining very high over 3 weeks. The exact diffusion rate of antibiotic varies by the brand of PMMA cement, the concentration of antibiotic in the bead, the surface area of the bead, and the type of antibiotics. High local concentrations of antibiotic from antibiotic-impregnated PMMA beads have not caused tissue toxicity or been shown to limit wound healing. The antibiotics added to bone cement should be bactericidal, broad-spectrum antibiotics that are particularly effective against gram-positive cocci and gram-negative rods. In addition, the antibiotics should be thermo-stable (so as not to degrade during exothermic polymerization reaction), and water-soluble. The antibiotics should also have a low rate of developing resistant pathogens, and low allergic potential. Antibiotics are generally used in a ratio of approximately 1 to 2 g of antibiotic to 40 g of bone cement. The aminoglycosides and vancomycin are some of the better choices for antibiotic bead use, because of their broad spectrum of activity, low incidence of reaction, and heat stability. The antibiotic beads are usually removed within 2 to 4 weeks to prevent overgrowth of granulation tissue.

Currently, there are limited reports describing the authors' surgical approach for diabetic limb salvage, including the radical surgical debridement, decreasing soft tissue and bone defect, and stabilization with an external fixation device. Diabetes mellitus has been considered as a relative contraindication for the application of an external fixation device, because of a high incidence of a pin tract infection or irritation; however, the Ilizarov method is also less invasive and can be used in septic conditions with excellent results [22–24].

In conclusion, diabetic limb salvage with large soft tissue defects with exposed tendon, joint, or bone lies beyond the limits of conventional techniques. The proposed surgical protocol can be used in selected patients who have osteomyelitis and severe soft tissue defect after aggressive surgical debridement. Finally, the aforementioned techniques require an increased amount of surgical experience and availability for maximum outcomes.

References

[1] Hoar CS, Torres J. Evalution of of below-the-knee amputation in the treatment of diabetic gangrene. N Engl J Med 1962;266:440–3.

[2] Aksoy DY, Gürlek A, Çetinkaya Y, et al. Change in the amputation profile in diabetic foot in a tertiary reference center: efficacy of team working. Exp Clin Endocrinol Diabetes 2004;112: 526–30.

[3] Gibbons GW, Marccaccio EJ, Burgess ARN, et al. Improved quality of diabetic foot care, 1984 versus 1990. Reduced length of stay and costs, insufficient reimbursement. Arch Surg 1993;128:576–81.

[4] Zgonis T, Roukis TS. A systematic approach to diabetic foot infections. Adv Ther 2005;22: 244–62.

[5] Frykberg RG, Zgonis T, Armstrong DG, et al. Diabetic foot disorders: a clinical practice quideline (2006 revision). J Foot Ankle Surg 2006;45(5 Suppl):S1–66.

[6] Cooper PS. Application of external fixators for management of Charcot deformities of the foot and ankle. Semin Vasc Surg 2003;16:67–78.

[7] Cooper PS. Application of external fixators for management of Charcot deformities of the foot and ankle. Foot Ankle Clin 2002;7:207–54.

[8] Jolly GP, Zgonis T, Polyzois V. External fixation in the management of Charcot neuroarthropathy. Clin Podiatr Med Surg 2003;20:741–56.

[9] Baravarian B, Van Gils CC. Arthrodesis of the Charcot foot and ankle. Clin Podiatr Med Surg 2004;21(2):271–89.

[10] Farber DC, Juliano PJ, Cavanagh PR, et al. Single stage correction with external fixation of the ulcerated foot in individuals with Charcot neuroarthropathy. Foot Ankle Int 2002;23: 130–4.

[11] Roukis TS, Zgonis T. The management of acute Charcot fracture—dislocation with the Taylor's spatial external fixation system. Clin Podiatr Med Surg 2006;23(2):467–83.

[12] Papa J, Myerson M, Girard P. Salvage with arthrodesis, in intractable diabetic neuropathic arthropathy of the foot and ankle. J Bone Joint Surg Am 1993;75:1056–66.

[13] Oznur A. Management of large soft tissue defects in a diabetic patient. Foot Ankle Int 2003; 24(1):79–82.

[14] Oznur A, Tokgozoglu M. Closure of central defects of the forefoot with external fixation. J Foot Ankle Surg 2004;43(1):56–9.

[15] Oznur A, Ozer H. Ray amputation with limited incision. Foot Ankle Int 2006;27(5):382.

[16] Roeder B, Van Gils CC, Maling S. Antibiotic beads in the treatment of diabetic pedal osteomyelitis. J Foot Ankle Surg 2000;39(2):124–30.

[17] Kumagai SG, Mahoney CR, Fitzgibbons TC, et al. Treatment of diabetic (neuropathic) foot ulcers with two-stage debridement and closure. Foot Ankle Int 1998;19:160–5.

[18] Pinzur MS, Sage R, Schaegler P. Ray resection in the dysvascular foot. Clin Orthop Relat Res 1984;191:232–4.
[19] Smith DG, Stuck RM, Ketner L, et al. Partial calcanectomy for the treatment of large ulcerations of the heel and calcaneal osteomyelitis. J Bone Joint Surg Am 1992;74:4571–6.
[20] Roukis TS, Zgonis T. Skin grafting techniques for soft-tissue coverage of diabetic foot and ankle wounds. J Wound Care 2005;14:173–6.
[21] Pinzur MS, Sage R, Stuck R, et al. Amputations in the diabetic foot and ankle. Clin Orthop Relat Res 1993;296:64–7.
[22] Strauss MB, Bryant BJ, Hart JD. Forefoot narrowing with external fixator for problem cleft wounds. Foot Ankle Int 2002;23:433–9.
[23] Zgonis T, Oznur A, Roukis TS. A novel technique for closing difficult diabetic cleft foot wounds with skin grafting and a ring-type external fixation system. Operative Techniques Orthopaedics 2006;16:38–43.
[24] Zgonis T, Roukis TS, Frykberg RG, et al. Unstable acute and chronic Charcot's deformity: staged skeletal and soft tissue reconstruction. J Wound Care 2006;15:276–80.

ELSEVIER SAUNDERS

Clin Podiatr Med Surg 24 (2007) 529–546

CLINICS IN PODIATRIC MEDICINE AND SURGERY

Bioengineered Alternative Tissues and Hyperbaric Oxygen in Lower Extremity Wound Healing

Paul J. Kim, DPM[a,b,*], Matt Heilala, DPM[a,c], John S. Steinberg, DPM[a,d], Glenn M. Weinraub, DPM, FACFAS[a,e]

[a]*Foot and Ankle Institute, 918 Congress Avenue Ste 200, Austin, TX 78701, USA*
[b]*Arizona Podiatric Medicine Program, Midwestern University Division of Dentistry and Medicine, 19555 North 59th Avenue, Glendale, AZ 85308, USA*
[c]*4100 Lake Otis Parkway #312, Anchorage, AK 99508, USA*
[d]*Department of Plastic Surgery, Georgetown University School of Medicine, 3800 Reservoir Road, 1-Main-West, Center for Wound Healing, WA, DC 20007-2113, USA*
[e]*The Permanente Group, Kaiser Permanente, Department of Orthopaedic Surgery, 3555 Whipple Road, Building A, Union City, Hayward, CA 94587, USA*

Management of the diabetic wound has improved dramatically in the last decade. With the advent and clinical application of recombinant chemical and cellular mediators of wound healing and a better understanding of the importance of serial debridement, most foot wounds can be healed with little morbidity. Despite these advances, there remains the recalcitrant wound for which more heroic efforts seem warranted. Often, the primary impediments to healing include inadequate blood flow to the wound and an alteration in the local biologic milieu. For these patients, advanced wound healing technologies, orthobiologics, and bioengineered alternative tissues (BAT) may tilt the scales in the direction of definitive wound closure.

Numerous advancements have been made in the wound care arena. Specifically, the area of topically applied products has revolutionized the healing of chronic nonhealing wounds. BAT and topically applied platelet preparations are two of the newer technologies available. Both act to stimulate the conversion of a chronic wound to an acute wound and are used in the treatment of many problem wound types and locations.

* Corresponding author. Arizona Podiatric Medicine Program, Midwestern University Division of Dentistry and Medicine, 19555 North 59th Avenue, Glendale, AZ 85308.

E-mail address: pkimxx@midwestern.edu (P.J. Kim).

0891-8422/07/$ - see front matter
doi:10.1016/j.cpm.2007.03.011

There is growing interest in human and animal "skin" products for the healing of wounds in the lower extremity. Many different terms have been used to describe these new technologies, including *bioengineered skin*, *bioengineered skin substitutes*, *biological skin substitutes*, *tissue engineered skin*, and *bioengineered skin equivalents* [1–9]. The use of these different terms has added to the confusion over the numerous products available. Furthermore, some of the terms simply do not describe these products accurately. The authors propose a new umbrella term, *bioengineered alternative tissue,* that they believe is a more precise description. The term *bioengineered* describes chemical and biologic processes that are involved in the production of these products, including the infusion of certain components that promote wound healing. The term *alternative tissue* denotes the fact that these products are not autologous skin and should not be treated as such. This difference is the greatest point of confusion, which has often led to these products being wrongly used in lieu of a split-thickness or full-thickness skin graft. BAT products promote the conversion of a stagnant wound to an acute wound and are used in different wound types and at different wound stages than an autogenous skin graft procedure.

There are certain important considerations before the application of BAT products. The first consideration is timing. It is not so much a matter of which product should be used but when each product should be used. The products are not necessarily used in situations when a wound has been making good progress in healing; rather, they are used in situations when a wound is struggling or shows signs of impairment. An appropriate benchmark that defines a chronic wound is when a wound ceases to decrease 10% to 15% every week or 50% over a 1-month period [10]. Another important consideration is that the wound should be free of active infection. An active infection will make these products ineffectual. Further, sharp debridement of fibrotic and necrotic tissue about the wound edges and the wound base is essential to remove inhibitory factors such as proteases and collagenases [11,12]. BAT products rely on an environment that has an adequate blood supply; therefore, vascular studies examining the level of ischemia to the affected limb should always be considered when treating a chronic wound and applying BAT products. Optimization of the wound environment before the application of BAT products will ensure a successful wound closure.

Anatomy of skin

Fundamental to the use of BAT products is an understanding of the histology and biology of the skin and surrounding structures. Four important components should be considered in wound care: the epidermis, dermis, hypodermis (subcutaneous adipose tissue), and underlying tissue (Fig. 1). The epidermis is the most superficial component of skin. It has no direct vascular supply and is sloughed continuously. The dermis is often regarded as the most important skin component to wound healing. The hypodermis

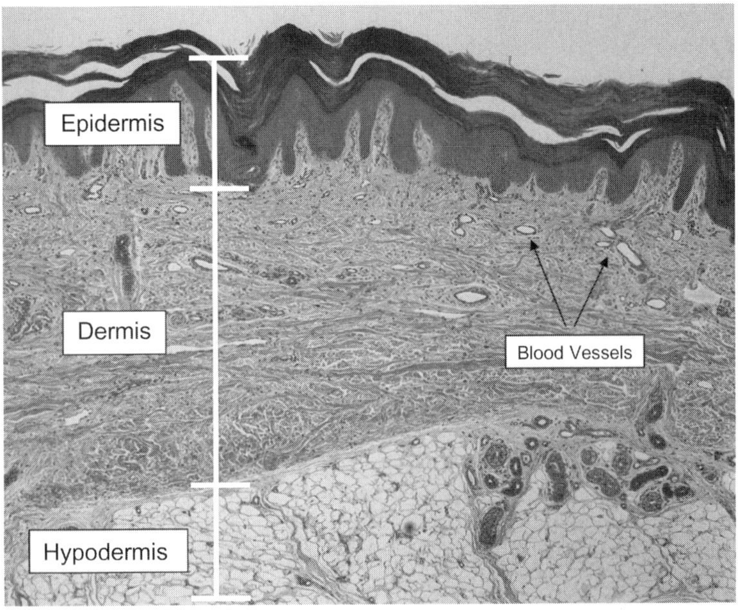

Fig. 1. A histologic cross section of human plantar skin at 6× magnification with hematoxylin and eosin staining techniques. (*Courtesy of* Linda Walters, PhD, Glendale, Arizona.)

contains adipose tissues where neurovascular bundles are located. The underlying tissues include fascia, tendon, and bone, all of which have the potential for granulation tissue formation.

Inflammatory cells and cells that make up the skin contain important growth factors (eg, epidermal growth factor [EGF], fibroblast growth factor [FGF], vascular endothelial growth factor [VEGF], platelet-derived growth factor [PDGF], transforming growth factor-beta [TGF-β]) that stimulate tissue repair and angiogenesis during the wound healing process. Living cell-based BAT products generally stimulate these processes in the wound bed or can deliver growth factors extrinsically when applied to the wound. Some BATs contain living fibroblasts and keratinocytes in addition to growth factors. When selecting a particular BAT product, it is important to keep in mind the different layers of tissue and their architecture. In many cases, a specific product choice can be made to match the wound depth and nature. When BAT products are used incorrectly, the results have a lesser degree of predicted success; therefore, the clinician may wrongly conclude that the product is ineffective or inferior. Proper selection of BAT products increases the likelihood of successful wound closure.

Categorization

Not all BAT products are the same. Each product has been specifically designed to interact with the wound environment in a unique way; however, some broad categories can assist in the proper selection of a BAT product (Table 1). The first category is "living tissue," which includes products such as Apligraf (Organogenesis, Canton, Massachusetts), Dermagraft (Advanced Biohealing, La Jolla, California), Epicel (Genzyme Tissue Repair Corp., Cambridge, Massachusetts), Laserskin/Vivoderm (Fida Advanced Biopolymers, Italy), and Orcel (Ortec International, New York, New York). These products are derived from living cell cultures which contain human living keratinocytes or fibroblasts imbedded within the product. Generally, these products should be reserved for superficial wounds. The other broad category of products is considered "bioactive adjuncts." Examples of this class of products include Integra (Integra Life Sciences, Plainsboro, New Jersey), Oasis (Healthpoint, Fort Worth, Texas), GammaGraft (Promethean LifeSciences, Pittsburgh, Pennsylvania), GraftJacket (Wright Medical Technology, Arlington, Texas), EZ-Derm (Brennen Medical, St. Paul, Minnesota), Alloderm (Life Cell Corp., Woodlands Texas), Biobrane (Dow Hickam/Bertek Pharmaceuticals, Sugar Land, Texas), and TransCyte (Advanced Biohealing, La Jolla, California). These products function as tissue scaffolds that allow for a supportive structural environment for cellular ingrowth. They generally should be used for deeper wounds in which the base of the wound can be built-up.

Table 1
Broad classification and brief description of commonly used bioengineered alternative tissue products

Classification	Description
Living tissues	
Apligraf	Living human dermal fibroblasts and epidermal keratinocytes in bovine collagen matrix
Dermagraft	Fibroblasts imbedded in polyglactin mesh
Laserskin/Vivoderm	Hyaluronic material imbedded with keratinocytes cultured from the patient
Epicel	Cultured autograft
Orcel	Neonatal fibroblasts and keratinocytes cultured and embedded onto bovine collagen
Bioactive adjuncts	
Integra	Bovine type I collagen, chondroitin-6-sulfate
Oasis	Porcine intestinal submucosa
GammaGraft	Gamma-irradiated human allograft
GraftJacket	Acellular collagen matrix derived from human allograft
EZ-Derm	Porcine collagen
Alloderm	Cadaveric dermal skin
Biobrane	Peptides embedded in nylon mesh adhered to silicone backing
TransCyte	Nylon mesh fabric seeded with fibroblasts (fibroblasts eventually destroyed, leaving growth factors and proteins behind)

Sequential application of different BAT products or repeated applications of the same product may be necessary to ultimately close a wound (Fig. 2). This decision should be made based on the percent decrease in wound dimensions or the degree of granulation tissue noted in the wound bed. BAT products can promote complete epithelialization of a wound; however, a split-thickness skin graft may be more effective and efficient in achieving final closure.

Clinical outcomes

The literature is replete with case reports and small uncontrolled studies examining the efficacy of these products. Some products have little to no research supporting their use for chronic wounds in the lower extremity. The focus herein is on BAT products that have been more rigorously studied in the peer-reviewed literature.

The two most commonly used BAT products in the living tissue category are Apligraf and Dermagraft. Apligraf is a bilayered tissue construct that microscopically resembles true skin. It is composed of bovine collagen and living human cells (keratinocytes and fibroblasts) derived from neonatal foreskin. After application, the living cells contained in the graft continue to produce matrix proteins and growth factors which aid in the healing

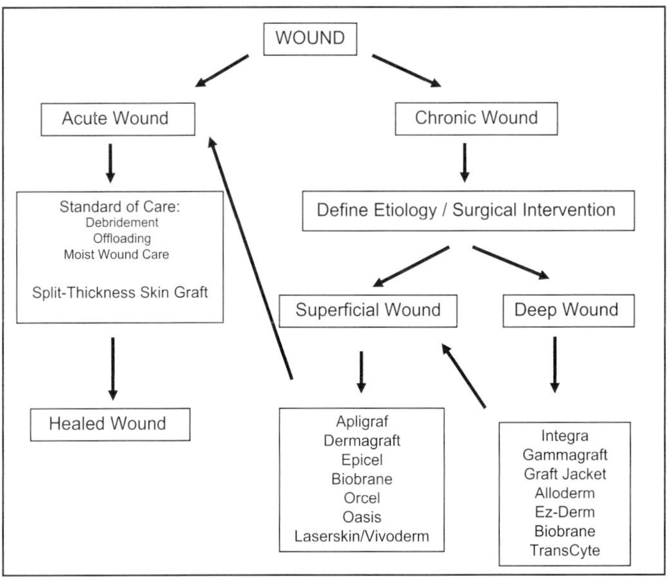

Fig. 2. Decision algorithm for the use of BAT. This simple decision tree algorithm depicts the thought process involved in the use of BAT. Superficial wound, a wound that involves the epidermis and dermis; deep wound, a wound that involves the hypodermis or deeper tissues.

process. This product is approved by the US Food and Drug Administration (FDA) for the treatment of chronic venous ulcers and diabetic foot ulcerations (Fig. 3, case example). The efficacy of Apligraf in the promotion of wound healing in the lower extremity has been supported by published case reports and clinical trials [13–21]. The largest and most comprehensive study was published by Veves and colleagues [21]. In that prospective, multicenter, randomized trial, Apligraf was compared with saline-moistened gauze in a total of 208 diabetic patients with neuropathic wounds. There was a significant increase in the number of healed wounds and a decrease in the median time to complete healing in the Apligraf group when compared with the saline-moistened gauze group. Other investigators report that Apligraf may also be economically prudent for the healing of chronic wounds in the lower extremity [17,19].

Dermagraft is also a member of the living cell BAT category. This BAT product was not available at the time of this submission, although it is scheduled to return to the market in 2007. Dermagraft is obtained from growing, living allogeneic fibroblasts on a polyglactin mesh. Similar to Apligraf, fibroblasts are obtained from neonatal foreskin and, after implantation, remain viable and continue to secrete matrix proteins and growth factors. The polyglactin mesh is biodegradable and is reabsorbed after 3 to 4 weeks. Dermagraft has been reported to have positive efficacy in healing wounds in the lower extremity [22–26]. Marston and colleagues [27] examined 314 patients with chronic diabetic foot ulcers of greater than 6 weeks' duration in a prospective, single-blind, randomized controlled study. The

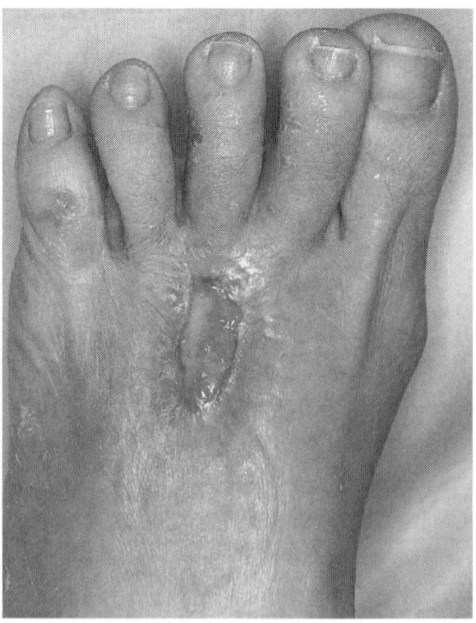

Fig. 3. Apligraf case example.

patients treated with Dermagraft experienced a significantly greater decrease in ulcer size and ulcer-related adverse events when compared with the conventional therapy group. In addition, they reported closure of 30% of the ulcers treated with Dermagraft at 12 weeks versus an 18.3% closure with saline-moistened gauze therapy alone.

Other BAT products in the living tissue category are not as well researched, and there are limited trials published in the peer-reviewed literature. These products include Laserskin (Vivoderm), Epicel, and Orcel. Laserskin is constructed from material made of hyaluronic acid and is perforated using a laser and subsequently seeded on both sides with autologous keratinocytes from a biopsy of the patient's own skin. The pores within this product enhance drainage of fluid from the wound bed. Lobmann and colleagues [28] examined the long-term outcome of using Laserskin on chronic wounds of 14 diabetic patients. They reported a 79% wound closure rate at 64 days post graft application. Epicel is a cultured autograft composed of living keratinocytes derived from a biopsy of the patient's own skin that is subsequently cultured for 3 weeks. It has no dermal component and is suited for more superficial wounds. Orcel is made of allogeneic neonatal fibroblasts and keratinocytes which are cultured onto opposite sides of a matrix of cross-linked bovine collagen. The matrix contains viable cells that secrete growth factors and cytokines to promote healing. The authors were unable to uncover any published trials evaluating the efficacy of Epicel or Orcel in treating chronic wounds of the lower extremity.

The bioactive adjuncts category encompasses many products which serve as scaffolds for wound healing. These BAT products contain no living cells. Two of the products that fall into this category include Integra and GraftJacket. The prototype in this category is Integra. Integra is a nonliving matrix composed of bovine type 1 tendon collagen and chondroitin-6-sulfate, which has historically been used in the management of acute burn wounds [29–34]. Integra has more recently been used by wound care specialists in the treatment of chronic ulcerations in the lower extremity with good success (Fig. 4, case example) [35,36]. The ability of Integra to fill large defects makes it ideal for deep wounds that may extend to deep fascia and bone [36–38]. GraftJacket is an acellular collagen matrix derived from cadaveric skin. The allogeneic human tissue is processed using technology that removes the epidermis and all cellular components while preserving the matrix and biochemical components. This product has been shown to be effective in the treatment of deep foot wounds in diabetic patients [39,40]. A prospective, randomized controlled study by Brigido [40] reported that a single application of GraftJacket resulted in a significant decrease in wound area, depth, and volume in comparison with a wound gel.

Other BAT products that fall into the category of bioactive adjuncts include GammaGraft, Alloderm, and Oasis. GammaGraft is a gamma-irradiated cadaveric allograft. This product contains both epidermal and dermal components and is stored in a penicillin/gentamicin solution. GammaGraft

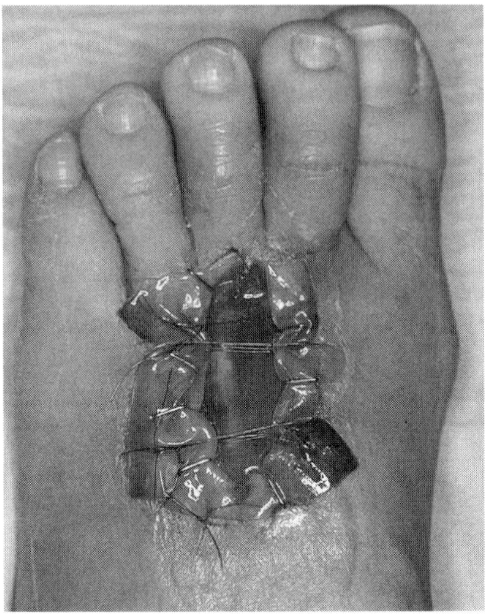

Fig. 4. Integra case example.

has been reported to have good results in smaller wounds on the dorsal aspect of the foot and lower leg [41]. Alloderm is an acellular, nonliving dermal replacement composed of human cadaveric skin in which the epidermis has been removed by salt processing. The majority of research has evaluated the efficacy of Alloderm in the treatment of full-thickness burns, where it has been found to exhibit excellent elasticity and good pigmentation with minimal wound contracture and scarring [42,43].

Oasis is composed of porcine small intestine submucosa that provides a scaffold for the growth of new tissue. It is an acellular product containing collagen and growth factors. Mostow and colleagues [44] in a randomized clinical trial examined the efficacy of Oasis in 120 patients with chronic venous ulcers of the lower extremity. They reported that 55% of the ulcers in the group treated with Oasis plus compression healed completely compared with 34% of the ulcers in the group who were treated with compression therapy alone. In addition, none of the subjects treated with Oasis experienced recurrence at 6-month follow-up. Niezgoda and colleagues [45] directly compared Oasis with Regranex (Johnson & Johnson, Somerville, New Jersey) in a randomized, controlled, multicenter trial. A higher percentage of patients who had treatment with Oasis went on to complete healing when compared with the Regranex group, although the difference was not statistically significant.

The BAT products Biobrane, EZ-Derm, and TransCyte are not used as frequently as the products already mentioned. As a result, there are less published studies examining their clinical efficacy in chronic wounds of the lower extremity. Biobrane is a bilayered membrane consisting of nylon mesh fabric adhered to a thin layer of silicone. Peptides embedded within the mesh promote wound bed adherence and fibrovascular ingrowth. The product is intended mainly as a temporary wound cover and has been used for the temporary coverage of freshly excised full-thickness wounds. EZ-Derm is composed of cross-linked porcine collagen. TransCyte consists of a nylon mesh fabric coated with porcine dermal collagen seeded with cultured neonatal human fibroblasts on a silicone backing. During the manufacturing process, the fibroblasts secrete proteins and growth factors, after which the cryopreservation process kills all the living cells. This product is not currently available; its manufacturing operations were shared with Dermagraft.

Processed platelet technology

Topical application of autologous blood products on chronic wounds has gained popularity. Specifically, there have been increasing reports in the medical literature on the use of platelet rich plasma (PRP) and other platelet preparations. The authors reviewed the current literature pertaining to the use of these products in the promotion of healing of chronic wounds. To better evaluate the efficacy of these products, the discussion herein includes the anatomy and physiology of platelets in the wound environment, the important components of this technology and its application, and clinical outcomes.

Anatomy and physiology

Platelets are a critical component in the wound healing process and actively participate by acting as physical barriers, recruiting and regulating inflammatory cells, and secreting growth factors and other bioactive proteins. The latter component is especially important. Individual platelets contain intracellular structures known as alpha granules. These alpha granules contain components including growth factors, clotting factors, and other proteins involved in wound healing. After activation by thrombin, platelets aggregate to the area of injury and release the contents of their alpha granules to initiate clotting to begin the healing process. The platelet aggregate (platelet plug) serves as a barrier to the external environment. PDGF is one of the key components released by the alpha granules. PDGF is involved in the formation of connective tissue and promotes revascularization and has been shown to promote granulation tissue [46]. PDGF is also involved in epithelialization, wound contraction, and remodeling. Furthermore, platelets release TGF-β and platelet-derived angiogenesis factor (PDAF), which have key roles in wound matrix production by promoting collagen production and new capillary formation.

Platelets are involved in many steps of the wound healing process. Their inherent functions in the human body have spurred the advent of products that attempt to recreate, stimulate, and activate these processes. The following sections discuss in further detail the technology of topically applied platelet preparations.

The technology

Similar to the use of BAT products, proper assessment and preparation of the wound should be conducted before the application of platelet preparations. This preparation includes infection control, routine débridement, and adequate off-loading through external devices (eg, multidensity inserts, removable walking cast) or surgical removal of bony prominences (eg, exostosectomy, reconstruction). Furthermore, underlying systemic conditions such as peripheral vascular disease and collagen vascular disease must be addressed. One may also consider obtaining laboratory studies including a coagulation panel to ascertain the number of platelets in the circulating system. Although a clear platelet deficiency may dissuade the use of these products, no absolute threshold has been established.

Different processing methods are used for platelet preparations. Platelet preparations called "platelet releasates" require processing in a laboratory. In this process, the autologous platelets are first separated from other blood products. Next, growth factors including PDGF and TGF-β are extracted from the platelets and placed into a solution with other reagents. Generally, multiple containers are produced of this solution for daily topical application. Platelet preparations that are produced in the office, wound care center, or operating room are growing in popularity. The patient's whole blood is drawn (typically, 5–60 mL) and centrifuged to separate the blood products: PRP, platelet poor products (PPP), and erythrocytes. The PRP is preserved while the PPP and erythrocytes are discarded. The PRP is then activated using thrombin. Additional reagents including calcium chloride are mixed into the solution. The now activated PRP is then applied (sprayed) topically using a hand-held device similar to a syringe and needle onto the wound surface (Fig. 5, case example). This platelet preparation should be applied within 10 to 30 seconds after activation for optimal results. The resultant viscous coagulum that forms readily adheres to the surface of the wound. A nonadherent dressing is applied over this wound followed by a bolster dressing (4 × 4 or other dressing material) and Coban (3M, St. Paul, Minnesota) or other dressing material. This process is repeated every 4 to 7 days. The area is left undisturbed until the following visit when sharp debridement may be necessary. Multiple applications may be necessary, with typical treatments requiring greater than 1 month.

Currently, multiple competing platelet preparation systems are used for external application on wounds in the lower extremity. Some of these systems include the Symphony II PCS (DePuy Spine, Raynham, Massachusetts), VivoStat System (Vivolution, Birkeroed, Denmark), SmartPrep

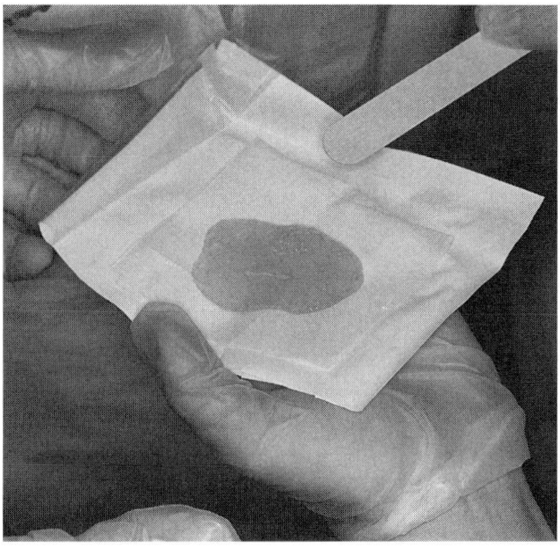

Fig. 5. AutoloGel case example.

(Harvest Tech Corp., Plymouth, Massachusetts), AutoloGel (Cytomedix, Rockville, Maryland), and Magellan (Medtronic, Minneapolis, Minnesota). The differences in these systems are subtle and revolve around the centrifuge constructs and additive properties within the respective reagents.

Clinical outcomes

The published peer-reviewed clinical research on the use of processed platelet technologies on chronic wounds in the foot and ankle includes mostly small case studies or studies that are uncontrolled. Herein, the focus is on larger human trials involving chronic wounds in the lower extremity.

One of the larger studies using processed platelet technology was published by Glover and colleagues [47]. This retrospective study examined 3830 patients with chronic wounds using platelet releasate technology versus comprehensive wound care alone. Significantly higher healing rates and lower amputation rates were reported with the use of platelet releasate. Margolis and colleagues [48] supported these results in their study published in 2001. This retrospective cohort study compared the healing rate of diabetic neuropathic foot ulcers using platelet releasate versus standard wound care. Platelet releasate was more effective than standard wound care, with a greater effect reported in larger and deeper wounds. A more recent study published by Driver and colleagues [49] supports the use of platelet preparations on diabetic foot ulcers. This prospective, randomized, controlled, double-blinded, multicenter study compared a PRP preparation versus a normal saline gel. A greater percentage of the PRP group healed versus the control group. Other studies support these reports for the use of topical platelet preparations [50–55].

Hyperbaric oxygen therapy in diabetic limb salvage

Despite recent advances in wound healing understanding and technology, there remains the recalcitrant wound for which more heroic efforts seem warranted. Often, the primary impediment to healing is inadequate blood flow to the wound. Paramount is the lack of oxygen delivery to the compromised tissues. Although advances have made revascularization of the limb more feasible and less invasive, a minority of these patients continue to have nonhealing wounds with poor perfusion. For these patients, a novel discovery of the nineteenth century may have a role.

Hyperbaric oxygen is a well-studied technology of selected indication that is poorly understood by the public and most medical professionals. A concise overview of the physiology and contemporary applications of hyperbaric oxygen therapy (HBOT) is provided herein to assist the foot and ankle specialist in discerning whether this modality may have a role in complex wound management.

Historically, the concept of atmospheric pressure and its effect on systemic gas partial pressure was seen clinically in caisson workers of the 1850s. Working in hyperatmospheric environments and quickly returning to normal atmospheres led to decompression illness and even air gas embolism as seen in divers ascending too rapidly. Bert [56] in 1878 proposed the "bubble theory" to explain this physiologically. Recompression of these symptomatic patients in a chamber, described by Moir [57] in 1889, was found to ameliorate much of these debilitating symptoms known as the "bends." Boerema [58], recognized by many as the father of hyperbaric medicine, published an article entitled "Life Without Blood" in 1960 which demonstrated the effective delivery of oxygen to tissues in live pigs in the complete absence of blood cells. These initial discoveries led to the further application of basic physics principles to hyperoxygenate tissues to stimulate healing.

Definition

HBOT involves high-dose oxygen inhalation while the entire body, not simply the extremity, is pressurized above normal atmospheric pressure. It is accomplished by placing the whole patient within a chamber that is pressurized by air or 100% oxygen. In air-pressurized chambers, the subject breaths 100% oxygen in a mask, a sealed hood donned over the head and neck, or an endotracheal tube. If oxygen is used as the pressurization gas, a separate oxygen delivery method is not required because the patient simply breaths freely in the chamber. The chamber is either a monoplace, a room for one patient, or a multiplace, a room for more than one patient. Most chambers are monoplace. For simplicity, many chambers are oxygen pressurized, although concerns of catastrophic fire and explosion exist, and such events have occurred resulting in the immediate death of the patient and a large crater in the building in which the chamber was housed. Air-pressurized chambers also have a fire risk, although they are equipped with fire suppression water deluge systems that are useless in monoplace chambers.

Basic physiology and mechanism of action

Extensive basic science work performed over the last 40 years has firmly established the framework and rationale for the medicinal application of HBOT. As Davis and Hunt [59] have stated, "There is no longer any question as to whether or not elevation of problem wound oxygen is efficacious—it is." Key statements and mechanisms that have gained consensus by the Undersea and Hyperbaric Medicine Society, established in 1967, are as follows:

- Problem wound oxygen tension is usually below 20 mm Hg and is often 0 mm Hg.
- A gradient of 40 mm Hg from wound to periwound tissues is necessary to induce macrophage angiogenesis factor production.
- Intermittent correction of wound hypoxia encourages fibroblastic replication and collagen synthesis to support neovascularization.
- Raising wound oxygen levels above 30 mm Hg significantly increases white cell kill capability and can be additive to antibiotic therapy.
- Anaerobic microorganisms that lack superoxide dismutase or catalase are killed or rendered ineffective by oxygenated wounds.
- Oxygen tension as measured directly in wound and periwound tissues is often induced to levels higher than 1000 mm Hg during and immediately following HBOT.

General indications

The Undersea and Hyperbaric Medicine Society established a committee on HBOT in 1976. The critical analysis of existing and proposed uses for HBOT remains its central role. The first report of the society published in 1977 is reviewed and revised every 3 years. This publication is used as a credible guideline for third-party payers and HBOT practitioners. The current list of accepted indications for HBOT is as follows:

- Air or gas embolization
- Carbon monoxide poisoning or carbon monoxide complicated by cyanide poisoning
- Clostridial myositis and myonecrosis (gas gangrene)
- Crush injury, compartment syndrome, and other acute traumatic ischemias
- Decompression sickness
- Enhancement of healing in selected problem wounds
- Exceptional blood loss (anemia)

Intracranial abscess
Necrotizing soft tissue infections
Refractory osteomyelitis
Delayed radiation injury (soft tissue and bony necrosis)
Skin grafts and flaps (compromised)
Thermal burns

Obstacles to and applications of hyperbaric oxygen therapy in diabetic limb salvage

Great advancements have been made in the multidisciplinary approach to diabetic wound management. HBOT is no longer a new technology, yet its use even in modern centers is uncommon at best. Costs and logistics seem to be a continued impediment to patient access. Concerns of overuse have further impeded its role. One session or "dive" often costs $750 to $2000. Ten to fifteen dives is a typical initial series to determine response. A full course of therapy is generally 30 to 60 treatments, five per week over 6 to 12 weeks.

Understanding that "HBO is a drug," Sheffield [60] suggested that proper patient and wound screening are essential for the responsible use of HBOT. Pressurizing a human is fraught with potential complications such as oxygen toxicity, barotrauma (ears), visual disturbances and cataract formation, tension pneumothorax, decompression sickness, and gas embolization. In the hope of preventing such reactions and complications, medical screening including a chest radiograph and ear examination is necessary before treatment. In addition to a general medical work-up, local wound screening must occur. Toward that end, several key features must be established:

The wound has not been responsive to standard more time- and cost-effective treatments.
The absence of an infected or a noninfected bio-burden is confirmed by wound exploration, debridement, and occasionally imaging.
Confirmation of periwound hypoxia is performed by transcutaneous oximetry ($TcPO_2$).
Confirmation of normal patient respiratory/ventilatory capacity is performed with a reference $TcPO_2$ chest lead.
A response or elevation of periwound oxygen tension is established with a 100% oxygen challenge or with a "test dive."
Revascularization of the dysvascular extremity is not feasible.

Unfortunately, some patients are treated with HBOT for "problem wounds" before appropriate wound screening. The end result is a catastrophic financial burden and a continued nonhealing wound. This problem intuitively would occur less at more formalized centers that involve foot and ankle specialists who may assist in covering the "basics" of diabetic wound healing, such as effective off-loading and aggressive debridement when necessary. This observation underscores the important role of the podiatric surgeon in the continued use of HBOT. A simple statement summarizes the aforementioned criteria and indication for HBOT in the treatment of the diabetic lower extremity wound: HBOT is indicated in the hypoxic wound when the vasculature cannot feasibly be reconstructed or when vascular interventions have failed and persisting wound hypoxia is the remaining primary cause of delayed healing or nonhealing. Another relative indication that is worthy of consideration is the desire to rapidly cover exposed vital tissues and structures such as healthy bone, joint, or tendon following debridement. In such instances, HBOT is used as a "granulation machine" in the otherwise vascular healing wound. The caveat to such uses is that third-party payers may not accept this as an accepted indication in the formal guidelines set forth by the Undersea and Hyperbaric Medicine Society publication; therefore, coverage is often left to appeals on behalf of the critical nature of the extremity at risk.

Combination treatments

New approaches to treatment of the complex wound have set the stage for a multitude of combination techniques. Subatmospheric or vacuum-assisted closure therapy, bioengineered allograft tissues, topically applied recombinant growth factors, and autogenous platelet gels are among the recent modalities and technologies that are occasionally used in conjunction with HBOT. A factor limiting which additional products may be present during a "dive" is whether the substance is a potential fuel source for combustion in an oxygen-rich environment. Petrolatum-based nonadherant and latex-containing dressing materials are forbidden in the hyperbaric oxygen chamber.

Summary

HBOT was derived out of a marriage of the observation of physical phenomena and illness occurring incidentally in the diving and industrial communities and the innovations of many brilliant theorists and researchers over two centuries. Continued scrutiny of its application and safety by organizations such as the Undersea and Hyperbaric Medicine Society will likely broaden its potential indication. In contradistinction, its role in treating the diabetic foot will likely narrow as methods of revascularization and infection management become more sophisticated, less costly, and more effective.

Ultimately, the success of these advanced healing products may depend on factors that lie outside the control of the clinician. Psychosocial and economic influences may dictate which of the products are chosen for the patient. Nevertheless, a working knowledge of each of these products and a thorough evaluation of the available published research will assist the clinician in the appropriate selection.

Proper wound bed preparation and a stable wound environment are often the most important steps to achieving successful wound healing. It is imperative that product application be delayed until the wound base is properly prepared to receive it.

Clearly, the horizon is bright when one looks at the future of bioengineered technology. Many new products are under development, and we are refining the proper use of the currently available technologies. This experience should add up to faster, more reliable, and more predictable wound healing in many of the most complicated patients.

References

[1] Bello YM, Falabella AF, Eaglstein WH. Tissue-engineered skin, current status in wound healing. Am J Clin Dermatol 2001;2(5):305–13.

[2] Curran MP, Plosker GL. Bilayered bioengineered skin substitute (Apligraf): a review of its use in the treatment of venous leg ulcers and diabetic foot ulcers. BioDrugs 2002;16(6): 439–55.

[3] Claxton MJ, Armstrong DG, Boulton AJM. Healing the diabetic wound and keeping it healed: modalities for the early 21st century. Curr Diab Rep 2002;2(6):510–8.

[4] Dini V, Romanelli M, Piaggesi A, et al. Cutaneous tissue engineering and lower extremity wounds (part 2). Int J Low Extrem Wounds 2006;5(1):27–34.

[5] Harding KG, Morris HL, Patel GK. Science, medicine and the future: healing of chronic wounds. Br Med J 2002;324(7330):160–3.

[6] Jones I, Currie L, Martin R. A guide to biological skin substitutes. Br J Plast Surg 2002;55: 185–93.

[7] Kirsner RS, Falanga V, Eaglstein WH. The development of bioengineered skin. Trends Biotechnol 1998;16(6):246–9.

[8] Lee KH. Tissue-engineered human living skin substitutes: development and clinical application. Yonsei Med J 2000;41(6):774–9.

[9] Marston WA. Dermagraft, a bioengineered human dermal equivalent for the treatment of chronic nonhealing diabetic foot ulcer. Expert Rev Med Devices 2004;1(1):21–31.

[10] Sheehan P, Jones P, Caselli A, et al. Percent change in wound area of diabetic foot ulcers over a 4-week period is a robust predictor of complete healing in a 12-week prospective trial. Diabetes Care 2003;26(6):1879–82.

[11] Attinger CE, Bulan EJ. Debridement: the key initial step in wound healing. Foot Ankle Clin 2001;6:627–60.

[12] Brem H, Sheehan P, Boulton AJM. Protocol for treatment of diabetic foot ulcers. Am J Surg 2004;187(Suppl):1S–10S.

[13] Akopian G, Nunnery SP, Piangenti J, et al. Outcomes of conventional wound treatment in a comprehensive wound center. Am Surg 2006;72(4):314–7.

[14] Brem H, Balledux J, Bloom T, et al. Healing of diabetic foot ulcers and pressure ulcers with human skin equivalent. Arch Surg 2000;135(6):627–34.

[15] Brem H, Balledux J, Sukkarieh T, et al. Healing of venous ulcers of long duration with a bilayered living skin substitute: results from a general surgery and dermatology department. Dermatol Surg 2001;27(11):915–9.

[16] Falanga VJ. Tissue engineering in wound repair. Adv Wound Care 2000;13(S2):15–9.

[17] Fivenson D, Scherschun L. Clinical and economic impact of Apligraft for the treatment of nonhealing venous leg ulcers. Int J Dermatol 2003;42:960–5.

[18] Long RE, Falabella AF, Valencia I, et al. Treatment of refractory, atypical lower extremity ulcers with tissue-engineered skin (Apligraf). Arch Dermatol 2001;137(12):1660–1.

[19] Redekop WK, McDonnell J, Verboom P, et al. The cost effectiveness of Apligraf treatment of diabetic foot ulcers. Pharmacoeconomics 2003;21(16):1171–83.

[20] Sams HH, Chen J, King LE. Graftskin treatment of difficult to heal diabetic foot ulcers: one center's experience. Dermatol Surg 2002;28(8):698–703.
[21] Veves A, Falanga V, Armstrong DG, et al. Graftskin, a human skin equivalent, is effective in the management of noninfected neuropathic diabetic foot ulcers: a prospective randomized multicenter clinical trial. Diabetes Care 2001;24:290–5.
[22] Hanft JR, Surprenant MS. Healing of chronic foot ulcers in diabetic patients treated with a human fibroblast-derived dermis. J Foot Ankle Surg 2002;41(5):291–9.
[23] Allenet B, Parée F, Lebrun T, et al. Cost-effectiveness modeling of Dermagraft for the treatment of diabetic foot ulcers in the French context. Diabetes Metab 2000;26:125–32.
[24] Grey JE, Lowe G, Bale S, et al. The use of cultured dermis in the treatment of diabetic foot ulcers. J Wound Care 1998;7(7):324–5.
[25] Newton DJ, Khan F, Belch JJF, et al. Blood flow changes in diabetic foot ulcers treated with dermal replacement therapy. J Foot Ankle Surg 2002;41(4):233–7.
[26] Omar AA, Mavor AID, Jones AM, et al. Treatment of venous leg ulcers with Dermagraft. Eur J Vasc Endovasc Surg 2004;27:666–72.
[27] Marston WA, Hanft J, Norwood P, et al. The efficacy and safety of Dermagraft in improving the healing of chronic diabetic foot ulcers, results from a prospective randomized trial. Diabetes Care 2003;26(6):1701–5.
[28] Lobmann R, Pittasch D, Mühlen I, et al. Autologous human keratinocytes cultured on membranes composed of benzyl ester of hyaluronic acid for grafting in nonhealing diabetic foot lesions: a pilot study. J Diabetes Complications 2003;17:199–204.
[29] Boyce ST, Kagan RJ, Meyer NA, et al. The 1999 clinical research award: cultured skin substitutes combined with Integra artificial skin to replace native skin autograft and allograft for the closure of full-thickness burns. J Burn Care Rehabil 1999;20(6):453–61.
[30] Heitland A, Piatkowski A, Noah EM, et al. Update on the use of collagen/glycosaminoglycate skin substitute: six years of experience with artificial skin in 15 German burn centers. Burns 2004;30:471–5.
[31] Michaeli D, McPherson M. Immunologic study of artificial skin used in the treatment of thermal injuries. J Burn Care Rehabil 1990;11(1):21–6.
[32] Ryan CM, Shoenfeld DA, Malloy M, et al. Use of Integra artificial skin is associated with decreased length of stay for severely injured adult burn survivors. J Burn Care Rehabil 2002;23(5):311–7.
[33] Stern R, McPherson M, Longaker MT. Histologic study of artificial skin used in the treatment of full-thickness thermal injury. J Burn Care Rehabil 1990;11(1):7–13.
[34] Wisser D, Rennekampff HO, Schaller HE. Skin assessment of burn wounds covered with a collagen based dermal substitute in a 2 year-follow-up. Burns 2004;30:399–401.
[35] Silverstein G. Dermal regeneration template in the surgical management of diabetic foot ulcers: a series of five cases. J Foot Ankle Surg 2006;45(1):28–33.
[36] Molnar JA, DeFranzo AJ, Hadaegh A, et al. Acceleration of Integra incorporation in complex tissue defects with subatmospheric pressure. Plast Reconstr Surg 2004;113(5):1339–46.
[37] Violas P, Abid A, Darodes P, et al. Integra artificial skin in the management of severe tissue defects, including bone exposure, in injured children. J Pediatr Orthop B 2005;14(5):381–4.
[38] Wilensky JS, Rosenthal AH, Bradford CR, et al. The use of bovine collagen construct for reconstruction of full-thickness scalp defects in the elderly patient with cutaneous malignancy. Ann Plast Surg 2005;54(3):297–301.
[39] Martin BR, Sangalang M, Wu S, et al. Outcomes of allogenic acellular matrix therapy in treatment of diabetic foot wounds: an initial experience. Int Wound J 2005;2(2):161–5.
[40] Brigido SA. The use of an acellular dermal regenerative tissue matrix in the treatment of lower extremity wounds: a prospective 16-week pilot study. Int Wound J 2006;3(3):181–7.
[41] Rosales MA, Bruntz M, Armstrong DG. Gamma-irradiated human skin allograft: a potential treatment modality for lower extremity ulcers. Int Wound J 2004;1(3):201–6.

[42] Walden JL, Garcia H, Hawkins H, et al. Both dermal matrix and epidermis contribute to an inhibition of wound contraction. Ann Plast Surg 2000;45(2):162–6.
[43] Lattari V, Jones LM, Varcelotti JR, et al. The use of a permanent dermal allograft in full-thickness burns of the hand and foot: a report of three cases. J Burn Care Rehabil 1997; 18(2):147–55.
[44] Mostow EN, Haraway GD, Dalsing M, et al. OASIS Venus Ulcer Study Group. Effectiveness of an extracellular matrix graft (OASIS Wound Matrix) in the treatment of chronic leg ulcers: a randomized clinical trial. J Vasc Surg 2005;41(5):837–43.
[45] Niezgoda JA, Van Gils CC, Frykberg RG, et al. Oasis Diabetic Ulcer Study Group. Randomized clinical trial comparing OASIS wound matrix to Regranex gel for diabetic ulcers. Adv Skin Wound Care 2005;18(5):258–66.
[46] Mustoe TA, Pierce GF, Morisima C, et al. Growth factor induced acceleration of tissue repair through direct and inductive activities in a rabbit dermal ulcer model. J Clin Invest 1991; 87:694–703.
[47] Glover JL, Weingarten MS, Buchbinder DS, et al. A 4-year outcome-based retrospective study of wound healing and limb salvage in patients with chronic wounds. Adv Wound Care 1997;10(1):33–8.
[48] Margolis DJ, Kantor J, Santanna J, et al. Effectiveness of platelet releasate for the treatment of diabetic neuropathic foot ulcers. Diabetes Care 2001;24(3):483–8.
[49] Driver VR, Hanft J, Fylling CP, et al. A prospective, randomized, controlled trial of autologous platelet-rich plasma gel for the treatment of diabetic foot ulcers. Ostomy Wound Manage 2006;52(6):68–87.
[50] Atri SC, Misra J, Bisht D, et al. Use of homologous platelet factors in achieving total healing of recalcitrant skin ulcers. Surgery 1990;108(3):508–12.
[51] Knighton DR, Ciresi K, Fiegel VD, et al. Classification and treatment of chronic nonhealing wounds: successful treatment with autologous platelet-derived wound healing factors. Ann Surg 1986;204(3):322–30.
[52] Knighton DR, Ciresi K, Fiegel VD, et al. Stimulation of repair in chronic, nonhealing, cutaneous ulcers using platelet-derived wound healing formula. Surg Gynecol Obstet 1990;170:56–60.
[53] Steed DL, Goslen JB, Holloway GA, et al. Randomized prospective double-blind trial in healing chronic diabetic foot ulcers: CT-102 activated platelet supernatant, topical versus placebo. Diabetes Care 1992;15(11):1598–604.
[54] Crovetti G, Martinelli G, Issi M, et al. Platelet gel for healing cutaneous chronic wounds. Transfus Apher Sci 2004;30:145–51.
[55] Saldalamacchia G, Lapice E, Cuomo V, et al. A controlled study of the use of autologous platelet gel for the treatment of diabetic foot ulcers. Nutr Metab Cardiovasc Dis 2004;14: 395–6.
[56] Bert P. Bubble theory. In: Bert P, editor. Barometric pressure: researches in experimental physiology [English translation of 1943 edition]. Columbus (OH): College Book Company; 1878.
[57] Paul Sheffield. Lecture and Manual, Hyperbaric Medicine: A Historical Perspective. Moir E, 1889. HMTT San Antonio, TX, December 5–11, 1999.
[58] Boerema I, Meyene NG, Brummelkamp WH, et al. Leven zonder bloed [life without blood]. Ned Tijdschr Geneeska 1960;104:949–54 [in Dutch].
[59] Davis JC, Hunt TK. Problem wounds, the role of oxygen. 1988.
[60] Sheffield PJ. Director of Research and Education, Course Director, Hyperbaric Medicine Team Training, Nix Hospital. San Antonio (TX), December 5–11, 1999.

ELSEVIER
SAUNDERS

Clin Podiatr Med Surg
24 (2007) 547–568

CLINICS IN
PODIATRIC
MEDICINE AND
SURGERY

Advanced Plastic Surgery Techniques for Soft Tissue Coverage of the Diabetic Foot

Thomas Zgonis, DPM, FACFAS[a,*],
John J. Stapleton, DPM, AACFAS[a],
Thomas S. Roukis, DPM, FACFAS[b]

[a]*Department of Orthopaedics/Podiatry Division, University of Texas Health Science Center at San Antonio, 7703 Floyd Curl Drive, MC 7776, San Antonio, TX 78229, USA*
[b]*Department of Surgery, Madigan Army Medical Center, 9040-A Fitzsimmons Avenue, MCHJ-SV, Tacoma, WA 98431, USA*

Coverage of open diabetic foot soft tissue defects represents a challenge to the reconstructive surgeon [1–10]. Primary closure without undo tension is often not feasible secondary to the size, location, and proximity of vital neuron-vascular-tendinous structures to the wound, as well as the general inelasticity of the skin of the foot, especially the plantar area, and the diabetic integument [11]. Healing through secondary intention often leads to an unstable scar prone to repeated ulceration, particularly in neuropathic plantar wounds and those at the junction of plantar and dorsal skin surfaces [12]. Obtaining stable, durable, and functional wound closure of a diabetic foot wound or open pedal amputation through plastic surgical techniques is essential to limit the potential for repeated ulceration, infection, and "supra-pedal" amputation [13]. Myriad conservative and surgical techniques can be used to obtain wound closure. The authors discuss their approach and present operative pearls for their most commonly employed plastic surgical techniques to provide adequate soft tissue coverage of diabetic foot wounds. Emphasis is placed on the techniques necessary to perform these procedures and the surgical thought process involved in closing diabetic foot wounds.

* Corresponding author.
E-mail address: zgonis@uthscsa.edu (T. Zgonis).

doi:10.1016/j.cpm.2007.03.002 *podiatric.theclinics.com*

Surgical rationale

The goal of wound healing in the diabetic foot is to obtain durable wound closure to salvage a stable and functional limb while minimizing operative risks [14–16]. The decision for the type of wound closure in the diabetic foot depends on several factors (Box 1).

Box 1. Factors that influence wound closure procedures

Wound
Location
Depth
Size
Tissue extensibility/contracture
Exudate
Bacterial colonization

Vascular
Arterial insufficiency
Venous insufficiency
Lymphedema

Deformity
Charcot neuroarthropathy (stable versus unstable)
Underlying bone prominence
Equinus

Previous infection
Superficial (soft tissue)
Deep (bone or joint involvement)

Host
Controlled or uncontrolled diabetes mellitus
Renal insufficiency
Coronary artery disease
Congestive heart failure
Anemia
Hypertension
Malnutrition
Tobacco, alcohol, or drug dependency
Ambulatory and functional status
Age of the patient (life expectancy)
Psychosocial status
Obesity
Compliance

A reconstructive ladder from least complex to most complex assists the surgeon in the decision-making process (Box 2) [16]. In reality, this process represents more of an "elevator" than a ladder, which would require climbing each rung in succession, because some procedures are not appropriate for certain patients, require a protracted period of time, or are not possible at certain institutions [14,15].

Management of complex diabetic foot wounds that have been present for many months or years begins with the medical management and stabilization of the patient. The exception is when diabetic foot wounds become severely infected, mandating urgent or emergent surgery to prevent limb loss or death [17–21]. When the patient presents with a severe diabetic foot infection that is life- or limb-threatening, surgery is performed acutely to eradicate infection, and soft tissue reconstruction is delayed until the patient is medically stabilized and the characteristics of the wound are optimized [17–21]. The overall management of diabetic foot wounds is best handled through a multidisciplinary approach, which includes treatment by some or all of the following depending on the specific arrangements in the hospital: a foot and ankle surgeon, vascular surgeon, plastic surgeon, internist, endocrinologist, cardiologist, physiatrist, wound care nurse, physical therapist, psychologist, and nutritionist [1,2,21–23]. The roles of each provider need to be made clear from the initial admission of the patient and redefined on a regular basis to avoid misunderstandings, repeated services, delays in care, and excess financial cost. Using a team approach, the multiple comorbidities commonly found in patients with diabetes should be addressed and coordinated with regard to the timing of surgery. The timing of the surgery can be as significant as the quality of the surgery. The surgeon should address obvious issues that could compromise the surgical outcome before surgical reconstruction, such as infection, vascular insufficiency, poor cardiac output, and anemia [12]. Numerous techniques are used to obtain wound closure in the diabetic foot. The procedure chosen must be tailored to each patient and circumstance to obtain soft tissue

Box 2. Soft tissue reconstructive elevator for the foot and ankle

Simple

Healing by secondary intention
Primary wound closure
Skin grafting (split versus full-thickness)
Local fascial or fasciocutaneous flaps
Local muscle or musculocutaneous flaps
Pedicled composite flaps
Composite vascularized osteocutaneous flaps
Free tissue transfer with microvascular anastomosis

Complex

coverage that is durable and mechanically sound [3,5,13,16,24,25]. The simplest and least invasive modalities should be used first when feasible. Complex surgical reconstructions should be reserved for the "fully optimized" patient; simpler procedures should be considered for patients with underlying comorbidities that may necessitate protracted and complicated management.

Surgical débridement

The most important initial step in treating diabetic foot soft tissue defects is to perform a timely and complete surgical débridement [26]. This process entails the surgical excision of all nonviable or infected soft tissue and bone so that the margins and base of the soft tissue defect are healthy and viable. Gentle retraction and meticulous soft tissue handling should be employed to preserve the viable tissue adjacent to the defect; however, the débridement should not be limited because of the size or location of the index wound, because proper soft tissue reconstruction can only be performed after successful débridement and wound preparation regardless of its size, depth, or location. Deep bone and soft tissues obtained intraoperatively under aseptic technique should be cultured to ensure the patient is placed on appropriate culture-specific, targeted antibiotics [27]. Wounds that are chronic but appear healthy also should be débrided to convert the wound to an acute wound to allow progression through the normal healing phases [26]. The authors initially perform radical sharp débridement of infected or nonviable wounds to the level of viable bleeding tissue in the operating room unless a deep space abscess is present, at which time it must be drained immediately regardless of the patient's location, nothing-by-mouth status, and other medical issues.

Surgical wound débridement should be performed without the use of a tourniquet to appropriately evaluate the viability of the regional soft tissue and underlying structures. If there is exposed bone or a suspicion of underlying osteomyelitis, bone cultures are obtained at the index of surgery through the use of a bone trephine or rapid resection of the involved joints followed by application of a polymethylmethacrylate antibiotic loaded bone cement (PMMA-ALBC). This procedure initiates the filling of the defect until the final reconstructive surgery is performed and a bone graft used.

After adequate surgical débridement, the wound is irrigated with copious amounts of saline to reduce the number of bacteria present in the wound. The authors' technique involves several steps. First, the limb is placed inside an irrigation basin that has a notch cut out of it to accept the lower limb. The basin is covered by a radiograph cassette cover with a suction tube placed to remove the irrigation. Next, the wound is irrigated with 3 L of sterile saline using a pulse lavage system (Interpulse System; Stryker Instruments, Kalamazoo, Michigan). A Gram stain and aerobic and anaerobic cultures are then obtained from the depths of the wound to determine what bacterial species remain to further aide in medical and surgical decision making. Either bacitracin or Neosporin is infiltrated into the remaining 3 L of sterile saline, and the wound is again irrigated using the pulse lavage system to afford regional asepsis. At this point, the outer gloves of the operative team are changed, and all instruments used in the initial débridement are removed from the surgical field to reduce the potential for further wound contamination. Meticulous hemostasis is achieved with a combination of electrocautery with bipolar cautery and ligation using metallic ligation clips, because this is the least reactive foreign substance available and does not require the protracted series of steps necessary to perform suture ligation that can entrap vital structures beyond the vessel intended for ligation.

The authors have found that the use of PMMA-ABLC beads is a simple means of promoting regional asepsis, filling dead spaces, and maintaining a moist environment within the wound because the antibiotics readily leach from the beads over several days into the blood coagulum. PMMA-ABLC beads (Fig. 1A) are most commonly fashioned by one of the surgical members at the time the wound is being irrigated, because, at that point, the final defect is appreciated, allowing for "economy of motion" in the operating room that saves time. The PMMA-ABLC beads are placed into the defect to cover all vital structures including bone and are covered by gently approximating the skin edges (Fig. 1B, C) and covering them with petroleum-impregnated gauze, or by placing an adhesive barrier alone or negative pressure therapy. The wound is left undisturbed for 72 hours but evaluated by partially removing the dressing to examine the skin edges for maceration and necrosis.

Following the initial bedside dressing change and wound inspection under clean conditions, serial débridement in the operating room is performed as needed to obtain a stable wound free of necrotic tissue and cardinal signs of infection. At each dressing change, the skin about the foot, ankle, and lower leg is cleansed with a surgical scrub brush impregnated with antibiotic, and the wound is irrigated with 1 L of sterile saline. A useful technique is to use a 1-L intravenous bag of sterile saline for irrigation. It is not uncommon for a patient to be brought back to the operating room several times for débridement before the wound is optimized for definitive closure. Failure to achieve an adequately débrided wound will likely lead to failure of any attempt at soft tissue reconstruction [1,2,12,13,26]. The authors typically use this time to access tissue perfusion and compare it with tissue perfusion that was evident intraoperatively to determine the need for vascular intervention. In poorly perfused wounds, expediting vascular intervention to prevent further tissue loss is essential to limb salvage [23,28]. The authors typically use a power hydrodissection tool (Versajet Hydrosurgery System; Smith & Nephew, Memphis, Tennessee) (Fig. 2) during serial débridement to remove any remaining nonviable tissue or granulation tissue where bacterial colonization may be evident. This device creates a localized vacuum effect (Venturi effect) that allows for hydration of the wound, precise débridement preventing excessive soft tissue loss, and irrigation. McGlamry elevators or uterine curettes are cost effective and useful in débriding

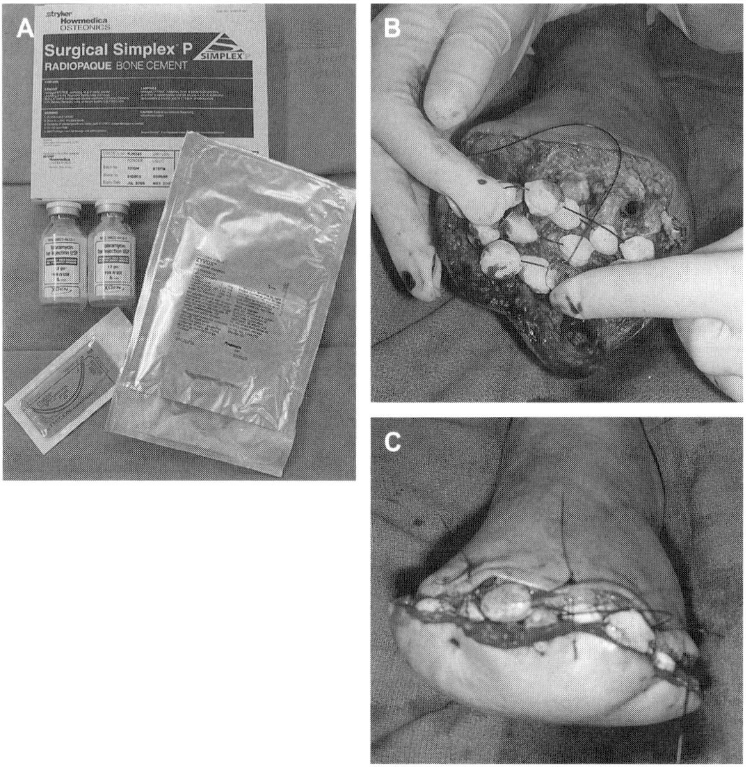

Fig. 1. (*A*) Components used to create PMMA-ABLC. (*B*) PMMA-ABLC beads measuring between 5 and 10 mm in diameter have been applied to a No. 2 nylon suture that allows for postoperative MRI if needed, which would not be possible if metallic wire was used. The nylon material is a monofilament and is much less likely to harbor bacteria when compared with umbilical tape, which is commonly used by some surgeons. The beads are gently placed within the wound. (*C*) Widely spaced sutures using 2-0 nylon have been placed to prevent migration of the PMMA-ABLC beads without undue tension.

granulation tissue for final wound bed preparation. After appropriate wound bed preparation, negative pressure therapy can be used to facilitate granulation tissue until definitive soft tissue reconstruction is performed [24].

Split-thickness skin grafting

Split-thickness skin grafts offer many advantages in the management of diabetic foot wounds (Box 3) [12,16,29–31]. The grafts can be applied to wounds with exposed healthy granulation tissue, dermis, fascia, muscle, peritenon, paratenon, and periosteum [12,29,31]. A split-thickness skin graft should not be used in wounds with greater than 5 mm of exposed bone or tendon, in adipose tissue, or in weight-bearing areas [29,31,32]. The authors

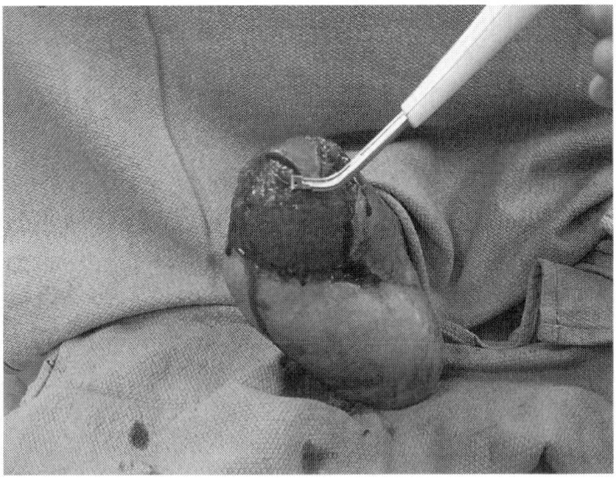

Fig. 2. The use of a Hydrosurgery system to provide a precise débridement, preventing excessive soft tissue loss and creating a suitable wound bed for application of a split-thickness skin graft.

often use deep fascia, surrounding tissue, periosteum, or muscle to obtain closure of exposed bone before application of the split-thickness skin graft. Our technique involves suturing the dermis of the wound edge to the deeper subcutaneous tissues to prevent deep cavities and uneven surfaces, creating a smaller wound for insetting of the graft. This technique is particularly useful before split-thickness skin grafting the donor site of the reverse flow sural artery flap. The main prerequisites for split-thickness skin grafting are the presence of a granular wound bed with no drainage, malodor, periwound erythema, or edema. Granulation tissue is an indicator of skin graft readiness and survival and is usually not present if the wound bed is poorly perfused or contaminated. The most superficial layer of granulation tissue should be gently débrided to reduce the bacterial count in the interstices of this tissue before insetting the skin graft [33]. Skin grafts will fail in the presence of any bacteria species with a concentration greater than 10^5 or in the presence of beta-hemolytic streptococcus, *Pseudomonas* species, and

Box 3. Advantages of split-thickness skin grafting in the diabetic foot

- "Easy take" in the foot and lower extremity
- Better chance of survival in vascular compromised patients
- Simple to perform and easily available
- Reliable and minimally invasive
- Can cover large open wounds and amputations
- Cost effective if it needs to be repeated
- Useful for soft tissue defects on non–weight-bearing areas
- Closing donor sites for local flaps or pedicle flaps

methacillin-resistant *Staphylococcus aureus* [33]. Appropriate asepsis of the wound bed and granulation tissue with the use of a silver-impregnated hydrogel is a useful means of maintaining a moist wound bed and providing regional asepsis without inhibiting cellular activity within the wound [34,35].

After débridement and preparation of the recipient diabetic foot wound, the harvest site is prepared again with Betadine or alcohol. The area is marked to ensure the appropriate size needed and infiltrated with 1% lidocaine with 1:100,000 epinephrine. The donor site can be infiltrated after harvest of the split-thickness skin graft to avoid the creation of an uneven surface while using the power dermatome. The area is then lubricated with mineral oil or sterile saline. An assistant maintains constant traction on the proximal and distal aspect of the area that the graft is to be harvested from. This traction is an extremely important step because any laxity in the tissue will make passage of the dermatome more difficult and lead to multiple "hops and skips" over the skin, creating an irregular graft and unsightly scar (Fig. 3A, B). A power air-driven dermatome using a 2-in blade set at 0.0018 in is routinely used in the diabetic foot. The harvested skin graft is then placed on a dermal carrier and meshed at a 1:1.5 ratio using a commercially available mesher. The graft can also be fenestrated manually using a surgical scalpel (ie, pie crusting). Meshing and pie crusting increase the surface area of the graft while permitting drainage that reduces the potential to form a hematoma or seroma [31,32].

At this point, the authors use autogenous platelet-rich and poor plasma (Accelerate; Exactech, Gainesville, Florida). Platelet-poor plasma (ie, fibrinogen) is applied to the recipient and donor site (Fig. 4A, B) [31,36]. The donor site is then covered with a petroleum-impregnated gauze dressing, absorptive pads, and elastic bandage. The donor site is not exposed for 2 to 3 weeks' time to allow adequate re-epithelialization to occur and to limit the pain and repeated trauma of more frequent dressing changes. The

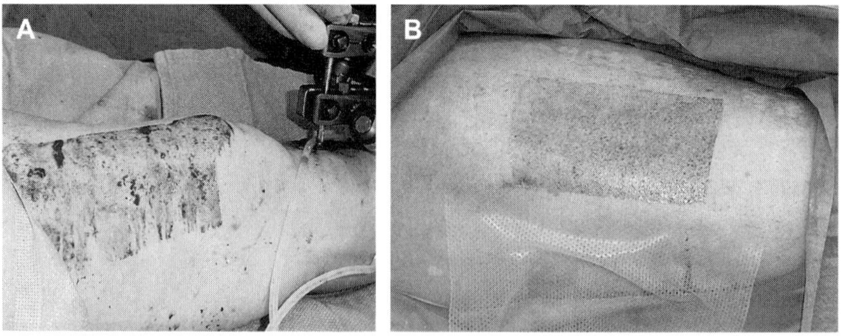

Fig. 3. (*A*) Example of a poorly placed and irregular split-thickness skin graft donor site due to improper tension during harvest of the graft. (*B*) Example of a properly placed and performed split-thickness skin graft donor site associated with appropriate tension by the surgical assistant.

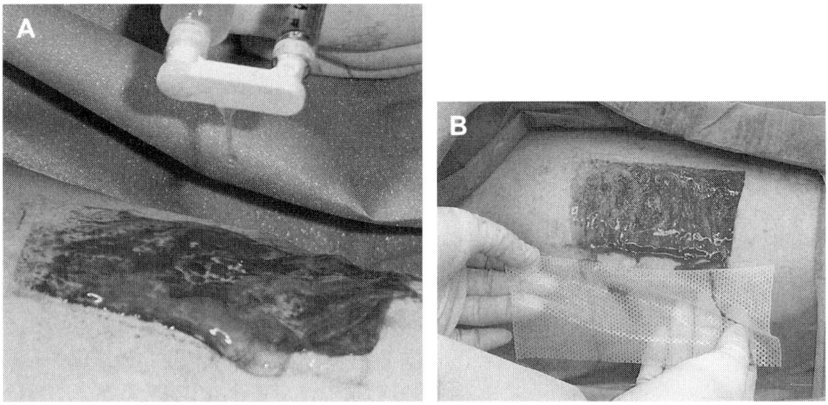

Fig. 4. (*A*) Platelet-poor plasma is shown being applied to the split-thickness skin graft donor site where it has already begun to "gel." (*B*) Final appearance of a split-thickness skin graft donor site from the thigh that has been covered with platelet-poor plasma before dressing application.

petroleum-impregnated gauze is simply trimmed and allowed to shed over time as the skin epithelializes.

The split-thickness skin graft is then secured to the recipient site with skin staples or sutures (Fig. 5A). Platelet-rich plasma (ie, platelet-derived concentrated growth factors) is then applied to the secured graft (Fig. 5B). A bolster or stent dressing is applied to prevent motion at the graft interface until the skin graft has been completely inosculated [37–39]. The authors apply a specialized hydrogel-impregnated gauze pad (Theragauze Absolute Non-Stick Moist Wound Care; Soluble Systems, Newport News, Virginia) directly over the graft site followed by a layer of silicone-impregnated dressing (Mepitel; MöIncycke Health Care, Norcross, Georgia) that is stapled to the perimeter of the graft. Surgical sponges or pieces of sterile cotton cast padding are then soaked in saline and applied over the site (Fig. 5C), followed by folding of the silicone-impregnated dressing edges that are stapled to the saline-soaked padding underneath (Fig. 5D). This method represents a simple, cost-effective bolster dressing that is easier to apply and remove when compared with traditional multiple suture type dressings. The bolster dressing should be removed several weeks after application to avoid the inadvertent loss of skin grafts during dressing changes; however, it is acceptable to evaluate the graft application site before this time if cardinal signs of infection are present. Additionally, negative pressure therapy can be employed if the application site is highly irregular or covers a large surface area [40–44].

Local flaps

Local flaps are extremely useful in soft tissue reconstruction of diabetic plantar wounds. These flaps provide durability by replacing "lost" soft

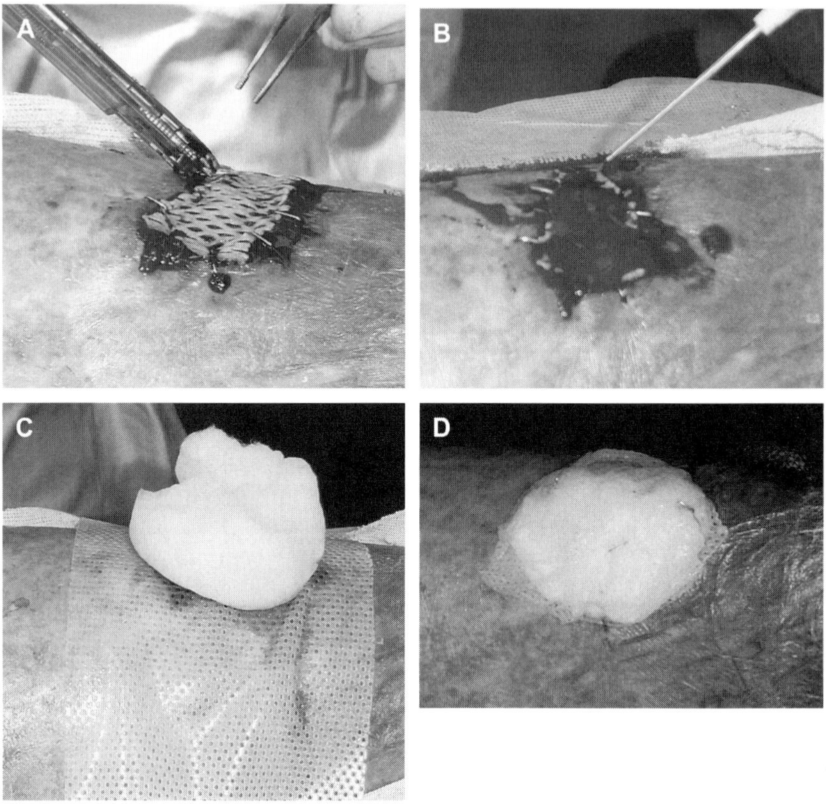

Fig. 5. (*A*) Split-thickness skin graft stapled in place over a properly prepared wound bed that has been covered with a thin layer of platelet-poor plasma. (*B*) Platelet-rich plasma applied to the split-thickness skin graft. (*C*) A silicone-impregnated dressing has been applied over a hydrogel-impregnated gauze dressing, stapled about its perimeter, and covered with saline-soaked cast padding. (*D*) The edges of the silicone-impregnated dressing have been folded over the saline-soaked cotton padding and stapled in place.

tissue with "like" soft tissue. Using local flaps on the plantar aspect of the foot in diabetic patients with neuropathy limits the formation of an unstable scar that is prone to future skin breakdown when healing occurs by secondary intention [12]. Local flaps include the epidermis, dermis, subcutaneous tissue, and, in certain unique circumstances, the fascia and underlying muscle [45]. Local flaps based on the required dissection offer the advantage of excellent exposure to surgically address underlying skeletal deformity without creating additional incisions [46].

Local flaps are vascularized by a cutaneous artery, a musculocutaneous perforating artery, or a septocutaneous perforating artery [47–49]. The vast majority of these septofasciocutaneous perforating vessels are found between the digital slips of the plantar aponeurosis in the plantar forefoot and along the intermuscular septum of the abductor hallucis, flexor digitorum brevis, and abductor digit minimi in the plantar midfoot and distal rearfoot [50,51]. These vessels have been shown to be more closely spaced together in the plantar forefoot and distal midfoot and more widely spaced apart in the plantar proximal midfoot and rearfoot [50,51]. Identification of perforators can be established and marked out by using a hand-held Doppler probe on the operative field [50]. Although the blood supply to a local flap may appear random, this does not imply that incision placement and flap design are random. Knowledge of the vascular anatomy of the foot and known angiosomes is essential for proper flap placement and design. Local flaps are typically based on geometric designs, the mobility of the soft tissues, the nature of their movement, and the angiosomes of the foot. Local flaps can be advanced, transposed, or rotated to provide soft tissue coverage of the defect [45]. The safest design of a local flap is where the movement of the flap occurs over the area of greatest skin elasticity or lines of maximum extensibility and toward the nearest dominant perforating artery [12]. The surgeon should be aware that necessary resection of bone secondary to osteomyelitis or deformity often creates soft tissue laxity permitting flap movement that would otherwise be unavailable [46]. As a result, flap designs commonly used in the diabetic foot are based on the anatomic location of the soft tissue defect (Box 4).

To ensure viability of the flap, meticulous gentle surgical technique must be performed throughout the procedure. Traction should only be used when needed, and delicate instrumentation is important to prevent inadvertent tissue ischemia. Local flaps are routinely created by undermining in the suprafascial plane by releasing the tethering effects of the mooring ligaments while preserving the perforating vessels to the flap. Undermining should be kept to a minimum to permit adequate mobility of the flap. Excessive undermining

Box 4. Local flap designs by anatomic location

Digits and forefoot
Single and bilobed flaps
Toe fillet flap
Rhomboid flaps
Double-Z rhomboid flaps
V-Y advancement flaps

Midfoot and distal rearfoot
Rotational flaps—arc shaped
Transpositional flaps—tongue shaped
T flaps
V-Y advancement flaps

and dissection can violate perforating vessels and jeopardize the viability of the flap by creating regional ischemia, venous congestion, or both. Meticulous hemostasis is essential to prevent hematoma formation deep to the flap that can serve as a nidus for infection or result in thrombosis of the perforating vessels and thereby adversely affect flap viability. For this reason, the flaps are generally dissected and raised under tourniquet control. Before insetting the flap, the tourniquet is deflated to ensure adequate hemostasis and flap viability. The flap is then sutured using a minimum amount of deep sutures to prevent ischemia to the undersurface of the flap. The authors prefer to use a combination of staples and 2-0 nylon suture.

The postoperative care of local flaps is extremely important and mandates close observation to detect complications early to prevent flap failure. The patient must be placed on bed rest with the involved extremity elevated on one pillow with the heel off of the weight-bearing surface of the bedding. This positioning can also be accomplished by using external fixation to offload the local flap. The flap is checked every 2 hours during the first 24 hours for signs of ischemia and venous congestion (Fig. 6A, B).

Muscle flaps

Local intrinsic foot muscle flaps can be useful in covering plantar, medial, and lateral soft tissue defects in the diabetic foot, especially when there is exposed hardware, bone, joint capsule, or tendon, and are particularly useful in the treatment of osteomyelitis [12,46,52,53]. They provide increased local blood flow to the area, enhancing the deliverance of antibiotics and white blood cells and facilitating the healing process. Muscle flaps can be harvested to include the cutaneous portion supplied by the musculocutaneous perforating vessels; however, in the foot, this is often difficult, and muscle flaps are often harvested in isolation followed by coverage with a split-thickness skin graft.

The most common types of muscle flaps in the foot include the abductor hallucis, flexor digitorum brevis, abductor digiti minimi, and the extensor

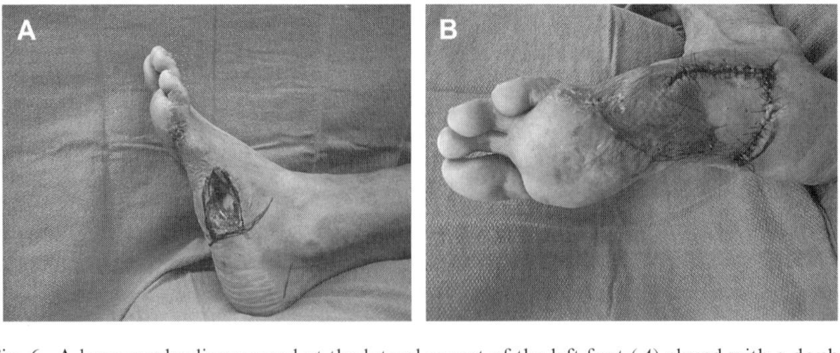

Fig. 6. A large nonhealing wound at the lateral aspect of the left foot (*A*) closed with a double local rotational advancement flap (*B*).

digitorum brevis [12,52–54]. These muscle flaps are classified as type II because they contain a dominant vascular pedicle and several more distal minor pedicles allowing for easy rotation and various modifications [12,52–54]. Dissection is routinely performed from distal (ie, insertion) to proximal (ie, origin), allowing mobilization of the distal portion of the muscle to provide coverage. The surgeon needs to understand how far proximal dissection can be performed for each muscle. Anatomic dissections on cadavers can provide the surgeon with a better understanding of the extensibility, as well as the limitations, of intrinsic foot muscle flaps. A detailed knowledge of the muscle vasculature expedites harvest and permits modifications while minimizing complications. An example of a modification would be to harvest the muscle from proximal (ie, origin) to distal (ie, insertion), relying on the distal perforators and collateral circulation through retrograde flow to maintain muscle viability.

Muscle flaps must be handled delicately, especially in diabetic patients with calcified vessels and muscle atrophy. Intraoperative use of a Doppler ultrasound probe and loupe magnification should be used to minimize intraoperative complications associated with disruption or failure to include the dominant vascular pedicle. Insetting the muscle should be done without excessive tension or torsion on the dominant vascular pedicle so that blood flow and muscle viability are not compromised. The muscle is rotated in one fluent motion, and the amount of time that it is handled is kept to a minimum. The muscle is then sutured to the dermis and fascia at the perimeter of the defect. The vascular inflow should be assessed with a Doppler ultrasound probe after insetting the muscle. If the inflow is compromised, the muscle must be repositioned to ensure adequate blood flow. A split-thickness skin graft is then applied along with a bolster dressing as described previously (Fig. 7A–C).

Pedicle flaps

Pedicle flaps differ from local flaps in that they require isolation of an identifiable, named neurovascular bundle supplying the composite block of tissue intended to be transferred. The creation of a pedicle flap requires separation of either the source vessels or septofasciocutaneous perforating vessels. A pedicle flap may be fasciocutaneous, adipofascial, or musculocutaneous in certain circumstances. As a result of the collateral network of vessels in the foot and lower leg, pedicle flaps may be created with an antegrade (ie, anatomic) or retrograde (ie, reverse) flow depending on the pressure gradients created from ligation of the source or septofasciocutaneous vessels. Pedicle flaps may be raised adjacent to a soft tissue defect, much like a local flap, or from a site at a distance from the soft tissue defect, much like a free flap. This choice offers the surgeon many reconstructive options in addressing soft tissue defects about the foot. Pedicle flaps should be created with the notion that the donor sites should not compromise weight-bearing areas of

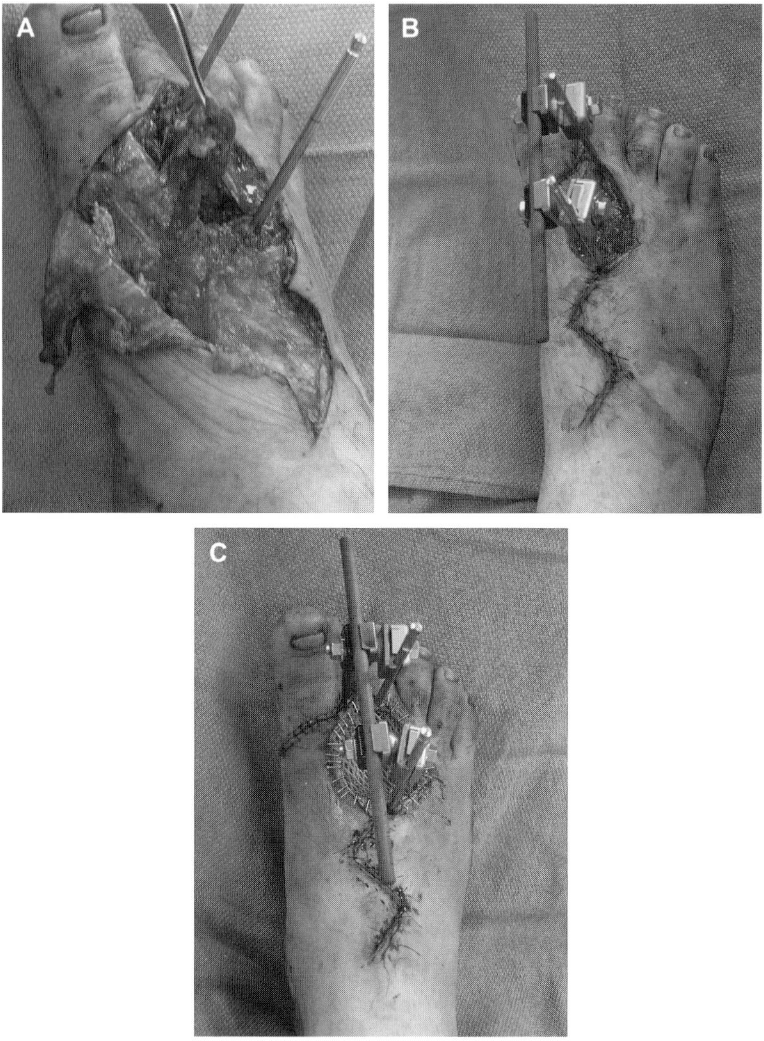

Fig. 7. Harvesting the insertion of the abductor hallucis muscle (*A*) to cover a severe soft tissue and bone defect at the second metatarsal shaft (*B*), followed by a split-thickness skin graft and external fixation for stabilization and daily monitoring (*C*).

the foot. The pedicle flaps most commonly used for diabetic foot wounds are the great toe fibular artery flap, the medial plantar artery flap, and the reverse flow sural artery flap [46]. These flaps provide soft tissue coverage of the forefoot, midfoot, and rearfoot regions, respectively [46].

The great toe fibular artery flap is an adipofasciocutaneous flap that can provide coverage to defects plantar to the metatarsal heads [55–58]. The flap is raised from the lateral aspect of the hallux and includes the digital artery from the first dorsal metatarsal artery and accompanying vein and nerve.

This flap offers the advantage of covering defects as lateral as the fifth metatarsal head [55,57]. The donor site can be closed primarily or coverage obtained with a split-thickness skin graft or full-thickness (ie, pinch) graft. Primary closure of the donor site is facilitated by removing the lateral one third of the proximal and distal phalanges of the hallux, which does not affect function and creates enough laxity in the soft tissues to afford tension-free primary closure [57].

The medial plantar artery flap is useful for soft tissue defects about the dorsal medial or plantar lateral midfoot and heel. This flap is the "work horse" for soft tissue reconstruction in patients who have a wound in conjunction with a diabetic Charcot neuroarthropathy "rocker-bottom" deformity [46]. This flap is often used in conjunction with arthrodesis or ostectomy procedures to address the underlying osseous Charcot deformity. Flaps raised from the instep of the foot are supplied by two vessels: (1) the collateral flow from the dorsalis pedis and (2) perforators off the superficial branch of the medial plantar artery [59–63]. When the medial plantar artery flap is raised with a medially based peninsula (ie, skin island), both angiosomes are preserved; however, if needed, the flap may be converted to an island based off the medial plantar artery, eliminating one source of vascular supply to increase mobilization of the pedicle [60]. The medial plantar artery is commonly raised with antegrade flow but can be raised with retrograde flow when used for more plantar distal soft tissue defects [61,62]. The dissection required for raising the medial plantar artery flap offers the surgeon a direct approach from the plantar aspect of the foot to address any underlying osseous deformity (Fig. 8A, B).

The reverse flow sural artery neurofasciocutaneous flap is useful for coverage of defects around the heel, ankle, and lower leg [12,64–68]. The flap can be of various sizes, with the largest sural artery flap reported, 12 cm × 15 cm, offering the advantage of providing soft tissue coverage to areas that previously required free tissue transfer with microvascular anastomosis [69]. The flap is raised from the posterolateral aspect of the leg based on the arterial supply from the median superficial sural artery and arteria nervorum of the medial sural nerve that anastomose distally with the fasciocutaneous branches off the perforators of the peroneal artery, resulting in retrograde blood flow. Venous drainage is obtained from venae comitantes to the median superficial sural artery and the lesser saphenous vein. The sural artery flap has been shown to have high complication rates, particularly in patients with diabetes, arterial insufficiency, venous insufficiency, and multiple comorbidities [70]. Venous congestion resulting in flap necrosis is the most frequent complication encountered, with a reported incidence of up to 70% in patients with multiple comorbidities [70]. For this reason, many technical pearls are used to minimize the complications commonly associated with this pedicled flap (Box 5) [71–73].

The authors use the noninvasive vascular laboratory preoperatively to mark the course of the lesser saphenous vein including measurement of

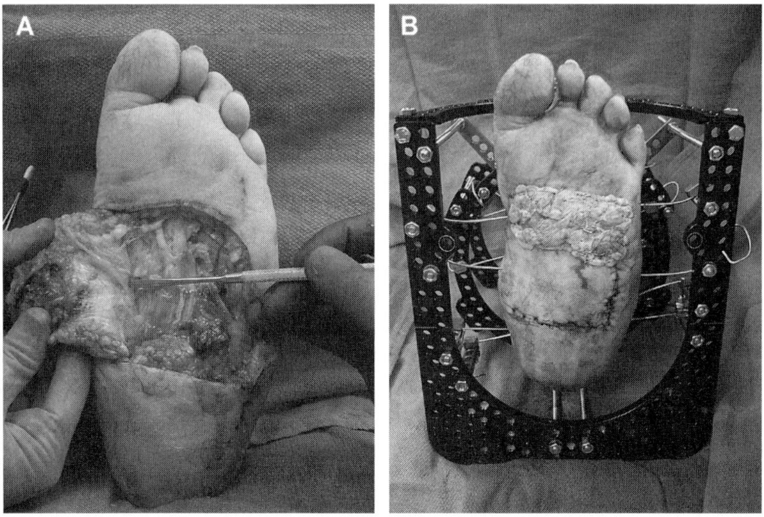

Fig. 8. A medial plantar artery flap for soft tissue coverage at the plantar lateral column of a Charcot foot (*A*), followed by a lateral column arthrodesis, circular multiplane external fixator, and skin grafting to the non–weight-bearing donor site (*B*).

the diameter of the vein. This examination allows precise incision and donor site placement, minimizing unnecessary dissection and reducing operative time. The next step is to mark the level of the most distal peroneal arterial perforator, which is usually found 5 cm proximal to the distal tip of the lateral malleolus between the fibula and Achilles tendon. This position is confirmed using a hand-held Doppler ultrasound probe on the operative field. The flap is then designed based on the size of the defect. Maximizing the

Box 5. Technical tips for the reverse flow sural artery flap

- Mark the course of the lesser saphenous vein.
- Confirm placement of the last septocutaneous perforator from the peroneal artery with a hand-held Doppler ultrasound probe.
- Make a "Z" incision over the pedicle components.
- Use loupe magnification.
- Use a cutaneous tail over the pedicle components.
- Delay the sural artery flap in a compromised flap or patient.
- Use split-thickness skin grafting over the pedicle components.
- Use external fixation to off-load the flap, prevent motion, and mandate elevation of the limb.
- Perform close observation in the postoperative period.
- Medicinal leeches should be readily available.

distance the most proximal edge of the flap is created from the popliteal fossa has been shown to decrease complication rates, because the blood supply is more robust and venous drainage more complete the further from the popliteal fossa the cutaneous portion of the flap is raised. The authors typically use a Z-incision from the flap to the level of the soft tissue defect.

Dissection of the flap under loupe magnification begins proximal to distal initially to ligate and include with the composite block of tissue the median superficial sural artery and the lesser saphenous vein along with identification of the sural nerve. These structures have great variability in their relationship, and great care should be taken to identify and include each structure to limit the potential for complications. The flap is raised either supra- or subfascial. At this point, dissection is performed from distal to proximal isolating the well-identifiable pedicle components. Incorporating a cutaneous tail or extension over the pedicle components has been shown to decrease complications associated with tension over the pedicle site and should be considered in compromised patients [69]. The tourniquet, if used, should be released to evaluate the viability of the cutaneous and adipofascial portions of the flap before insetting. In scenarios of questionable flap viability, a delayed procedure can be performed to open choke vessels to increase blood flow to the flap, which involves applying a petroleum-based gauze dressing between the underlying superficial posterior muscles and deep surface of the flap and gentle reapproximation of the skin edges over nonsuction drains positioned at gravity [73–75].

The flap is evaluated several times daily for signs of necrosis, ischemia, venous congestion, and infection. After 7 to 10 days of delay, the patient is returned to the operating theater, and the flap is re-elevated and inset into the defect. Following a delayed procedure, the tissues within the flap are usually more edematous and less pliable, which can create a mismatch between the dimensions of the flap and the defect intended to be covered. Liberal use of split-thickness skin grafts to provide coverage of any exposed tissue not covered by the flap should be employed rather than attempting to undermine the perimeter of the wound or create tension on the flap to cover the defect. The flap is then inset without torsion or tension to the pedicle components and secured using skin staples and sutures as described previously. Closure over the pedicle components is achieved primarily or more commonly via a split-thickness skin graft. If less than 5 cm, the donor site can be closed primarily. Larger defects are closed using a split-thickness skin graft from the ipsilateral extremity. The literature has shown that the use of external fixation to off-load this flap decreases the likelihood of complications and flap failure [70,72]. The foot can be positioned in slight plantar flexion minimizing tension across the pedicle component.

Numerous techniques are employed to prevent complications associated with the reverse flow sural artery flap to achieve successful soft tissue coverage of the most challenging wounds in the diabetic foot. Postoperatively, close monitoring as described previously is paramount to ensure a successful

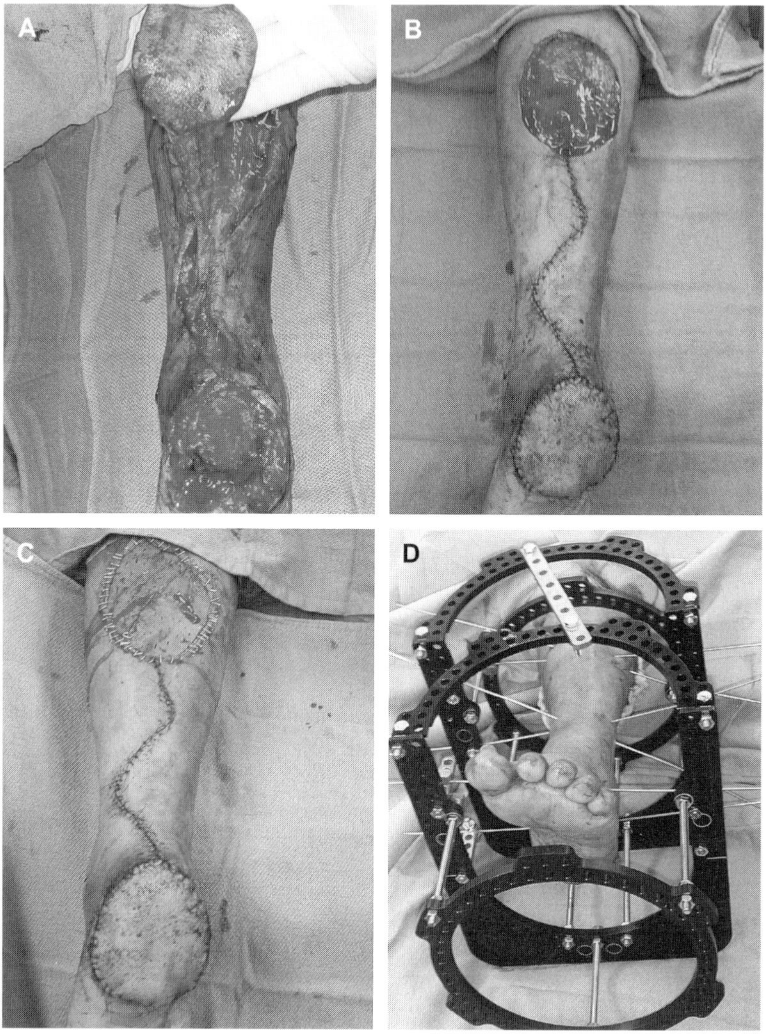

Fig. 9. Harvesting the reverse flow sural pedicle flap (*A*) to cover a large defect on the posterior aspect of the calcaneus (*B*). Harvesting is followed by a split-thickness skin graft to the donor site (*C*) and an off-loading external fixation device (*D*).

outcome. In this regard, the authors have found it essential to have medicinal leeches available for immediate use and employ them at the first sign of venous congestion. This complication is verified by a bluish hue to the flap when compared with the adjacent surrounding tissues, by dark almost purple blood expressed following perforation of the cutaneous portion of the flap with a No. 11 blade, and by coolness of the cutaneous portion of the flap when compared with adjacent tissue. Once identified, one medicinal leech per area the size of a silver dollar should be employed every 6 to 8 hours for the next 7 to 10 days or until the venous congestion has resolved following recannulization of the venous outflow. A significant amount of blood loss should be anticipated if leeches are necessary. The acute protracted nature of the blood loss can cause significant hemodynamic instability for the patient who is already compromised. Additionally, a significant inflammatory response occurs following the administration of blood product, which can have a detrimental effect on flap viability. For these reasons, the authors prefer to have the patient obtain an appropriate volume of blood product several days before performing the flap to allow for proper oxygenation of the flap, to create a reserve should the need for medicinal leeches occur, and to limit the need for post-flap blood product resuscitation. Obviously, this soft tissue reconstruction procedure should not be taken lightly or be performed by inexperienced surgeons, and many "fine-points" exist that are beyond the scope of this article (Fig. 9A–D).

Summary

A stepwise approach using the reconstructive elevator in the surgical management of diabetic foot wounds is essential for functional limb salvage. A multidisciplinary team consisting of surgical and medical disciplines is needed to adequately manage these wounds. The surgeon should have experience and knowledge in evaluating the diabetic foot wound to determine when and how to intervene. Nontraditional thinking incorporated with sound plastic surgical techniques is leading to the successful management of these surgical challenges. The goal of limb salvage is to provide the patient with a limb that is stable, mechanically sound, and resistant to further breakdown while resuming an ambulatory status. Custom shoes, in-shoe orthoses, and bracing are used postoperatively as adjuncts to soft tissue reconstruction to assist in achieving this long-term goal.

References

[1] Frykberg RG, Armstrong DG, Giurini J, et al. Diabetic foot disorders: a clinical practice guideline. American College of Foot and Ankle Surgeons. J Foot Ankle Surg 2000;39(Suppl 5):S1–60.

[2] Frykberg RG, Zgonis T, Armstrong DG, et al. Diabetic foot disorders: a clinical practice guideline (2006 revision). J Foot Ankle Surg 2006;45(Suppl 5):S1–66.

[3] Kantor J, Margolis DJ. Treatment options for diabetic neuropathic foot ulcers: a cost-effectiveness analysis. Dermatol Surg 2001;27(4):347–51.

[4] Margolis DJ, Kantor J, Santanna J, et al. Risk factors for delayed healing of neuropathic diabetic foot ulcers: a pooled analysis. Arch Dermatol 2000;136(12):1531–5.

[5] Margolis DJ, Kantor J, Berlin JA. Healing of diabetic neuropathic foot ulcers receiving standard treatment: a meta-analysis. Diabetes Care 1999;22(5):692–5.

[6] Margolis DJ, Allen-Taylor L, Hoffstad O, et al. Diabetic neuropathic foot ulcers: predicting which ones will not heal. Am J Med 2003;115(8):627–31.

[7] Margolis DJ, Allen-Taylor L, Hoffstad O, et al. Healing diabetic neuropathic foot ulcers: are we getting better? Diabet Med 2005;22(2):172–6.

[8] Margolis DJ, Allen-Taylor L, Hoffstad O, et al. Diabetic neuropathic foot ulcers: the association of wound size, wound duration, and wound grade on healing. Diabetes Care 2002;25(10):1835–9.
[9] Brem H, Sheehan P, Rosenberg HJ, et al. Evidence-based protocol for diabetic foot ulcers. Plast Reconstr Surg 2006;117(Suppl 7):193S–209S [discussion: 210S–11S].
[10] Brem H, Sheehan P, Boulton AJ. Protocol for treatment of diabetic foot ulcers. Am J Surg 2004;187(5A):1S–10S.
[11] Sommerlad BC, McGrouther DA. Resurfacing the sole: long-term follow-up and comparison of techniques. Br J Plast Surg 1978;31(2):107–16.
[12] Jolly GP, Zgonis T, Blume P. Soft tissue reconstruction of the diabetic foot. Clin Podiatr Med Surg 2003;20(4):757–81.
[13] Cohen BK, Zabel DD, Newton ED, et al. Soft-tissue reconstruction for recalcitrant diabetic foot wounds. J Foot Ankle Surg 1999;38(6):388–93.
[14] Bennett N, Choudhary S. Why climb a ladder when you can take the elevator? Plast Reconstr Surg 2000;105(6):2266.
[15] Gottlieb LJ, Krieger LM. From the reconstructive ladder to the reconstructive elevator. Plast Reconstr Surg 1994;93(7):1503–4.
[16] Levin LS. The reconstructive ladder: an orthoplastic approach. Orthop Clin North Am 1993;24(3):393–409.
[17] Pinzur MS, Sage R, Abraham M, et al. Limb salvage in infected lower extremity gangrene. Foot Ankle 1988;8(4):212–5.
[18] Scher KS, Steele FJ. The septic foot in patients with diabetes. Surgery 1988;104(4):661–6.
[19] Tan JS, Friedman NM, Hazelton-Miller C, et al. Can aggressive treatment of diabetic foot infections reduce the need for above-ankle amputation? Clin Infect Dis 1996;23(2):286–91.
[20] Wieman TJ. Principles of management: the diabetic foot. Am J Surg 2005;190(2):295–9.
[21] Zgonis T, Roukis TS. A systematic approach to diabetic foot infections. Adv Ther 2005;22(3):244–62.
[22] Dargis V, Pantelejeva O, Jonushaite A, et al. Benefits of a multidisciplinary approach in the management of recurrent diabetic foot ulceration in Lithuania: a prospective study. Diabetes Care 1999;22(9):1428–31.
[23] Sumpio BE, Aruny J, Blume PA. The multidisciplinary approach to limb salvage. Acta Chir Belg 2004;104(6):647–53.
[24] Argenta LC, Morykwas MJ. Vacuum-assisted closure: a new method for wound control and treatment. Clinical experience. Ann Plast Surg 1997;38(6):563–76 [discussion: 577].
[25] Hanft JR, Surprenant MS. Healing of chronic foot ulcers in diabetic patients treated with a human fibroblast-derived dermis. J Foot Ankle Surg 2002;41(5):291–9.
[26] Attinger CE, Bulan E, Blume PA. Surgical debridement: the key to successful wound healing and reconstruction. Clin Podiatr Med Surg 2000;17(4):599–630.
[27] Zgonis T, Jolly GP, Buren BJ, et al. Diabetic foot infections and antibiotic therapy. Clin Podiatr Med Surg 2003;20(4):655–69.
[28] Sumpio BE, Lee T, Blume PA. Vascular evaluation and arterial reconstruction of the diabetic foot. Clin Podiatr Med Surg 2003;20(4):689–708.
[29] Donato MC, Novicki DC, Blume PA. Skin grafting: historic and practical approaches. Clin Podiatr Med Surg 2000;17(4):561–98.
[30] Ratner D. Skin grafting: from here to there. Dermatol Clin 1998;16(1):75–90.
[31] Roukis TS, Zgonis T. Skin grafting techniques for soft-tissue coverage of diabetic foot and ankle wounds. J Wound Care 2005;14(4):173–6.
[32] Attinger C. Use of skin grafting in the foot. J Am Podiatr Med Assoc 1995;85(1):49–56.
[33] Robson MC. Wound infection: a failure of wound healing caused by an imbalance of bacteria. Surg Clin North Am 1997;77(3):637–50.
[34] Pospisilova A. [A new generation of dressings in the treatment of leg ulcers]. Cas Lek Cesk 1998;137(9):264–6.

[35] Dissemond J. [Modern wound dressings for the therapy of chronic wounds]. Hautarzt 2006;57(10):881–7.
[36] Roukis TS, Zgonis T, Tiernan B. Autologous platelet-rich plasma for wound and osseous healing: a review of the literature and commercially available products. Adv Ther 2006;23(2):218–37.
[37] Orengo I, Lee MW. Surgical pearl: the "unsuture" technique for skin grafts. J Am Acad Dermatol 1998;38(5 Pt 1):758–9.
[38] Larson PO. Foam-rubber stents for skin grafts. J Dermatol Surg Oncol 1990;16(9):851–4.
[39] Weiner LJ, Moberg AW. An ideal stent for reliable and efficient skin graft application. Ann Plast Surg 1984;13(1):24–8.
[40] Llanos S, Danilla S, Barraza C, et al. Effectiveness of negative pressure closure in the integration of split thickness skin grafts: a randomized, double-masked, controlled trial. Ann Surg 2006;244(5):700–5.
[41] Weinfeld AB, Kelley P, Yuksel E, et al. Circumferential negative-pressure dressing (VAC) to bolster skin grafts in the reconstruction of the penile shaft and scrotum. Ann Plast Surg 2005;54(2):178–83.
[42] Chang KP, Tsai CC, Lin TM, et al. An alternative dressing for skin graft immobilization: negative pressure dressing. Burns 2001;27(8):839–42.
[43] Blackburn JH 2nd, Boemi L, Hall WW, et al. Negative-pressure dressings as a bolster for skin grafts. Ann Plast Surg 1998;40(5):453–7.
[44] Nakayama Y, Iino T, Soeda S. A new method for the dressing of free skin grafts. Plast Reconstr Surg 1990;86(6):1216–9.
[45] Paragas LK, Attinger C, Blume PA. Local flaps. Clin Podiatr Med Surg 2000;17(2):267–318.
[46] Zgonis T, Roukis TS, Frykberg RG, et al. Unstable acute and chronic Charcot's deformity: staged skeletal and soft-tissue reconstruction. J Wound Care 2006;15(6):276–80.
[47] Attinger CE, Evans KK, Bulan E, et al. Angiosomes of the foot and ankle and clinical implications for limb salvage: reconstruction, incisions, and revascularization. Plast Reconstr Surg 2006;117(Suppl 7):261S–93S.
[48] Taylor GI. The angiosomes of the body and their supply to perforator flaps. Clin Plast Surg 2003;30(3):331–42 [v].
[49] Taylor GI, Palmer JH. The vascular territories (angiosomes) of the body: experimental study and clinical applications. Br J Plast Surg 1987;40(2):113–41.
[50] Roukis TS. The Doppler probe for planning septofasciocutaneous advancement flaps on the plantar aspect of the foot: anatomical study and clinical applications. J Foot Ankle Surg 2000;39(5):270–90.
[51] Colen LB, Replogle SL, Mathes SJ. The V-Y plantar flap for reconstruction of the forefoot. Plast Reconstr Surg 1988;81(2):220–8.
[52] Attinger CE, Ducic I, Zelen C. The use of local muscle flaps in foot and ankle reconstruction. Clin Podiatr Med Surg 2000;17(4):681–711.
[53] Attinger CE, Ducic I, Cooper P, et al. The role of intrinsic muscle flaps of the foot for bone coverage in foot and ankle defects in diabetic and nondiabetic patients. Plast Reconstr Surg 2002;110(4):1047–54 [discussion: 1055–57].
[54] Yoshimura Y, Nakajima T, Kami T. Distally based abductor digiti minimi muscle flap. Ann Plast Surg 1985;14(4):375–7.
[55] Buncke HJ Jr, Colen LB. An island flap from the first web space of the foot to cover plantar ulcers. Br J Plast Surg 1980;33(2):242–4.
[56] Colen LB, Buncke HJ. Neurovascular island flaps from the plantar vessels and nerves for foot reconstruction. Ann Plast Surg 1984;12(4):327–32.
[57] Roukis TS, Zgonis T. Modifications of the great toe fibular flap for diabetic forefoot and toe reconstruction. Ostomy Wound Manage 2005;51(6):30–2 [34, 36].
[58] Morain WD. Island toe flaps in neurotrophic ulcers of the foot and ankle. Ann Plast Surg 1984;13(1):1–8.

[59] Miyamoto Y, Ikuta Y, Shigeki S, et al. Current concepts of instep island flap. Ann Plast Surg 1987;19(2):97–102.
[60] Shaw WW, Hidalgo DA. Anatomic basis of plantar flap design: clinical applications. Plast Reconstr Surg 1986;78(5):637–49.
[61] Butler CE, Chevray P. Retrograde-flow medial plantar island flap reconstruction of distal forefoot, toe, and webspace defects. Ann Plast Surg 2002;49(2):196–201.
[62] Bhandari PS, Sobti C. Reverse flow instep island flap. Plast Reconstr Surg 1999;103(7): 1986–9.
[63] Narsete TA. Anatomic design of a sensate plantar flap. Ann Plast Surg 1997;38(5):538–9.
[64] Jolly GP, Zgonis T. Soft tissue reconstruction of the foot with a reverse flow sural artery neurofasciocutaneous flap. Ostomy Wound Manage 2004;50(6):44–9.
[65] Jeng SF, Wei FC. Distally based sural island flap for foot and ankle reconstruction. Plast Reconstr Surg 1997;99(3):744–50.
[66] Donski PK, Fogdestam I. Distally based fasciocutaneous flap from the sural region: a preliminary report. Scand J Plast Reconstr Surg 1983;17(3):191–6.
[67] Huisinga RL, Houpt P, Dijkstra R, et al. The distally based sural artery flap. Ann Plast Surg 1998;41(1):58–65.
[68] Akhtar S, Hameed A. Versatility of the sural fasciocutaneous flap in the coverage of lower third leg and hind foot defects. J Plast Reconstr Aesthet Surg 2006;59(8):839–45.
[69] Yilmaz M, Karatas O, Barutcu A. The distally based superficial sural artery island flap: clinical experiences and modifications. Plast Reconstr Surg 1998;102(7):2358–67.
[70] Baumeister SP, Spierer R, Erdmann D, et al. A realistic complication analysis of 70 sural artery flaps in a multimorbid patient group. Plast Reconstr Surg 2003;112(1):129–40 [discussion: 141–2].
[71] Belfkira F, Forli A, Pradel P, et al. [Distally based sural neurocutaneous flap: clinical experience and technical adaptations. Report of 60 cases]. Ann Chir Plast Esthet 2006;51(3): 199–206.
[72] Noack N, Hartmann B, Kuntscher MV. Measures to prevent complications of distally based neurovascular sural flaps. Ann Plast Surg 2006;57(1):37–40.
[73] Tosun Z, Ozkan A, Karacor Z, et al. Delaying the reverse sural flap provides predictable results for complicated wounds in diabetic foot. Ann Plast Surg 2005;55(2):169–73.
[74] Erdmann D, Gottlieb N, Humphrey JS, et al. Sural flap delay procedure: a preliminary report. Ann Plast Surg 2005;54(5):562–5.
[75] Kneser U, Bach AD, Polykandriotis E, et al. Delayed reverse sural flap for staged reconstruction of the foot and lower leg. Plast Reconstr Surg 2005;116(7):1910–7.

ELSEVIER
SAUNDERS

Clin Podiatr Med Surg
24 (2007) 569–582

CLINICS IN PODIATRIC MEDICINE AND SURGERY

Amputation in Diabetic Patients

Hendrik Van Damme, MD, PhD*,
Raymond Limet, MD, PhD

Department of Cardiovascular Surgery, University Hospital Liège, B 4000 Liège, Belgium

A disproportionate number (more than 50%) of amputations occur in diabetic patients who only represent 5% to 10% of the general population [1–5]. Diabetic patients have a ten times higher risk of amputation when compared with non-diabetic age-adjusted controls. Diabetic patients are at higher risk for limb loss owing to a loss of protective sensation; reduced defense mechanisms, leading to an increased susceptibility to infection; and the presence of distal infrapopliteal arterial occlusive disease. As many as 80% of diabetic feet with trophic lesions lack protective sensation. The sensory neuropathy leads to an insensate foot and predisposes to skin breakdown by unrecognized trauma. Even today, many diabetic patients seek medical care too late when the foot infection or gangrene has evolved to an unsalvageable foot condition. In the series of Abou–Zamzam [4], a late presentation was involved in 25% of all amputations.

In recent years, the need for major amputations in diabetic patients has declined by 50%, mainly as a consequence of education programs [2,3]. This target was specified in 1992 in the Saint Vincent's Declaration [6]. Diabetic foot clinics provide preventive measures and institutional wound care for foot ulcers, such as the abrasion of callosities and adequate wide-toed shoes with cushioning weight-distributive insoles. Further reduction in limb loss has been possible by an aggressive policy toward distal revascularization of tibial and pedal arteries for limb salvage [7–9].

Diabetes-related amputations (major or minor) are characterized by a high failure rate. As many as 15% of transtibial below-knee amputations are ultimately converted to an above-knee amputation. Incisional wound-healing problems after minor toe or ray amputations are observed in 15% to 30% of cases [10–12]. Inadequate perfusion, compromised healing

* Corresponding author. C.H.U. Liège, B 35, Domaine Universitaire du Sart-Tilman, 4000 Liège, Belgium.

E-mail address: hvandamme@chu.ulg.ac.be (H. Van Damme).

0891-8422/07/$ - see front matter
doi:10.1016/j.cpm.2007.03.007

podiatric.theclinics.com

capacity, and an impaired response to infectious microorganisms lead to infected amputation wounds. Infection is often heralded by a loss of glycemic control. Prompt drainage and debridement are of utmost importance. The wound is left open, and serial wet-to-dry dressings are applied. The protracted wound-healing process often takes 2 or more months. Secondary healing of large infected wounds can be promoted by a vacuum-assisted closure device [13,14]. Secondary infection of an amputation wound should not automatically lead to a higher re-amputation [13,15,16]. Recurrent or new foot ulcerations are common in diabetic patients with advanced neuropathy and loss of protective sensory feedback [2,10].

A general rule is to limit amputation to minor ablation whenever possible [12,17]. This approach offers the best perspective of an autonomic gait and independent lifestyle. Only 15% of patients with a successful minor amputation require long-term placement in a nursing facility in comparison with 37% of those who undergo a major amputation [13]. The major disability after limb loss (30% to 50% of major amputees can no longer ambulate and remain wheelchair dependent) argues for foot-sparing surgical techniques.

Amputation conveys horror to the patient, who considers it a mutilating operation modifying his or her self-esteem. This psychologic barrier should be resolved by an overt conversation and comprehensive discussion with the patient. On the other hand, the vascular surgeon considers major amputation as a personal failure of his or her capacities. He or she excessively focuses on the end organ (the threatened limb) instead of the patient's well-being. Amputation should be regarded in a more positive light. It should be considered as a reconstructive procedure to restore independent ambulation. In that perspective, amputation contributes to the patient's well-being and disease-free survival.

Major, as well as minor, amputations in diabetic patients have four objectives: (1) to eradicate the presence of gangrene and necrotic tissue, (2) to control infection, (3) to relieve pain, and (4) to regain ambulation, allowing the patient to return to an independent existence in the community. This article discusses some aspects to improve the outcome and lower the wound failure rate of amputations in diabetic patients.

Minor amputations

Minor amputations include toe, ray, and partial foot amputations. To ensure a maximum chance of healing, minor amputations may need to be done by an experienced surgeon using a multidisciplinary team approach.

A noninvasive evaluation of the limb perfusion should be done before any minor amputation. Palpable foot arteries and pulsatile Doppler flow are present in purely neuropathic foot ulcers. A segmental perfusion pressure of 70 mm Hg or more is required for optimal wound healing. Transcutaneous oxygen measurement at the dorsum of the foot should ideally be

30 mm Hg or more; however, an oximeter is not always readily available, and the measured values are variable. None of the noninvasive investigation methods (transcutaneous oxygen tension, photoplethysmography, pulse wave recordings) are totally effective for the assessment of the wound healing potential [16]. Clinical judgment remains crucial, and overreliance on noninvasive tests may result in needless above-knee amputation.

When there is clinical evidence of an ischemic component, arterial imaging (angio-MRI is the first choice) should be performed. When required and when feasible, adjunctive distal revascularization should always be done before minor toe, ray, or transmetatarsal amputation [8,10,12,13,17]. Fig. 1 illustrates a failed first toe amputation in a dysvascular diabetic patient. Nehler and colleagues [16] observed a 50% failure rate of partial foot amputations in diabetic patients with a "presumed" adequate forefoot perfusion in whom no adjunctive revascularization was done. Holstein and colleagues [18] reported the best outcome for minor amputations in patients with purely neuropathic ulcers and palpable ankle pulses (an 86% limb salvage and 68% survival rate at 2 years). Patients who had non-reconstructible distal vascular disease had less favorable outcomes than patients who benefited from adjunctive revascularization (2-year limb salvage rate of 17% versus 85%, 2-year survival rate of 16% versus 55%). Miller and colleagues [19] found that unsuccessful revascularization (11% of all bypass procedures) was the most significant predictor of nonhealing and major amputation in cases of transmetatarsal amputation and bypass occlusion (30% required an above-knee amputation). For other researchers, the fear that patients with a failed revascularization will end up with a higher amputation level seems nonjustified [20].

A *single toe amputation* should be performed atraumatically, leaving the base of the first phalanx. Large-based equal dorsal and plantar skin flaps allow tension-free closure. The flexor tendon is pulled out before transection,

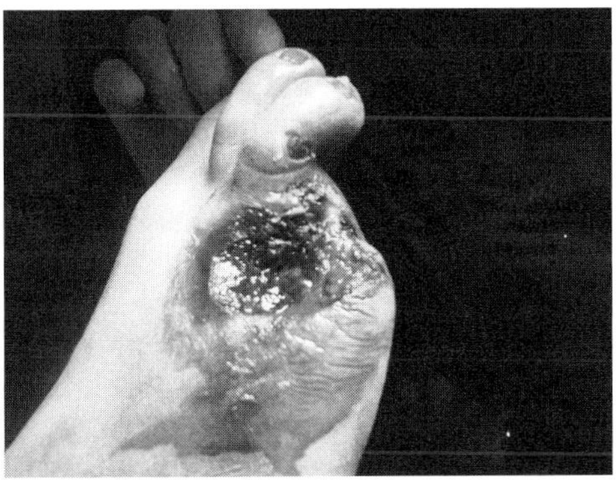

Fig. 1. Necrosis of the wound edges of a first toe amputation in a dysvascular diabetic patient. The foot ultimately was salvaged by a popliteopedal bypass and a first ray amputation.

allowing its retrieval. Preservation of the metatarsophalangeal joint results in a better gait and better foot stability, particularly in first and fifth toe amputations. Sharp scalpel dissection should be subperiosteal on the phalanx to avoid entry into the adjacent metatarsophalangeal joint. Amputation of the second toe is preferentially a ray amputation, with removal of the metatarsal head to avoid hallux valgus (desaxation of the great toe, which is no longer laterally supported by the second toe). It results in a harmonic narrowing of the forefoot. Leaving a fifth lesser toe isolated (after resection of the fourth toe) exposes it to injury and subluxation. It should preferentially be removed prophylactically together with the adjacent fourth toe. A general rule for all amputations is to avoid protracted foot dependency, respecting relative bed rest and foot elevation, because pedal edema will compromise wound healing. Mechanical off-loading of the foot is necessary in the first weeks to avoid wound dehiscence. The skin sutures are left in place for 3 weeks.

Minor amputations should be avoided in the acute phase of foot cellulitis. Stabilization of any infectious process by strict bed rest and off-loading of the inflamed foot, by intravenous broad-spectrum antibiotics, and by local drainage and sharp debridement should be attempted before any minor amputation [12,15,21,22]. These steps allow one to reduce the bacteriologic burden and permit primary healing of the subsequent minor amputation. In the patient who has residual foot cellulitis or evidence of even limited deep infection, the amputation wound is left open [13,15]. Repetitive wound packing with povidone-iodine meshes allows eradication of the underlying residual infection. A prolonged course of selective antibiotic therapy is mandatory to avoid reinfection. In rare instances of intractable spreading sepsis (wet gangrene) or systemic toxicity, primary open amputation should be considered at a toe level or ray level to avoid progression to an ascending infection [16]. Bercelli and colleagues [13] obtained a 70% limb salvage rate by open forefoot amputation in cases of overt osteomyelitis with tenosynovitis. Healing by secondary intention was obtained after a mean of 4.7 months, with a frequent (43%) need for repeat operative revisions. The healing time could be shortened to 1.6 months with a staged procedure. The open limited guillotine amputation of the wet gangrenous toe or forefoot is followed 7 days later by a re-resection and closure without increasing the risk of reinfection or major amputation [13].

A ray amputation removes the toe and adjacent metatarsal head. A dorsal longitudinal racquet incision encircling the base of the corresponding toe exposes the distal shaft of the metatarsal. The transection of the metatarsal shaft is preferentially done with an oscillating saw and is bevelled toward the plantar side. The intrinsic muscles are spared. Incision on the weight-bearing plantar surface should be avoided. Ray amputations are mainly done for plantar erosion of a prominent metatarsal head with evidence of osteomyelitis. They illustrate conservative forefoot surgery, preserving overall foot balance. A first ray amputation, with loss of the medial column, will result in a progressive planovalgus desaxation of the forefoot. A custom-made shoe insert is essential to support the modified medial foot arch [12]. If the toe is not involved, isolated metatarsal head resection allows eradication of the offending bone and secondary closure of the plantar eroded ulcer. Wieman and colleagues [23] reported an 88% success rate in a series of 101 consecutive metatarsal head resections for chronic plantar ulcers present for a mean of 7 months.

Hallux valgus deformity and associated osteomyelitis of the first metatarsophalangeal joint can be treated by isolated excision of the first metatarsophalangeal joint (including the underlying sesamoid bones), leaving the great toe in place (Fig. 2). The flail toe will secondarily fix by fibrosis and scarring. In this way, the patient experiences the foot surgery as less mutilating. An 8% reinfection rate was reported by Murdoch [24] in a series of 90 hallux amputations. At 3-year follow-up, new neuropathic foot ulcers developed in 52% of the patients. Most of them were unaware of, or were not compliant with, preventive measures. If the patient wears protective shoes with custom-molded insoles, the recurrence rate can be lowered to 26%.

Minor amputations result in foot deformities with modified pressure points and altered foot biomechanics. There is a substantial risk of "transfer ulcers" as a result of abnormal exaggerated pressure on adjacent areas. Nehler and colleagues [16] reported a 25% incidence of new noncontiguous ulcers within 1 year in patients with toe amputations. Wieman and colleagues [23] observed new ulcers elsewhere on the same foot in 43% of cases 1 year after metatarsal head resection. In the series of Yeager, 32% of the patients who healed after forefoot surgery primarily performed for neuropathic ulcers required repeat foot surgery during a 2-year follow-up [10]. The best

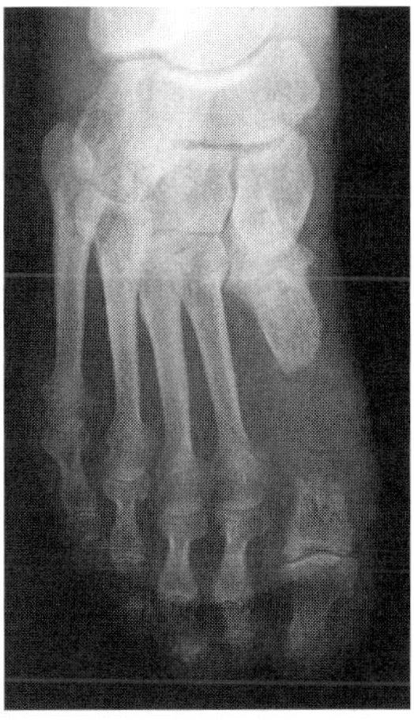

Fig. 2. Plain radiograph of excision of the first metatarsophalangeal joint for osteomyelitis. The first toe could be preserved (a so-called "flail" toe).

preventive method to maintain pedal skin integrity is to wear adapted good-fitting shoes with adequate custom-molded insoles, distributing pressure equally over the modified foot sole. The patient should wear these orthotic shoes and insoles for any ambulation, at home as well as outdoors. Regular attendance at the diabetic foot clinic will result in optimal implementation of preventive measures to avoid skin breakdown at the site of amputation and on the contralateral insensate foot. Overweight and the self-neglect of non-compliant patients are additional causes of recurrent pressure ulcers on the modified foot.

Chronic neuropathic ulceration can be managed by a pressure-relief procedure. The offending bony protuberance can be resected (ostectomy) with an oscillating saw through an incision that does not impinge on the weight-bearing surface of the foot. Typical resectable bony prominences are the bunion of a hallux valgus and the collapsed midfoot of a Charcot rocker-bottom foot deformity (calcaneocuboid or talonavicular dislocation). Adequate off-loading by a total contact cast is necessary for 8 weeks. In the Charcot foot, some authorities advocate correction of the bony architecture of the foot, necessitating an arthrodesis with screws and autologous iliac crest bone grafts to fill the gaps and to enhance the union [25]. This aspect of reconstructive surgery on a Charcot foot is beyond the scope of this review article.

When three or more toes require amputation, a *transmetatarsal amputation* is preferred and ensures a better foot static. Transmetatarsal amputation should preserve the whole length of the metatarsal shafts to maintain the medial and lateral foot arch. The metatarsal transection just proximal to the heads should be beveled toward the plantar side. The plantar fascia and fat pad should be left intact to preserve adequate vascularization of the plantar flap. The majority (70%) of transmetatarsal amputations are performed in diabetic patients. A 75% primary healing rate can be expected [9–11]. In half of the remaining cases, secondary wound healing is possible by repetitive debridement and moist wound dressing, eventually completed by a negative pressure dressing system [13,14]. Negative pressure wound therapy of complex diabetic foot wounds enhances granulation tissue formation in the wound bed and leads to a faster healing rate. The median time to obtain 75% to 100% granulation coverage was 42 days under negative pressure wound therapy compared with 84 days under standard wound care [14]. Negative pressure wound therapy facilitates wound closure and lowers the re-amputation rate when compared with standard wound care (3% versus 11%). For technical aspects of vacuum-assisted closure therapy, the reader is referred to a recent randomized study published in 2005 [14].

Patients on renal dialysis have a poor healing potential; in 60% of these patients, forefoot amputations will fail to heal, with half of the nonhealing forefoot amputations requiring conversion to below-knee amputation [13]. Griffith and colleagues [26] could not find a correlation between healing time (a mean of 5 months) and creatinine clearance; however, that study was a small heterogeneous series of 40 diabetic foot ulcers treated by local debridement or partial foot amputation. The mean creatinine clearance was as high as 51 mL/min, which is far better than that in patients with end-stage renal disease.

When forefoot gangrene extends too proximally, an adequate plantar soft tissue envelope is no longer available to cover the transected metatarsal shafts. A tarsometatarsal *Lisfranc amputation* is the alternative. The base of the first, second, and fifth metatarsal should be left in place because of tendinous insertions, ensuring midfoot stability. There is an inherent risk of muscle imbalance when these tendons (tibialis anterior and peroneal muscles) are sectioned. An equinus deformity can be partially corrected by lengthening of the Achilles tendon. In the midtarsal *Chopart amputation* (Fig. 3), the tibialis anterior muscle should be reattached to the talus to avoid equinus retraction by the triceps surae muscle. When extensive forefoot gangrene or infection precludes midfoot amputation, a *Symes ankle disarticulation* is an ultimate technique that preserves the hindfoot structures (heel pad and ankle). All foot bones, including the calcaneus, are resected. By subperiosteal dissection of the bones, the calcaneal periosteum is preserved and allows fixation of the heel pad over the transected distal tibia epiphysis through drill holes over the anterior margin of the tibia. In this way, the heel pad is firmly attached in its centralized mid position and its slippage is avoided. No weight bearing is allowed during 8 weeks. Proponents of this technique state that preservation of the heel pad allows an intact proprioreceptive feedback, supposing the absence of neuropathy and a sensate heel. Patients with a Symes amputation can walk short distances without fitting a prosthesis. The *Pirogoff amputation* preserves the calcaneum, which is tilted into the tibiofibular fork at the place of the resected

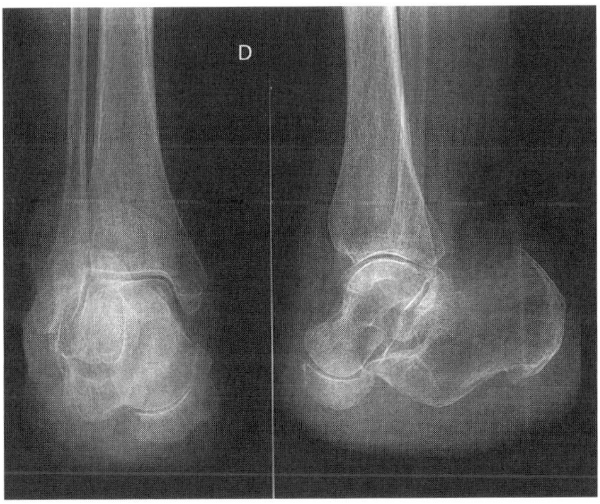

Fig. 3. A mediotarsal Chopart amputation. A rigid ankle-foot orthosis is required to avoid ankle sprain.

talus (Fig. 4). Osteosynthetic fixation is required to obtain bone consolidation. The patient should wear a rigid ankle-foot orthosis to sustain the modified ankle after Lisfranc, Chopart, Symes, or Pirogoff amputation.

The authors are reluctant to consider proximal foot amputations (midtarsal, Chopart) or ankle disarticulations (Symes, Pirogoff) in diabetic patients. The loss of proprioreception and sensory protection exposes the patient to new pressure ulcers. The vascularization of the hindfoot is not always optimal for these extensive dissections, and wound-healing problems are an inherent risk. A typical open forefoot amputation can be secondarily covered by a free muscle flap transfer to provide cushioning at the pressure areas of the modified foot. Once more, there is a considerable risk of recurrent pressure ulceration on the insensate muscle flap.

Partial foot amputations result in a 70% to 80% limb salvage rate at 5 years and allow almost all patients to resume an independent gait [9,15]. The functional result is far superior than that obtained following below-knee amputations [9,12]. The operative mortality rate is less than 1%, and the 5-year survival rate attains 43% [16]. Continued surveillance of the patient at the diabetic foot clinic is essential. In the past, minor foot amputations were often considered a precursor to major leg amputation. Up to one third of limited forefoot amputations evolved to a major amputation over a 3-year period [13,19,21]. Implementation of a multidisciplinary wound care team limits the need for re-amputation at a higher level.

Diabetic osteomyelitis

Erosion of metatarsophalangeal joints (particularly the first toe) or interphalangeal joints (claw toes) is often (up to 60%) complicated by

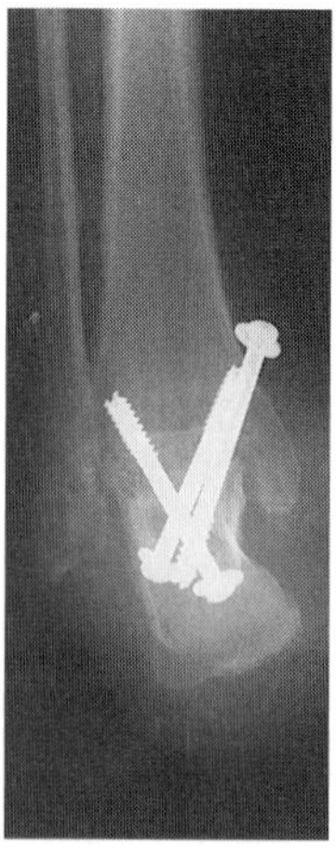

Fig. 4. A Pirogoff amputation. The calcaneus has been tilted into the tibiofibular joint and fixed with screws.

osteomyelitis or osteoarthritis [22]. There is a contiguous spread of bacteria from the plantar ulcer or interdigital web infection with involvement of the bone cortex and marrow. Shone and colleagues [27] reported a 23.5% incidence of osteomyelitis associated with foot ulcers and radiologic evidence of bone destruction. The diagnosis of bone involvement in a plantar pressure sore is classically done by the probe-to-bone test (associated with a 53% to 89% positive predictive value [27,28]). The most reliable imaging technique is MRI [27], which reveals bone marrow edema, periosteal elevation, and surrounding cellulitis. On T2-weighted images, there is high signal intensity along with contrast (gadolinium) enhancement. Osteomyelitis may not be evident on plain radiographs during the first months. Differential diagnosis with Charcot's neuropathic osteoarthropathy is not always evident. Bone biopsy is the reference criterion standard for the diagnosis of osteomyelitis, but it is not widely applied.

Patients with osteomyelitis constitute the most difficult subgroup of patients with a threatened diabetic foot. Traditional management requires off-loading and bed rest, intravenous antibiotic therapy, wide sharp debridement of nonviable and infected tissue, and surgical removal of the infected bone once the acute inflammatory phase has subsided [21,28]. Whenever possible, concurrent vascular reconstruction should be done in cases of impaired foot perfusion. Restoration of an adequate pulsatile blood flow to the foot arteries improves focal delivery of antibiotics and promotes tissue healing [8,15]. Host defense mechanisms do not operate optimally in the osseous environment, and gram-positive cocci incorporate into an impermeable glycocalyx. The reinfection rate has been reported to attain 40% [16]. Control of hyperglycemia and infection are interdependent. Optimization of glycemic control is essential and often requires a temporary shift toward insulin injections. Dialyzed patients with osteomyelitis at the forefoot level have the worst outcome, with 32% of these cases evolving to limb loss.

Some authorities question the rule of surgical bone excision in patients who have osteomyelitis and suggest conservative management [29]. A prolonged course of 6 to 12 weeks of culture-guided antibiotic coverage associated with debridement of the ulcer results in successful eradication of the infection in 70% of cases [29]. A protracted course of supervised nursing care of the underlying foot ulcer is required.

Major limb amputation

The goal of amputating as conservatively as possible to preserve a functional foot is not applicable in all cases. The decision to attempt limb salvage or to proceed with primary amputation should be based on a judicious evaluation of the patient's health status and the optimal risk-benefit ratio [30]. In a dysvascular patient with non-reconstructible distal arterial occlusive disease and foot gangrene, minor amputation will not heal or will require lengthy wound care with an inherent negative impact on the quality of life. For these patients, foot-sparing surgery should be considered hazardous. A primary below-knee amputation is the best option and should be preferred to serial, overambitious desperate attempts at foot salvage. A failed distal bypass may ultimately necessitate a less functional above-knee amputation.

Nonambulatory, bed-ridden patients with poor health who have foot gangrene or chronic foot infection are best served by a palliative above-knee amputation which will almost always heal and which shortens the hospital stay [20,31]. Other indications for primary above-knee amputation are the finding of severe dysvascularity with no detectable flow in a totally occluded popliteal artery in a patient with non-reconstructible infrapopliteal arterial disease, flexion-contracture of the knee, and elderly patients with limited mental capacity who are unable to follow an arduous rehabilitation program. Elderly frail patients are medically incapable of withstanding multiple operations [30]. The morbidity of limb-saving interventions exceeds any long-term benefit for these patients presenting with end-stage overt atherosclerosis. Major amputation raises concerns in almost any patient with a tremendous burden of comorbidities [30]. Underlying disease causes some postoperative morbidity (pneumonia, myocardial infarction, stroke, urinary retention) in half of major amputations [30,31]. The operative mortality rate is as high as 17% [7] (14% after above-knee amputations and 6.6% after below-knee amputations in the authors' experience [12], approaching mortality rates reported in recent series [5,32,33]). The mortality rate is higher for patients on renal dialysis (relative risk, 3.75) [33]. Two thirds of the postoperative deaths are of cardiovascular origin. The life expectancy of amputees is rather limited (a 30% rate of 5-year survival) [1,32–34].

Delayed wound healing is more frequent after transtibial amputation (20% to 45%) when compared with transfemoral amputation (10% to 25%) [1,5,31,35]. Nevertheless, diabetic patients heal better after transtibial below-knee amputation than do non-diabetic patients with end-stage peripheral arterial occlusive disease, because diabetic occlusive disease is almost infrapopliteal (88% versus 70% healing rate). As many as 15% of below-knee amputations ultimately require a conversion to above-knee re-amputation [1,4,5,32]. This risk is highest (25%) in dialyzed patients. Wound infection and stump necrosis are the most common causes leading to re-amputation at a higher level. The Burgess technique is the most common type of below-knee amputation. To minimize the risk of wound problems, the surgeon should perform atraumatic gentle handling of the skin and debulking of the deep muscles and soleus muscle to allow tension-free suturing of the posterior myofasciocutaneous flap. The tibial section should be bevelled with an oscillating saw to avoid sharp edges (oblique transection from proximal anterior to distal posterior). The peroneal bone (fibula) should be transected 2 cm more proximal than the tibia. If the fibula is sectioned too high, the amputation stump becomes conical and less suitable for prosthetic wearing. Nerves should be sectioned proximally under traction, allowing them to retract away from the end of the stump to minimize nerve-end irritation and neurinoma formation. A suction drain is left in place for 48 hours. Skin sutures are left in place for 3 weeks.

A distal transtibial amputation preserving two thirds of the length of the lower limb, as done in young trauma patients, is not indicated for diabetic patients. The blood supply to the distal third of the leg is poor, and the tibia is exposed to excessive pressure with the risk of neuropathic pressure ulceration.

A Gritti-Stokes through-knee amputation leaves the quadriceps function intact. The full length of the femur offers a maximum lever for ambulation. In elderly patients, the atrophic skin at the level of the femoral condyles and patella is vulnerable and suboptimal for prosthetic fitting.

Today, there is a general awareness of the importance of retaining the knee joint. Saving the knee joint gives a better perspective to prosthetic rehabilitation and preserves walking capability [1,5,35]. For elderly patients who are unable to wear a prosthesis, preservation of the knee joint facilitates sitting, turning, and transfer activities. Other authorities prefer primary above-knee amputation to avoid healing problems and reintervention in fragile elderly patients [31]. Rehabilitation with mobilization of the knee joint, balance exercises, and muscle strengthening should be started on day 1. An early exercise program is necessary to ensure retention of a full range of proximal joint motion.

The level of amputation (below-knee versus above-knee) is a major, but not the exclusive, determinant of the ability of the amputee to ambulate autonomically with his or her prosthesis [31,35]. On average, 60% of below-knee amputees become full prosthetic users (autonomic outdoors ambulation) compared with 30% of above-knee amputees. In the authors' experience, 69% of below-knee amputees and 55% of above-knee amputees recover an autonomic gait with a limb prosthesis [12]. Above-knee amputees consume more oxygen per meter walked (35 mL/kg/m) than below-knee amputees (25 mL/kg/m), explaining their more limited walking capability. These metabolic requirements are high when compared with the low energy expenditure 0.15 mL/kg/m oxygen update per meter walked by a control person [36].

In a recent study, Nehler and colleagues [31] reported that fewer than one half of the surviving amputees used their prosthesis and fewer than one third ambulated outdoors despite an arduous rehabilitation program. Preoperative factors associated with not wearing the prosthesis after lower limb amputation were analyzed by Nehler [31] and Taylor [34]. A major determinant is the patient's ambulatory status before the lower limb amputation. Nonambulatory patients at baseline remain nonambulatory after major limb amputation, even if they become pain free. The chance that these patients with limited functional fitness preoperatively will ambulate with their prosthesis is ten times lower when they are compared with patients normally ambulating preoperatively. Advanced age, dementia, and end-stage renal disease are detrimental factors predictive of a poor functional outcome, with a relative risk of 3 (odds ratio, 3) of not wearing the limb prosthesis. Less than 10% of octogenarian amputees regain autonomic gait with a limb prosthesis. The amputation will only relieve pain and avoid further deterioration of the patient's general health status. Diabetes itself is not deemed to be a risk factor predictive of poor functional outcome after lower limb amputation.

Summary

Whenever possible, a foot-sparing strategy should be followed. This approach includes staged procedures for infected wet gangrene of the forefoot. Susceptibility to infection, poor wound healing, loss of protective sensation, and limited tissue perfusion are determinant factors in the outcome of minor or major diabetes-related amputations. Special precautions can minimize the risk of failure of these amputations. When the chance of wound healing is low (non-reconstructible infrapopliteal arterial occlusive disease) or when the gangrene or infection extends beyond the midfoot, the concept of foot-sparing surgery is not reasonable and a major amputation should be preferred. This recommendation is also true for patients who are nonambulatory at presentation, for whom desperate foot salvage will not improve significantly their quality of life. Major amputation should no longer be considered as a failure in the management of the diabetic foot but rather as a valuable treatment option offering the patient a chance to return to functional independence and autonomic ambulation. All diabetic patients who undergo minor or major amputation should remain enrolled in a diabetic management program, including regular attendance at a diabetic foot clinic. Implementation of preventive measures and of foot care is essential to avoid new pressure ulcers and skin breakdown on the modified foot and on the opposite foot. The role of a well-structured multidisciplinary diabetic foot clinic cannot be overemphasized, particularly after amputation.

References

[1] Dormandy J, Heeck I, Vig S. Major amputations: clinical patterns and predictors. Semin Vasc Surg 1999;12:154–61.

[2] Apelgvist J, Larsson J. What is the most effective way to reduce incidence of amputation in the diabetic foot? Diabetes Metab Res Rev 2000;16(Suppl 1):S75–83.

[3] Meltzer D, Pels S, Payne W, et al. Decreasing amputation rates in patients with diabetes mellitus: an outcome study. J Am Podiatric Med Ass 2002;92:425–8.

[4] Abou Zamzam A, Teruys T, Killeen D, et al. Major amputations of the lower limb in a university hospital. Ann Vasc Surg 2003;17:86–90.

[5] Cruz C, Eidt J, Capps C, et al. Major lower limb amputations at a Veterans Affairs Hospital. Am J Surg 2003;186:449–54.

[6] Krans H, Posta M, Keen M. Diabetes care and research in Europe: the St. Vincent's Declaration Action Programme. International Diabetes Federation Europe, 1992.
[7] Lindholt J, Bovling S, Fasting H, et al. Vascular surgery reduces the frequency of lower limb major amputations. Eur J Vasc Surg 1994;8:31–5.
[8] Van Damme H. Crural or pedal artery revascularisation for limb salvage: is it justified? Acta Chir Belg 2004;104:148–57.
[9] Sheahan M, Hamdan A, Veraldi J, et al. Lower extremity minor amputations: the roles of diabetes mellitus and timing of revascularisation. J Vasc Surg 2005;42:476–80.
[10] Yeager R, Moneta G, Edwards J, et al. Predictors of outcome of forefoot surgery for ulceration and gangrene. Am J Surg 1998;175:388–90.
[11] Geroulakos G, May A. Transmetatarsal amputation in patients with peripheral vascular disease. Eur J Vasc 1991;5:655–8.
[12] Van Damme H, Rorive M, Martens de Noordhout B, et al. Amputations in diabetic patients: a plea for foot-sparing surgery. Acta Chir Belg 2001;101:123–9.
[13] Berceli S, Brown J, Irwin PH, Ozaki K. Clinical outcomes after closed, staged and open forefoot amputations. J Vasc Surg 2006;44:347–51.
[14] Armstrong D, Lavery L. Negative pressure wound therapy after partial diabetic foot amputations: a multicenter, randomised controlled trial. Lancet 2005;366:1704–10.
[15] Taylor L, Porter J. The clinical course of diabetics who require emergent foot surgery because of infection or ischemia. J Vasc Surg 1987;6:454–9.
[16] Nehler M, Whitehill T, Bowers S, et al. Intermediate-term outcome of primary digit amputations in patients with diabetes mellitus who have forefoot sepsis requiring hospitalisation and presumed adequate circulatory status. J Vasc Surg 1999;30:509–18.
[17] Chalmers R. Surgical techniques to save the diabetic foot. Diabetic Foot 2003;6:38–42.
[18] Holstein P, Sorensen S. Limb salvage experience in a multidisciplinary diabetic foot unit. Diabetes Care 1999;22:B97–103.
[19] Miller N, Dardik H, Wolodiger F, et al. Transmetatarsal amputation: the role of adjunctive revascularisation. J Vasc Surg 1991;13:705–11.
[20] Ebskov L, Hindso K, Holstein P. Level of amputation following failed arterial reconstruction compared to primary amputation: a meta-analysis. Eur J Vasc Endovasc Surg 1999; 17:35–40.
[21] Van Baal J. Surgical treatment of the infected diabetic foot. Clin Infect Dis 2004;39:S123–8.
[22] Frykberg R. An evidence-based approach to diabetic foot infections. Am J Surg 2003;186: 44S–54S.
[23] Wieman J, Mercke Y, Cerrito P, et al. Resection of the metatarsal head for diabetic foot ulcers. Am J Surg 1998;176:436–41.
[24] Murdoch D, Armstrong D, Dacus J, et al. The natural history of great toe amputations. J Foot Ankle Surg 1997;36:204–8.
[25] Stone C, Daniels T. Midfoot and hindfoot arthrodeses in diabetic Charcot arthropathy. Can J Surg 2000;43:449–55.
[26] Griffiths G, Wieman J. The influence of renal function on diabetic foot ulceration. Arch Surg 1990;125:1567–9.
[27] Shone A, Burnside J, Chipchase S, et al. Probing the validity of the probe-to-bone test in the diagnosis of osteomyelitis of the foot in diabetes. Diabetes Care 2006;29: 945.
[28] Jeffcoate W, Lipsky B. Controversies in diagnosing and managing osteomyelitis of the foot in diabetes. Clin Infect Dis 2004;39:S115–22.
[29] Pittet D, Wyssa B, Herter-Clavel C, et al. Outcome of diabetic foot infections treated conservatively. Arch Intern Med 1999;159:851–9.
[30] Nehler M, Hiatt W, Taylor L. Is revascularisation and limb salvage always the best treatment for critical limb ischemia? J Vasc Surg 2003;37:704–8.
[31] Nehler M, Coll J, Hiatt W, et al. Functional outcome in a contemporary series of major lower extremity amputations. J Vasc Surg 2003;38:7–14.

[32] Ploeg A, Lardenoye J, Vrancken-Peeters M, et al. Contemporary series of morbidity and mortality after lower limb amputation. Eur J Vasc Endovasc Surg 2005;29:633–7.

[33] Feinglass J, Pearce W, Martin G, et al. Postoperative and late survival outcomes after major amputation: findings from the Department of Veterans Affairs national surgical quality improvement program. Surgery 2001;130:21–9.

[34] Taylor S, Kalbaugh C, Blackhurst D, et al. Preoperative clinical factors predict postoperative functional outcome after major lower limb amputation: an analysis of 553 consecutive patients. J Vasc Surg 2005;42:227–35.

[35] Keagy B, Schwatrz J, Kotb M, et al. Lower extremity amputation: the control series. J Vasc Surg 1986;4:321–6.

[36] Waters R, Peny J, Antonelli D, et al. Energy cost of walking of amputees: the influence of level of amputation. J Bone Joint Surg 1976;58A:42–6.

ELSEVIER
SAUNDERS

Clin Podiatr Med Surg
24 (2007) 583–599

CLINICS IN
PODIATRIC
MEDICINE AND
SURGERY

Orthotic Management of Charcot Feet After External Fixation Surgery

Armin Koller, Dr med, MD[a,*], Stefan A. Meissner, MD[b], Maike Podella, MD[a], Raimund Fiedler, MD[a]

[a] *Department of Technical Orthopaedics, Münster University Hospital, Robert Koch 30, 48149 Münster, Northrhine-Westfaila, Germany*

[b] *Department of Orthopaedics, Münster University Hospital, Münster 48129, Germany*

Orthotic supply is essential in the treatment of neuropathic diabetic feet [1], including addressing plantar ulcers caused by pressure and shearing forces acting on soft tissues. Orthoses provide protection from harmful pressure above an individual threshold by means of partial or total unloading of the foot [2].

While there is a wide consensus that unloading is the most effective means of treatment, the etiology of Charcot foot remains largely unclear. The neurovascular theory is based on the assumption that the loss of sympathetic nerve function leads to enhancement of perfusion within the bone. The subsequent activation of osteoclasts would weaken trabecular structures and finally result in fractures. Although acute Charcot foot rarely develops in ischemic tissues, supporting the neurovascular theory [3]; however, this model does not explain the assumable laxity of ligaments and joint capsules that occasionally causes luxations without adequate trauma (ie "pathological luxation").

The neurotraumatic theory asserts that the loss of neurogenic joint control with repetitive stress leads to the initiation of an inflammatory response that results in destruction of cartilage and bone [4]. Jeffcoate and colleagues [5] recently hypothesized that an initial insult, even a minimal one, would suffice to trigger an inflammatory cascade through increased expression of proinflammatory cytokines, including tumor necrosis factor (TNF)α and interleukin 1β. Hence, elevated osteoclastogenesis would be a result of upregulation of the nuclear transcription factor (NF-κB) pathway.

* Corresponding author.

E-mail address: armin.koller@uni-muenster.de (A. Koller).

doi:10.1016/j.cpm.2007.03.012

podiatric.theclinics.com

In 1966, Eichenholtz [6] was the first to describe the natural history and radiological findings of the osteoarthropathic process, which he graduated into three stages. Stage I (developmental phase) is characterized by soft-tissue inflammation and edema, joint fragmentation, and osseous dislocation. Confusion with bacterial inflammatory processes is common in this stage. Stage II (coalescent phase) shows reduction of edema, bone callus proliferation, and fracture consolidation. Stage III (reconstructive phase) is marked by stabilization of the foot skeleton by osseous ancylosis and hypertrophic proliferation [7,8].

The quiescent or reparative Stages II and III can only proceed under protection from mechanical stress, because further fractures potentiate the inflammatory process [5]. Stress protection in the treatment of Charcot feet is almost synonymous with offloading or restricted weight bearing. Whereas vertical unweighting or a level pressure distribution are the key measures for successful treatment of plantar ulcers, orthoses for the treatment of Charcot feet have to be targeted at protection from joint movements by means of restricting bending and torque forces. There is no evidence that pressure by itself is harmful for Charcot joints; there is also a general lack of scientific evidence in terms of pressure-relieving interventions or treatment with orthoses and similar devices [9]. If the inflammatory process can be mechanically triggered, it seems to be wise to attenuate joint movements instead of load transmission on the foot.

The present article, therefore, aims to determine if an orthosis that is designed to immobilize the foot skeleton but to permit axial loading as far as possible is suitable for orthotic management of Charcot feet after external fixation surgery.

Material and methods

On the basis of the aforementioned considerations, and based on the authors' clinical experience, we have advanced the function and design of orthoses over the years in close collaboration with our orthopedic technicians. In the 1980s, we primarily applied bivalved Scotchcast (3M, St. Paul, Minnesota) orthoses. Skin lesions and clumsy motion were the major problems with this appliance. We therefore came to prefer individual orthoses based on a positive cast. The first model had an L-shape, front entrance, and a pretibial Velcro (Manchester, New Hampshire) fastener. The reduction of foot and ankle motion therein depended on correct handling of the fastener, which represents a general problem in orthotics. The current orthotic model features improved rigidity with rear entrance, solid heel holder, and a pretibial shell form-locking with the triangular shape of the tibia. The lower leg is virtually wedged from tibial head to heel so that the fastener around the calf is no longer the factor determining suspension in this orthosis. Furthermore, the foot is fixed through a tongue from synthetic leather. Donning the orthosis is shown on Fig. 1.

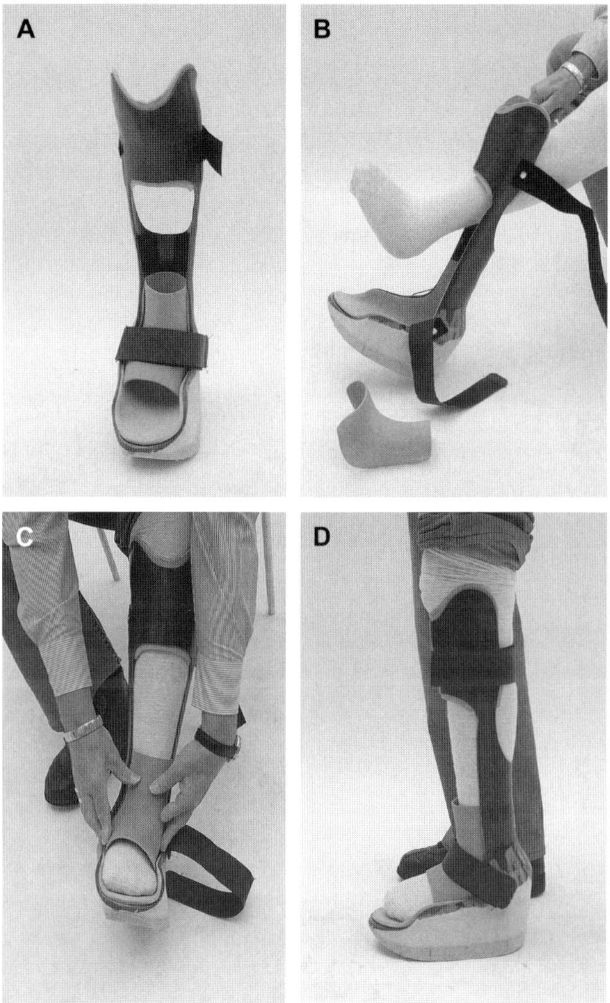

Fig. 1. (*A–D*) Donning the orthosis.

Manufacturing

For cast taking, the foot must be brought into corrected position. Particularly if the ankle joint is still flexible, exact adjustment of the foot is the key step in the production of the authors' orthotic device, because the vector of plantar forces is determined by this. Before suction molding of the interim orthosis made of polyethylene terephtalate glycol (PETG), a relatively thin soft pad made of 6 mm nonperforated ethylenvinylacetate (EVA) is wrapped around the foot and ankle of the model. As a clear-transparent material, PETG allows identification of pressure marks and modification of the orthosis using a hot air gun. Finally, the interim orthosis is reinforced with carbon fibers (Fig. 2).

The final orthosis is made from epoxy casting resin, and is fitted after edema regression. The rocker bottom is foamed from polyurethane and individually ground during dynamic gait analysis. In addition to an anterior and posterior rocker bar, the plateau of the sole is important for safe standing and stance phase stability. The comfortable rear and front cutouts make the orthosis lightweight (Fig. 3), with concomitant stability.

Design

The nonarticulated construction and the lack of weight-bearing at the tibial head characterize the Munster ankle foot orthosis (AFO). The full axial

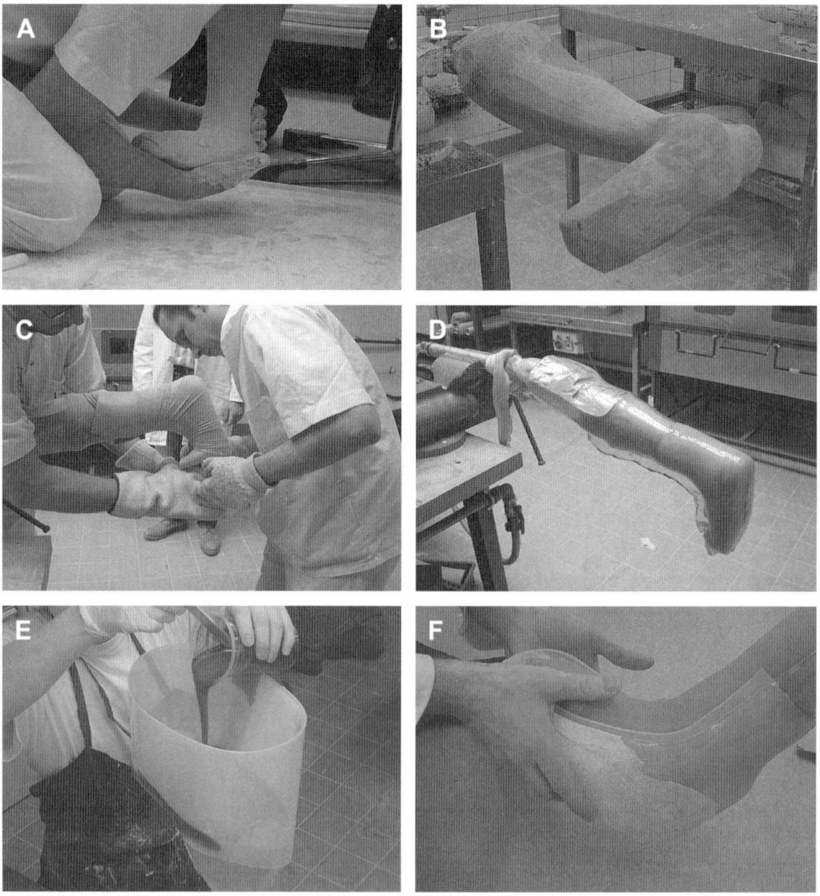

Fig. 2. Manufacturing of the orthosis. (*A*) Foot positioning. (*B*) Positive cast modification. (*C*) Extreme vibration attenuation (EVA) pad. (*D*) Suction molding with PETG. (*E*) Making of the polyurethane foamed rocker bottom. (*F*) First fitting.

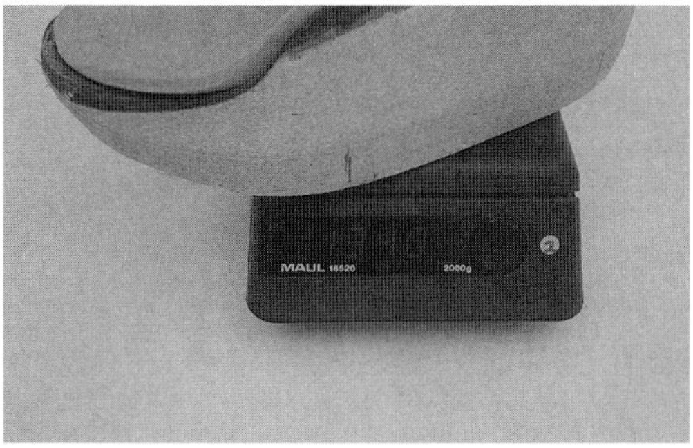

Fig. 3. Medium-weight orthosis weighing 1340 g.

load is used to facilitate bony fusion, particularly with neuroarthropathic processes at the rearfoot of Sanders Stages IV and V [10]. The rigid three-dimensional fixation of the foot serves for the reduction of shearing forces. An important point is the elimination of tibial rotary motion, because this is forwarded via the subtalar joint to the midtarsal joints. With regard to the neurotraumatic theory, this mechanical perturbation is undesirable. Therefore, a relatively thin pad appears to be more suitable to control motion of the foot, because the authors attach more importance to stability than to soft padding. Vulnerable bony prominences, of course, have to be protected against high pressure.

In contrast to shoes, even pressure distribution is of less importance. The design of the orthotic foot bedding is in fact responsible for a directed load transmission, to maintain the operative result or to counter deformity progression in cases of conservative treatment. Accentuated support of the longitudinal foot arch in the residual varus position of the ankle joint, for example, can even enforce foot malposition after resolution of soft tissue swelling. In this case, the ground reaction forces have to be transmitted through the lateral side of the foot to achieve deformity correction; an exaggerated arch support has to be avoided.

In any case, the nonarticulated construction and the tight-fitting shank of the AFO inevitably effect a reduction of plantar pressure, particularly during the heel strike and preswing phases of walking. Pressure measurements with Pedar (Novel, Munich, Germany) insoles demonstrate the mechanism in principle with a healthy test subject (Fig. 4). Note that the orthosis had to be penetrated for this purpose. Even in an orthosis made from pure PETG without any padding, plantar pressure peaks are reduced significantly. The pressure load at the base of the fifth metatarsal bone in the example mentioned above is caused by varus alignment of the orthosis. The model with additional pads and correct static adjustment does not feature noteworthy pressure peaks, although it is made without infracondylar support (see Fig. 4A–C).

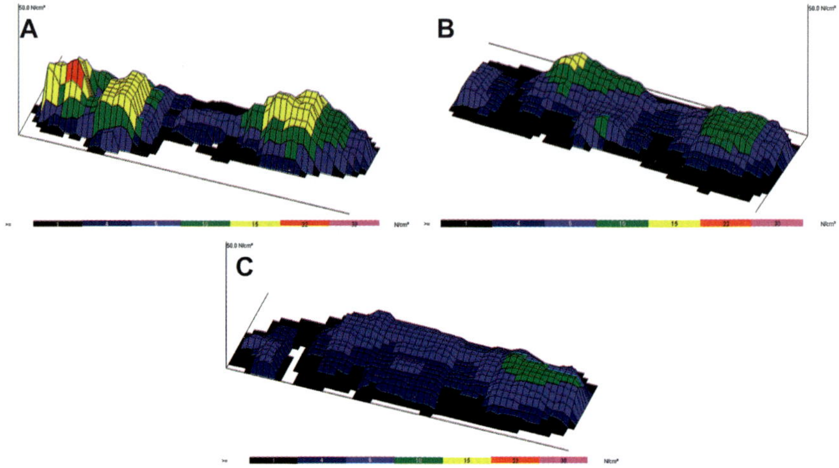

Fig. 4. (*A*) Shoe with molded insole (plantar orthosis for diabetics). (*B*) AFO orthosis without cushion (pure PETG). (*C*) AFO with thin cushion, correct static alignment, no infracondylar bearing.

The authors apply corrective forces mainly after deformity correction with external fixation. The following case illustrates that minor defective foot positions can also be corrected only by means of orthotics.

A 38-year-old female patient who formerly had diabetes Type I presented with varus deformity of the ankle joint and forefoot adduction of her right foot. Soft tissue around the ankle joint showed moderate swelling and warming. On plain radiographs, the ankle joint showed incongruity, and was graded Stage III in the Eichenholtz system. After combined pancreatic and renal transplantation, the authors considered the risk of infection carefully and tried to avoid operative deformity correction. By means of serial orthoses, a stepwise abduction of the forefoot was achieved (Fig. 5), so that a custom-made orthopedic shoe with high shank for stability of the ankle joint could be fitted at the end of treatment.

Although the Munster AFO was primarily intended for the conservative treatment of Charcot feet, it has meanwhile become the authors' main device for aftercare and mobilization after operative correction of foot deformities in diabetic neuroarthropathy. The authors' objective of external fixation is not exclusively arthrodesis in terms of bone fusion. Fibrous ancylosis in conjunction with the patients' polyneuropathy also allows for pain-free mobilization in orthoses [11].

The external fixation immobilizes the foot for just 6 to 8 weeks. After its removal, the subsequent plaster cast and antiedematous treatment for 2 to 3 days is followed by fitting of an interim orthosis. Since most of the patients with polyneuropathy are not able to reduce weight-loading of the foot in a controlled manner with the help of crutches, the authors allow full weight-bearing right from the start, but limit its duration to 15 to 30 minutes

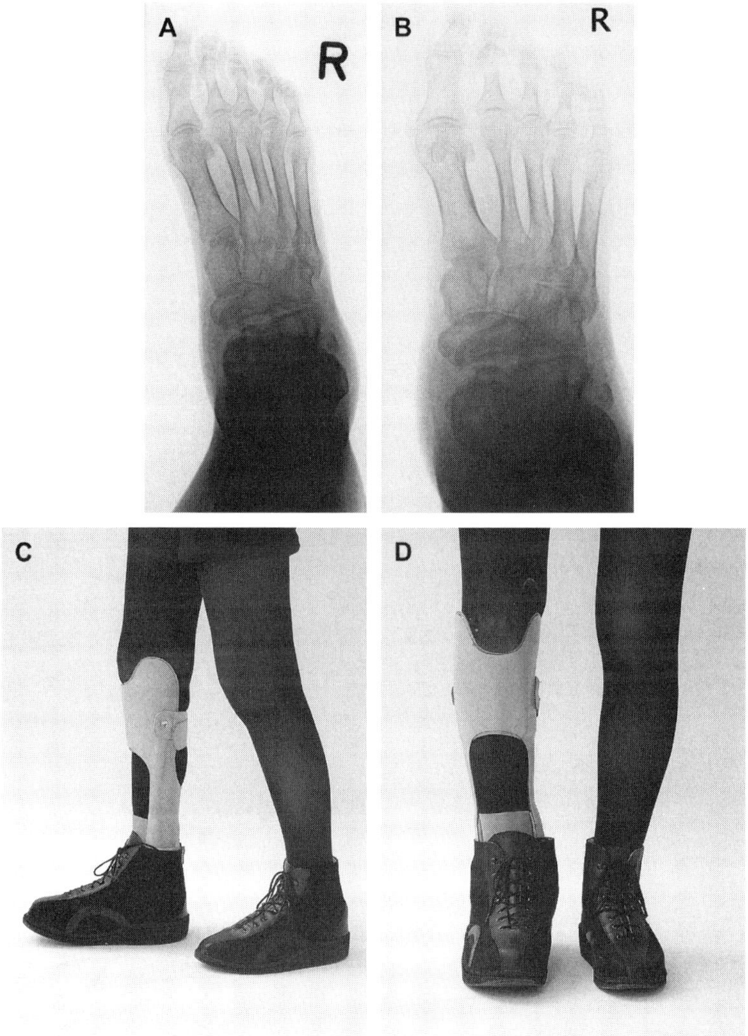

Fig. 5. (*A*) Forefoot adducted before treatment. (*B*) Normal alignment after treatment. (*C, D*) Orthosis with additional custom-made shoes.

at the beginning. Unless problems such as ulcers, pain, or swelling develop, the duration of weight-bearing is continuously stepped up.

The axial compression leads to compaction of the osseous structures of the hindfoot (Fig. 6). This can require a correction of the interim orthosis. After some days of full weight-bearing, it is occasionally detectable on radiographs that the distance between the bone fragments has declined. The final resin-casted orthosis is fabricated after 3 to 5 months, as soon as constant volume conditions of the soft tissue can be assumed.

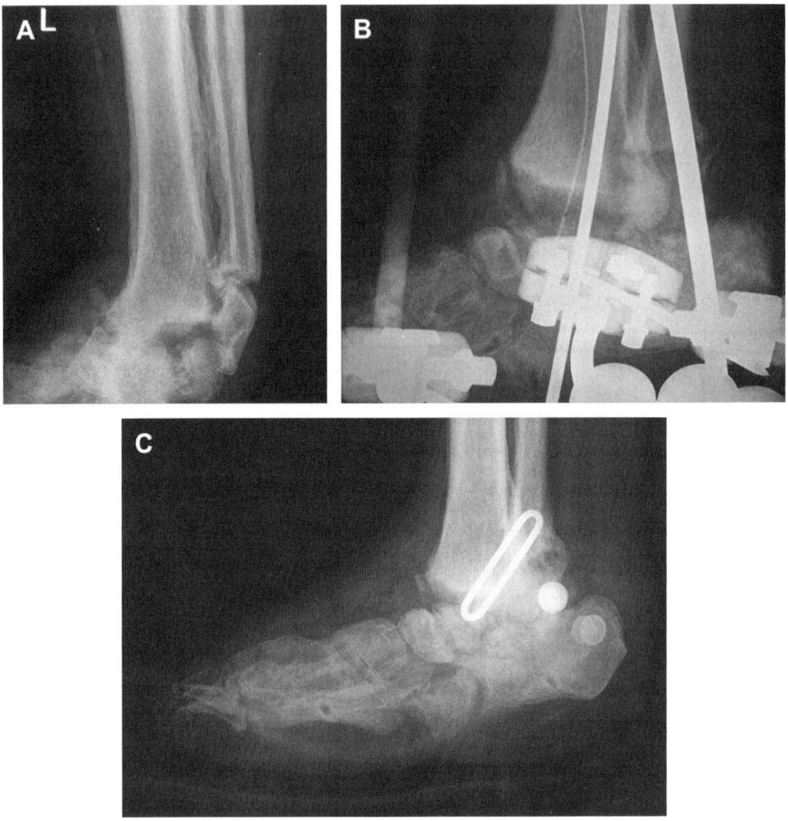

Fig. 6. (*A*) Destroyed talocrural joint with medial displacement of the foot. (*B*) Marked gap between distal tibia and foot. (*C*) Tibia impacting the foot under axial load.

Orthotic treatment is continued after external fixation surgery for 9 to 12 months, because the authors detected recurrent foot malpositions more frequently after too-short orthotic aftercare. Thus, orthotic treatment after fixation surgery of Charcot feet is an integral part of the treatment concept, and therefore requires close teamwork between surgeon and orthopedic technicians.

Nonoperative treatment aims and treatment steps should always be enunciated in cooperation between the team members as well. The authors' algorithm implies unloading Charcot feet of Eichenholtz Stage I completely, if necessary with additional protection by total contact casting (TCC). After a variable time frame of 5 to 8 weeks, during which edema fades away and Eichenholtz Stage II sets in, an interim orthosis can be fitted.

Conservative treatment does not aim at the correction of high-grade deformities, which are in the scope of surgery. Orthotic devices, rather, are to maintain the structure of the foot skeleton as it is found at the beginning of therapy, until the Charcot process has cooled off. Initiation of Eichenholtz

Stage III after a couple of months allows for the provision of custom made orthopedic shoes, if a considerable malposition of the foot does not exist. The authors prefer a smooth transition from orthoses to shoes. A fixing shoe with rolling sole (arthrodesis shoe) is initially worn for not more than 15 to 30 minutes. Unless skin lesions or a new episode of arthropathy occur, ambulation time in shoes may increase. The authors use neither temperature measurements nor bone scans to determine the point of time for termination of orthotic treatment [2,12].

Results

Two hundred Charcot feet in 187 patients (120 male, 67 female) with a mean age of 57.7 years were operated on consecutively following a standard schema at the authors' hospital between 1998 and 2006. Medium follow-up was 21.6 months (range 0.2–102.4 months). Indications for surgical treatment included high-grade deformities, deformities with progression under conservative treatment, instability, and infection. The mean body mass index was 31.8; the body mass index of 23 patients exceeded 40 and the maximum value was 59.7. In contrast to the 134 Type II diabetics with average illness duration of 12.6 (standard deviation [SD] 8.5) years and 27 Type I diabetics with average illness duration of 25.4 (SD 10.2) years, 30 patients (16%) were found to have polyneuropathy of nondiabetic genesis. Peripheral vascular disease (atherosclerotic) was verified in 24% of all patients through duplex sonography or arteriography. The absence of foot pulses alone did not fulfill the diagnostic criterion of atherosclertoic vascular disease (AVD). Nephropathy was found in 33.5% of all patients; 5.5% required dialysis.

During total follow-up, 44 feet (22%) developed new or recurrent ulcers within their orthosis or later within their shoes. In 8 of these 44 cases (18.2%) the ulcer was caused by recurrent deformity of the Charcot foot. Within the first year after surgery, only 13.5% (27 of 200) feet suffered from ulcers, 17.5% (35 of 200) did so within 2 years, and only in 2 feet of 200 (1%) did ulcers occur later than 5 years after surgery. As a consequence, 79.5% (35 of 44) of all ulcers observed were found within 2 years after operative intervention. The further development predominantly depended on the cause of lesion. Ulcers caused by recurrent foot deformity were treated surgically again with external fixation. Ulcers that arose newly or recurrently under orthotic supply could be successfully treated by modification or new fabrication of the device. None of the ulcers that had developed under orthotic supply led to amputation.

In 170 of 200 cases, the Eichenholtz stage at the start of treatment could be clearly determined: 77 cases were classified Stage II, the remainder of 93 cases were Stage III. For 60 cases of Stage II at the point of last surgical intervention, serial radiographs allowed calculating the time until the first radiograph showed Stage III. This period of time was 3.0 months on average (SD 3.4), including 6 to 8 weeks wearing the external fixation.

In order to evaluate mobility, patients were assigned to categories according to the K-levels for amputees (Medicare Classification System). The mean preoperative grade of mobility was 1.0 (SD 0.51) (K-level 1 = typical of the limited and unlimited household ambulator). At the time of last follow-up of patients supplied with an orthosis, the grade of mobility was 2.3 (SD 0.47) on average (K-level 2 = typical of the limited community ambulator), which corresponds to improvement of 1.3 (SD 0.74) grades of mobility.

Discussion

The total contact cast (TCC) is widely-accepted as the gold standard for pressure relief in the diabetic foot syndrome; however, this evaluation mainly applies to ulcer treatment. Off-loading devices for Charcot feet have not yet been examined in a randomized controlled trial (RCT). This is true for the TCC, as for any type of orthosis. In general, there is a lack of RCTs and subsequently a lack of evidence as to the relative effectiveness of orthotic devices [9]. Comparison of different types of orthoses for Charcot feet has hardly been possible on the basis of valid data. Orthotic management after reconstructive foot surgery in neuroarthropathy is therefore the responsibility of the surgeon, who makes special demands on his preferred device. And as long as reliable data about optimal orthotic after treatment are missing, knowledge about design, indication, advantages and disadvantages of different orthoses is needed to help with selection of a particular device. In the following, frequently used orthoses are contrasted with the TCC.

Total contact cast

The most significant advantage of the TCC is instant availability. It is cheap in fabrication and can be produced in most locations. Windowing of the cast allows treating wounds. The closed construction enforces good compliance.

The main disadvantage is that physical examination of the foot requires removal of the cast. For continued treatment, a new cast has to be applied. The reapplication of a split cast cannot be recommended because of too-high injury risk. Frequent replacements of the cast lead to significant expenditure of the time for the patient, and well-trained cast technicians, or physicians who are able to apply a TCC professionally and thereby reduce the risk of skin lesions are not omnipresent. A TCC limits the ability to walk to a greater extent than walkers or orthoses.

Charcot restraint orthotic walker

A Charcot restraint orthotic walker (CROW) (Fig. 7) is fabricated individually as well. The prior making of a plaster cast and a positive model

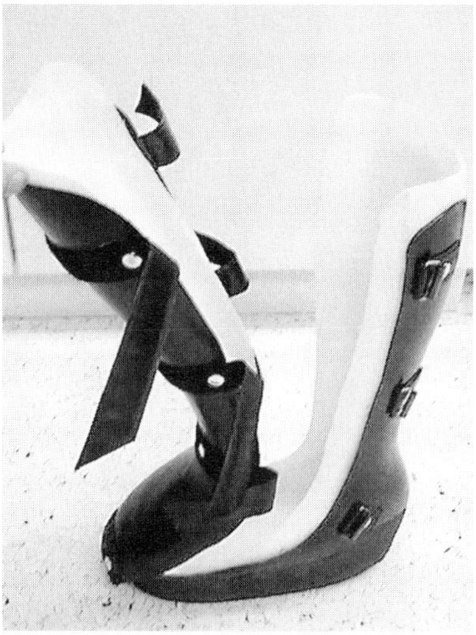

Fig. 7. CROW (*Courtesy of* Zentralverband Orthopädieschuhtechnik, Hannover, Germany; with permission.)

make a CROW fit more precisely than a TCC. It is a durable device, and the rocker bottom allows easier ambulation than with a TCC. For physical examination and ulcer treatment, the CROW can be removed without difficulty.

The removability of the CROW involves the risk of noncompliance. The load transmission on lower leg depends on the way of fastening the device. High pressure on soft tissues thereby enforces their atrophy, which can lead to worse fit of the orthosis and undesirable motions.

Prefabricated diabetic walker

The prefabricated diabetic walker (DW) (Fig. 8A–D) is also available immediately if it can be stored. The relatively low price gets even lower when the DW can be re-used for the next patient; however, regional legal regulations in product liability and infection prevention limit this option.

Depending on the model, mechanical stability decreases gradually. Product information by the manufacturer rarely gives any recommendations for the use in the treatment of Charcot foot. Particularly high-grade foot deformities are subject to restrictions, because in contrast to the CROW and TCC, the DW is not custom made. As an off-the-shelf orthosis, the DW has little scope for modifications. Lower legs with edema may be pressed into an unphysiologic shape. Air chambers may be damaged and loose function because patients may forget to inflate them, or in contrast, may cause skin lesions by overinflation of the air chambers.

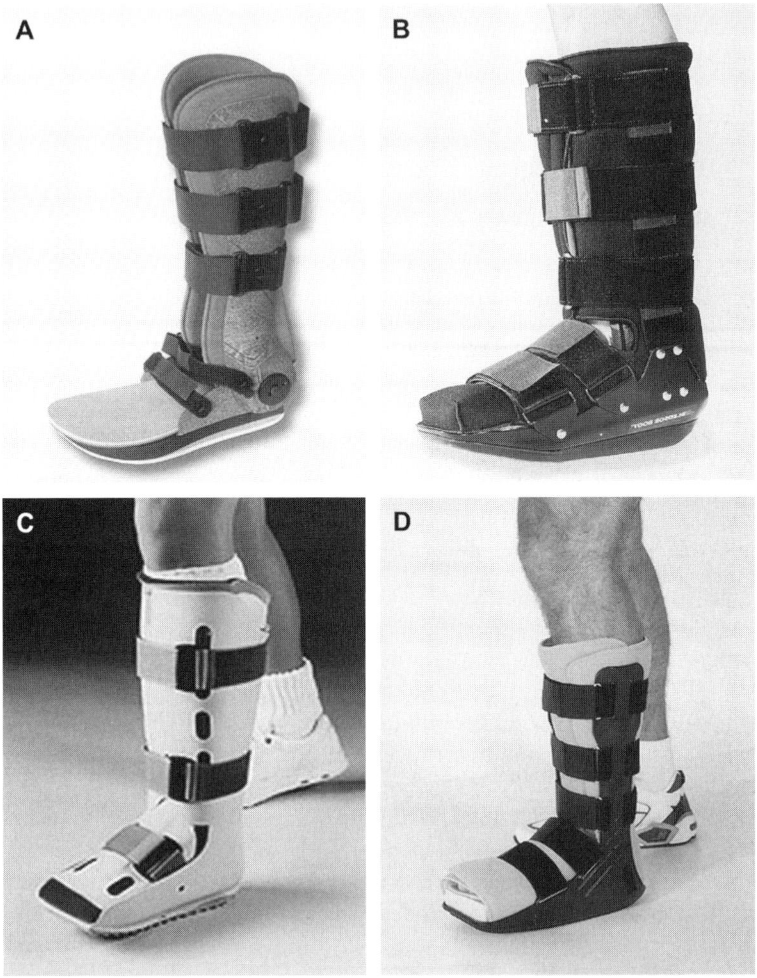

Fig. 8. DWs of various manufacturers. (*A*) (*Courtesy of* Helmut Rock, GmbH, Lenningen, Germany; with permisison) (*B*) (*Courtesy of* Bledsoe Brace System, Grand Prairie, TX; with permission) (*C*) (*Courtesy of* Aircast Inc., Vista, CA; with permission) (*D*) (*Courtesy of* Alimed, Inc., Dedham, MA; with permission.)

Load-relieving orthosis after Allgöwer

This device (Fig. 9A, B) allows complete off-loading of the foot concerned, which is not advantageous when complete off-loading is not necessary. Circular high pressure at the tibial head compromises lymphatic and venous draining and thereby increases the risk of edema. Furthermore, complete unloading results in enhanced demineralization of bone. Deformities can intensify because of muscular imbalance. A leg length adjustment of

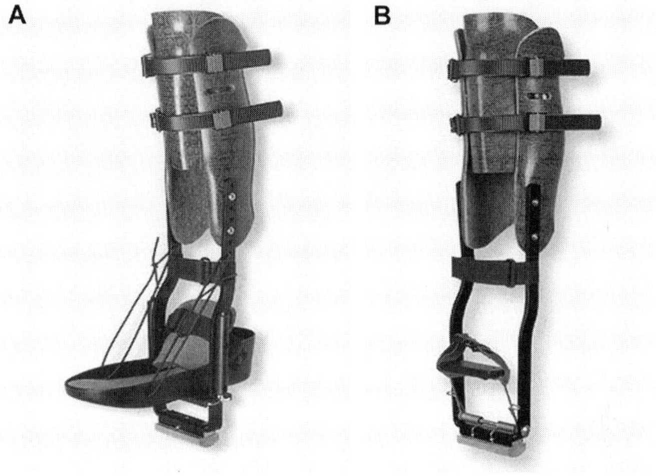

Fig. 9. Modular orthosis. (*A*) With footplate. (*B*) Without footplate. (*Courtesy of* Röck, Lenningen, Germany; with permission.)

at least 3 inches on the contralateral side is required, and limits mobility substantially.

Knee-ankle foot orthoses with ischial support

Knee-ankle foot orthosis (KAFO) (Fig. 10A, B) with ischial support offers full off-loading as well, which, however, is not universally necessary as previously mentioned.

Fabrication is very laborious and expensive. The adjustment takes twice so long as with a CROW. A KAFO is a significantly heavier device, and therefore even more disabling and stigmatizing. The compensation for leg length discrepancy is as complicated and difficult as in an orthosis of Allgöwer [13].

Münster ankle-foot orthosis

The Münster AFO follows the neurotraumatic theory and focuses attention on joint immobilization. Restriction of tibial rotation minimizes transmission of leg movements to the tarsus. Repetitive pressure on the plantar soft tissue and the foot skeleton appears to offer partial protection from further bone demineralization. Without noteworthy proximal constriction it is easier to control edema; compression stockings can be worn if necessary. Axial loading supports fragment fusion in the area of the hindfoot. Arthrodeses in the area of the midfoot are efficiently protected from bending moments. A lightweight construction is possible as is a heavy-duty version as shown in Fig. 11.

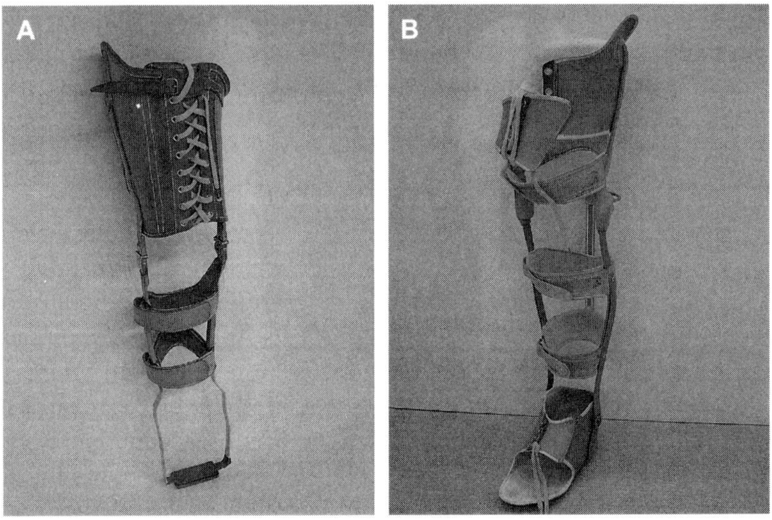

Fig. 10. (*A, B*) Two different models of KAFO with ischial support from the authors' outpatient clinic.

Just as the CROW and the DW, the authors' removable AFO bears the risk of noncompliance. When soft tissue shrinkage occurs, adjustments are necessary to ascertain continual function.

Mode of action and medical domain of the authors' orthosis are most comparable to the CROW. In contrast to the TCC and the DW, the Munster AFO is not designed to attenuate plantar pressure or load transmission to the foot skeleton. Immobilizing the foot joints, a principle used in the Munster design, was introduced by Morgan and colleagues [14]. They postulated that patellar tendon bearing braces and posterior shell ankle-foot orthoses would be inappropriate for that purpose, unlike the CROW. Almost 15 years ago, protection from cumulative microtrauma had been the keynote for orthotic treatment of Charcot feet. Subsequently, this idea has been replaced by the currently preferred relief of pressure or peak forces [15]. Orthoses effecting an insufficient reduction of load transmission to the midfoot or forefoot in the region of 20% were judged as improper, although the effects of load transmission on the movement of Charcot joints were not examined separately [16]. The authors are not aware of an RCT or any study that compared the efficacy of different types of orthoses in a larger cohort of Charcot feet. Even if the concept of joint immobilization appears to be consistent with up-to-date hypotheses about the etiology of neuroarthropathy [5], there is no evidence for this assumption. Nevertheless, the authors regard orthoses for total load relief as obsolete, apart from exceptional situations.

The novel conception to use axial forces to support fragment fusion in the area of the hindfoot is not concordant with the attempt to keep the vertical

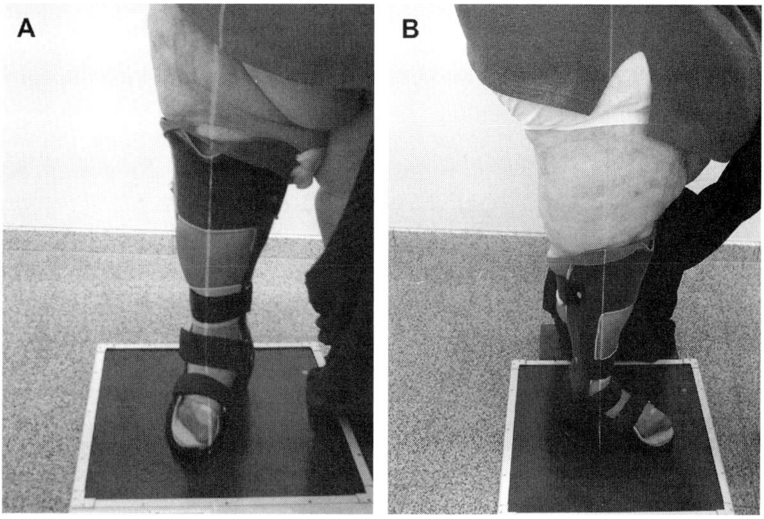

Fig. 11. (*A, B*) Verification of correct static alignment with the aid of L.A.S.A.R. Posture in a very obese female diabetic. (*Courtesy of* Otto Bock Health Care GmbH, Duderstadt, Germany; with permission.)

load as small as possible [16]. A solid arthrodesis is not mandatory for a favorable outcome. Because of the patients' neuropathy, a fibrous ancylosis with a plantigrade foot also allows for pain-free ambulation. It is the authors' opinion that axial load transmission to the hindfoot is not only unproblematic, but simply necessary to reach the goal of a robust connection between foot and lower leg.

In comparison to that, wedge osteotomies at the Lisfranc joint or triple-arthrodeses have a different requirement concerning orthotic aftertreatment. The AFO has to keep the arthrodesis stable and protect it from deleterious bending moments until complete bony fusion has occurred. In those selected cases, the authors wait for Eichenholtz Stage III to come in view on plain radiographs before surgery is performed. After 2 months in a non–weight-bearing cast, an interim orthosis is fitted for further 3 to 6 months–in an approach consistent with other authors [17–19].

When it comes to ulcers and the TCC, Wukich and Motko [20] detected 13 skin lesions in 13 patients in a prospective trial. Their calculation of 17% complications referred to 82 serial casts. Guyton [21] had 22 ulcers in a consecutive series of 398 total contact casts. Thirty percent of all patients suffered from at least one complication with serial casting. Charcot arthropathy represented the highest risk, whereas the use of a cast after deformity-correcting surgery in a neuropathic patient was rather safe. A frequently changed TCC was considered a safe method for immobilization of Charcot feet. In comparison with those two studies on TCC, the authors' rate of 13.5% within the first year after operation and 22% ulcers during the total follow-up correlates with a moderate risk for the authors' orthosis.

Moreover, the Munster AFO immobilizes the foot rather than the whole patient.

The authors assigned their patients to mobility categories on the analogy of K-levels for lower limb amputees. By operation and AFO, the medium score for patients wearing an orthosis (and not shoes) gained 1.3 points on average. At the time of last visit, the medium score was 2.3, slightly better than the typical "limited community ambulatory" (K-level 2). This simple scheme might be useful for comparison of patient groups with different types of orthoses or casts.

Until now, comparative studies on orthoses for the diabetic foot syndrome were predominantly performed with formulation of a biomechanical question. Parameters of interest were plantar pressure relief or attenuation of ground reaction forces in comparison to the TCC [22,23]. Some of the cohorts contained healthy subjects [24] or a very small number of patients who had Charcot feet [16]. With regard to the authors' understanding of the optimum effectiveness of AFOs for Charcot feet, the authors see a need for trials that examine the efficacy of joint immobilization in different types of orthoses. Even more interesting is the question whether a posited better effectiveness by better fixation of the foot has impact on the clinical outcome.

Summary

Orthoses with total load relief of the foot are out of place for the treatment of neuroarthropathy in the authors' department. TCC, CROW and DW are used, depending on the medical, social, and economic circumstances. There is not one single orthosis for the treatment of Charcot feet, but there are several models with advantages and disadvantages that the physician should be aware of. In a retrospective study of 200 Charcot feet, the AFO built in the authors' workshop turned out to be an efficient and comfortable appliance for orthotic treatment after reconstructive surgery. We prefer this type of orthosis because of its versatility and its safe application in a compliant patient.

Acknowledgment

The authors thank James M. Kelly, PhD at the University of Alabama at Birmingham for his comments on the manuscript, and Frank Schulz, certified prosthetist and orthotist at the Department of Technical Orthopedics at Münster University Hospital in Germany for his technical assistance and advice.

References

[1] Armstrong DG, Lavery LA. Acute Charcot's arthropathy of the foot and ankle. Phys Ther 1998;78:74–80.

[2] Boninger ML, Leonard JA Jr. Use of bivalved ankle-foot orthosis in neuropathic foot and ankle lesions. J Rehabil Res Dev 1996;33(1):16–22.

[3] Jeffcoate W. Vascular calcification and osteolysis in diabetic neuropathy—is RANK-L the missing link? Diabetologia 2004;47:1488–92.

[4] Rajbhandari SM, Jenkins RC, Davies C, et al. Charcot neuroarthropathy in diabetes mellitus. Diabetologia 2002;45:1085–96.

[5] Jeffcoate WJ, Game F, Cavanagh PR. The role of proinflammatory cytokines in the cause of neuropathic osteoarthropathy (acute Charcot foot) in diabetes. Lancet 2005;366:2058–61.

[6] Eichenholtz SN. Charcot joints. Springfield (IL): Charles C. Thomas; 1966.

[7] Jolly GP, Zgonis T, Polyzois V. External fixation in the management of Charcot neuroarthropathy. Clin Podiatr Med Surg 2003;20(4):741–56.

[8] Koller A, Fühner J, Wetz HH. [Radiological and clinical aspects of diabetic-neuropathic osteoarthropathy]. Orthopade 2004;33(9):972–82 [in German].

[9] Spencer S. Pressure relieving interventions for preventing and treating diabetic foot ulcers. Cochrane Database Syst Rev 2000;3:CD002302; doi: 10.1002/14651858.CD002302.

[10] Sanders LJ, Frykberg RG. Diabetic neuropathic osteoarthropathy: the Charcot foot. In: Frykberg RG, editor. The high risk foot in diabetes mellitus. New York: Livingstone; 1993. p. 297–336.

[11] Koller A, Hafkemeyer U, Fiedler R, et al. [Reconstructive foot surgery in cases of diabetic-neuropathic osteoarthropathy]. Orthopade 2004;33(9):983–91 [in German].

[12] McGill M, Molyneaux L, Bolton T, et al. Response of Charcot's arthropathy to contact casting: assessment by quantitative techniques. Diabetologia 2000;43:481–4.

[13] Allgöwer M. Siegeszug einer Konzeption? Helv Chir Acta 1958;45:537–40.

[14] Morgan JM, BiehlL WC, Wagner FW Jr. Management of neuropathic arthropathy with the Charcot restraint orthotic walker. Clin Orthop 1993;296:58–63.

[15] Saltzman CL, Hagy ML, Zimmerman B, et al. How effective is intensive nonoperative initial treatment of patients with diabetes and Charcot arthropathy of the feet? Clin Orthop 2005; 435:185–90.

[16] Saltzman CL, Johnson KA, Goldstein RH, et al. The patellar tendon-bearing brace as treatment for neurotrophic arthropathy: a dynamic force monitoring study. Foot Ankle 1992; 13(1):14–21.

[17] Johnson JE. Instructional course lectures, The American Academy of Orthopaedic Surgeons. J Bone Joint Surg Am 1998;80(11):1700–9.

[18] Marks RM. Complications of foot and ankle surgery in patients with diabetes. Clin Orthop 2001;153–61.

[19] Schon LC, et al. Charcot neuroarthropathy of the foot and ankle. Clin Orthop 1998;349: 116–31.

[20] Wukich DK, Motko J. Safety of total contact casting in high-risk patients with neuropathic foot ulcers. Foot Ankle 2004;25(8):556–60.

[21] Guyton GP. An analysis of iatrogenic complications from the total contact cast. Foot Ankle 2005;26(11):903–7.

[22] Armstrong DG, Stacpoole-Shea S. Total contact casts and removable cast walkers. Mitigation of plantar heel pressure. J Am Podiatr Med Assoc 1999;89(1):50–3.

[23] Hartsell HD, Brand RA, Frantz RA, et al. The effects of total contact casting materials on plantar pressures. Foot Ankle 2004;25(2):73–8.

[24] Hartsell HD, Fellner C, Saltzman CL. Pneumatic bracing and total contact casting have equivocal effects on plantar pressure relief. Foot Ankle 2001;22(6):502–6.

ELSEVIER
SAUNDERS

Clin Podiatr Med Surg
24 (2007) 601–610

CLINICS IN
PODIATRIC
MEDICINE AND
SURGERY

Addressing Psychosocial Aspects of Care for Patients with Diabetes Undergoing Limb Salvage Surgery

Thomas S. Roukis, DPM, FACFAS[a],
John J. Stapleton, DPM, AACFAS[b],
Thomas Zgonis, DPM, FACFAS[b,*]

[a]*Limb Preservation Service, Vascular/Endovascular Surgery, Madigan Army Medical Center, Tacoma, WA, USA*
[b]*Department of Orthopaedics/Podiatry Division, The University of Texas Health Science Center at San Antonio, 7703 Floyd Curl Drive, MC 7776, San Antonio, TX 78229, USA*

The term *psychosocial* refers to a person's psychologic development or well-being in the context of a social environment. An impressive array of psychosocial problems in patients with type 1 and type 2 diabetes mellitus have been documented in the scientific literature [1–8]. These psychosocial problems may be exacerbated by the presence of related foot pathologies or complications requiring extensive surgery or amputation [1,4,9–16]. Psychosocial problems present a challenge to the surgeon in terms of identifying the causative factors and establishing appropriate intervention to prevent complications that can be associated with "setting up the patient to fail" through a lack of or misunderstanding of the patient's psychosocial well-being [17]. An excellent surgeon-patient relationship needs to be established to understand the patient's psychosocial state to determine how major limb salvage surgery will challenge the patient and his or her support network.

Often these patients have already been treated by numerous health care professionals and have spent a tremendous amount of time, effort, and expense coping with their chronic condition. For this reason, adequate time spent to acquire a detailed history and physical is paramount to establish a proper initial encounter. The time allocated to obtain a thorough initial assessment is more efficient and effective than to face unrealized challenges

* Corresponding author.
E-mail address: zgonis@uthscsa.edu (T. Zgonis).

doi:10.1016/j.cpm.2007.03.008 *podiatric.theclinics.com*

during the recovery process such as unexpected complications, revisions, or prolonged disability [18]. Higher levels of postoperative physical and psychosocial morbidity are present with clinically depressed or emotionally unprepared patients. If patients are knowledgeable, motivated, and have an active role in their care, physical and psychologic outcomes are generally deemed more successful by the patient [17]. The authors and their support staff spend a significant amount of time obtaining a detailed psychosocial evaluation of all patients who are candidates for major limb salvage surgery. Once this has been established, it is easier to educate the patient about the surgical procedure, to involve the patient and their family in the decision-making process, and to continue a strong surgeon-patient relationship throughout the postoperative course. The authors have established a protocol to adequately assess and document pertinent psychosocial factors that should be addressed before and following surgical intervention in this patient population. This approach assists the surgeon in deciding when patients are suitable candidates for major limb salvage surgery. The surgeon involved in this type of work should organize a team that consists of, but is not limited to, internists, physiatrists, physical therapists, psychiatrists, psychologists, social workers, and nurses. Communication among these individuals is essential to adequately establish a long-term treatment plan to limit psychosocial morbidity.

Psychosocial evaluation

In our approach to the evaluation, we recognize that the diabetic patient about to undergo major limb salvage surgery is faced with a debilitating and limb-threatening physical illness that affects their physical and emotional functioning. When speaking with the patient, the surgeon must show that they are actively listening to all of the topics discussed. An atmosphere should be created in which the patient believes he or she has the undivided attention of their surgeon. The surgeon needs to address all questions honestly to avoid misunderstandings by the patient. The psychosocial evaluation includes an assessment of the patient's psychosocial history, interaction among their social network, and perspective of the surgery (Box 1).

The evaluation begins with the social history of the patient. Emphasis is placed on the individual's lifestyle, such as their educational achievement, employment, and vocational activities. A history of tobacco, alcohol, and drug use should include the quantity, frequency, and duration of usage. Previous cessation programs for substance abuse, misuse, or dependent use should be discussed; particular attention should be made to issues that the patient perceives as the reason for the failure or success of these programs. The surgeon should determine whether a cessation program or further intervention is needed before surgery, and a note indicating a need for heightened awareness of potential abuse issues following any intervention should be

Box 1. Potential psychosocial problems associated with diabetes mellitus

Psychologic problems
Depression
Anxiety
Stress
Difficulty coping
Loss of self-esteem

Social problems
Loss of income
Employment adjustment
Marital adjustment
Sexual dysfunction

Behavioral problems
Compliance issues
Tobacco, alcohol, or drug dependency
Self-neglect

included in each clinic update. A psychiatric history including previous or current intervention is essential to determine whether the patient suffers from mental health problems or personality disorders that could compromise informed involvement of the surgery process and the extended recovery.

The surgeon needs to determine the patient's compliance with other treatments. Often this can be difficult to access, particularly during an initial evaluation; however, a review of old clinic and surgical notes for other procedures, even those not directly involving the lower extremity, should be performed. Additionally, a private conversation with the family is warranted. The authors have frequently obtained a great deal of pertinent information from a detailed review of old medical and surgical notes and frank discussions with the family. The most appropriate approach is to let the patient and their family know that you do not want to set them up to fail, and that what they are about to embark on is fraught with potential complications that should be recognized, evaluated, and addressed before undergoing surgical intervention. Additionally, it is not unreasonable to demand a period of acceptable compliance by the patient before surgery by sending the patient to physical therapy or rehabilitation for gait training to assess their ability to remain strictly non–weight bearing using a gait aide. The patient should have several visits with the physical therapist, and their ability to arise from a seated position such as a commode, to travel a distance, and to ascend/descend stairs should be evaluated. If the patient is unable or unwilling to perform these tasks before surgery, it is highly likely that they will be noncompliant with the postoperative scenario, which would set them up to fail. The surgeon must talk to the patient and explain their concerns and the reason for the delay in surgical treatment to determine their compliance. Developing this sense of trust with the patient is fundamental for the surgeon.

Next the surgeon evaluates the patient's social network to determine whether there is adequate support or how surgical intervention may affect this interaction. Obtaining information on the family structure and family roles may be beneficial in assessing the challenges surgery may impose. A frank discussion about problem areas for the patient in regard to his or her family or social network is paramount and should be conducted early with the request that the patient's family be present for each office visit. Marital issues, financial burdens, and the health of other family members are factors to consider and discuss in detail. The perioperative period is a time during which a high degree of patient care is required, and the success of limb salvage surgery depends in part on the presence of a dedicated caregiver. A social worker should be consulted if the surgeon believes that there is no family member that can fulfill this role without fail. If a caregiver is available, the commitment level that is required to assist the patient throughout the surgical process to ensure an optimal outcome should be explained to them in detail. The surgeon cannot underestimate the importance of understanding the patient's social network preoperatively, because it will be presented with great challenges throughout the postoperative course [17].

The surgeon needs to determine the patient's perspective on surgical intervention. The surgeon should ask the patient what they expect from the surgery and what they will consider a successful outcome. It is helpful to have the patient write these perspectives down along with their version of the surgeon's answers so that this can be scanned into the patient's medical record. At times, what the surgeon and the patient believe is a successful outcome does not coincide. Occasionally, it may be predicted that the patient would fair better with an amputation of their lower extremity which, although not a panacea, would be a viable treatment option for diabetic foot-related complications [19]. The surgeon must identify these patients and discuss with them the thought process that led to this decision. Conversely, some patients would prefer a single-stage amputation to a series of reconstructive surgeries and a lengthy recovery course, and the surgeon should respect the patient's decision if it is made by a mentally competent patient who has been educated on all treatment options, as well as the short- and long-term outcomes. The surgeon should also determine what the patient perceives as the cause and the probable course of their current disability. This assessment will assist the surgeon in understanding if the patient comprehends the severity of their condition, or if further education and counseling on diabetes and the related complications is necessary. Discussion at this point also enables the surgeon to later elaborate on surgical possibilities and alternatives that will be in the best interest of the patient.

An adequate psychosocial evaluation provides the surgeon with necessary information to establish a comprehensive treatment plan based on the disease process and the patient as a whole.

Preoperative preparation and considerations

The preoperative evaluation is a particularly stressful time for the patient. The uncertainty of the procedure, hospitalization, office visits, restrictions in work and daily activities, financial burdens, and the prospect of a complicated postoperative course combine to exert a profound strain on the patient's psychosocial adjustment. For this reason, a thorough discussion of the surgical procedure and the postoperative course with related risks, benefits, and alternatives is paramount to have a well-informed and educated patient who can properly consent to surgery. Adequate time should be allocated to obtaining the informed consent. The authors typically bring the patient back for a separate visit to obtain surgical consent. This return visit allows the surgeon to better evaluate the patient's level of understanding of, and mental readiness toward, the planned surgery. Patient variables such as educational attainment, economic situations, culture, and cognitive function should be taken into consideration because they can have a profound effect on their overall decision-making capabilities. Social support through family, friends, or ancillary staff should be present at this visit to assist the surgeon in informing and educating the patient on the proposed surgery. The use of lay terminology, illustrations, and clinical pictures can provide clarification and reduce anxiety when discussing the surgical procedure. In addition, surgeons can set up meetings with patients who underwent similar surgery to help explain the proposed procedure. Although a certain degree of ambivalence is to be expected when deciding to undergo a major surgical procedure that is associated with numerous risks, a high level of uncertainty regarding the value of limb salvage should be explored further.

The surgeon should encourage the patient to ask questions. Patients may bring information they have gathered from the Internet, news media, family, friends, or other surgeons. It is important to acknowledge their efforts and, in a nonjudgmental way, to give patients guidance about the information or misinformation they have acquired. The surgeon also needs to have a list of trusted resources to give their patients to increase their understanding of their condition and surgical options. The surgeon should not only discuss the possible complications but also describe how they will be managed if encountered. Patients appreciate honesty when discussing surgical complications and are less likely to disrupt the continuity of their care in the face of a complication if they are well informed. Even with adequate preoperative preparation by the surgical team, there are incidences in which patients are reluctant to make a decision in regards to their treatment plan. These patients should be encouraged to obtain second and third opinions by other surgeons to prevent indecisive decisions and to ensure the commitment that is required on the patient's part throughout the surgical process. The authors explain that they should be at peace with their decision to undergo surgery and feel comfortable with whoever is performing their surgery.

From a psychosocial perspective, the surgeon needs to realize that rehabilitation begins as soon as surgery is considered an appropriate intervention. Early contact with the rehabilitative team can be beneficial in providing counseling, information, and advice, and in facilitating the development of realistic rehabilitation goals and expectations. This contact will eliminate fear and anxiety postoperatively when the patient faces this new challenge.

Despite all efforts to avoid major limb amputation, there are times when amputation is needed [20–23]. Avoidance of the realization that amputation may be a possibility in an attempt to be kind may lead to an angry and traumatized patient. For this reason, it is prudent to talk about when major limb amputation is indicated or in the best interest of the patient. The patient should feel that all means have been tried to create a stable, "braceable," or "shoeable" lower limb capable of withstanding the repetitive forces associated with weight bearing, and that the decision to amputate is a last resort if a functional lower limb can be restored. This assurance does not imply that the decision to amputate should be prolonged when it could affect the patient's life, particularly in the face of a severe infection or a nonfunctional lower limb that develops a repeated ulceration despite compliance (ie, the so-called "glass slipper foot"). The surgeon needs to discuss amputation in a simple and objective manner to avoid any perceived misconceptions by the patient to ensure psychosocial stability post amputation.

Postoperative considerations

Following limb salvage surgery, the patient can frequently be faced with additional challenges, multiple concerns, anxiety, and depression that need to be addressed and efficiently managed long after surgery. Ultimately, the success of limb salvage surgery remains dependent on the patient's ability to cope psychologically and to comply with the postoperative regimen. The next phase consists of the postoperative care during hospitalization and office visitation. During the initial postoperative period, the presence of the surgeon showing empathy, compassion, and understanding is vital. The surgeon needs to embrace the notion that the needs and communication challenges of the patient can vary greatly from the preoperative visits to postoperative visits. The presence of the surgical team during hospital rounds can be reassuring to the patient and should be a daily routine [24]. A critical skill to develop is to gather information during these visits in a caring methodical manner while not making the patient interaction feel rushed or incomplete. Satisfaction is higher for patients who believe they are the center of the interaction [25]. Residents and medical students who are part of the surgical team should be instructed to refrain from asking questions in front of the patient [24]. Teaching should be performed outside of the patient's room in an environment compliant with the Health Insurance Portability and Accountability Act (HIPPPA) to reduce the patient's anxiety and fear and to limit the potential for HIPPA violation [24]. This practice correctly portrays the notion that the patient's concerns are of primary importance. The authors find this environment to be established when hospital visits and conversations are started with an initial greeting by the senior member of the surgical team followed by open-ended questions directed to the patient that allow him or her to lead the conversation. Discussion in this manner is more revealing, and the patient is involved actively in the decision-making process of their treatment.

During the patient's hospitalization, rehabilitation facility and home health care needs should be established and secured before discharge. Clinical social workers and the rehabilitation team have a vital role in the care of the postoperative patient. Caring for and rehabilitating diabetic patients who undergo limb salvage surgery includes numerous unique clinical and personal challenges. A protocol with guidelines needs to be established by the surgical team in conjunction with these services so that a mutual understanding is established in regards to the postoperative care. Patients need ongoing support and validation throughout the postoperative period to ensure their psychosocial stability and functional recovery. In this regard, any pertinent information the rehabilitation team has to offer should be taken seriously and, if deemed appropriate, addressed thoroughly.

Discharge from the hospital should represent an accomplishment for the patient. Closure for hospital discharge is pivotal. It should include a prognosis for the patient along with a discussion of the remaining postoperative course. The patient should be given instructions for follow-up, medications, nutrition guidelines, ancillary services, ambulatory status, work and social restrictions, and instructions for hygiene. The postoperative diabetic patient should be given instructions on identifying infection and ways of contacting the surgical team if problems arise.

Office visitation should be performed in a routine fashion and on a regular basis to establish control of the postoperative care so that complications are avoided through early detection. The surgeon is given the opportunity to set the tone for an office visit on entering the examination room where the patient has been waiting. It is important to set a relaxed and non-threatening environment for the patient. A surgeon who looks startled, displays fear, or appears angry or frustrated can portray a sense of incompetence to the patient. Postoperative patients tend to feel vulnerable and in less control than usual. For this reason, showing patients they have one's respect and empathy is paramount. The authors have found it advantageous to have the patient seen first by the nursing staff. The nursing staff is trained to observe and relay to the surgeon the patient's demeanor, mood, questions, concerns, and any obvious problems with their surgery sites. The surgeon can then enter the room prepared to interact with the patient. The surgeon first needs to discuss the patient's concerns and then focus on the physical examination that will lead to further postoperative instruction refinement or treatment alterations.

The patient should be told at each visit their prognosis, and encouragement should be given to motivate them through particularly difficult times. It is helpful to remind the patient of the preoperative discussions regarding any known periods during the recovery that are difficult. For example, it seems almost universal that patients become tired of external fixation devices between the sixth and eighth postoperative week. The time needed for these devices should be explained to them during the preoperative period and brought up again during the postoperative time frame to show the patient that they are proceeding in a normal fashion, that their feelings are appropriate, and that they will resolve with removal of the device in the near future. If noncompliance is an issue, this needs to be discussed frankly with no fear of upsetting the patient. The authors routinely take pictures of the patient's lower limb surgical site with the dressings in place at the end of their clinical visit and again at the beginning of each clinical visit. Filthy, wet, obviously manipulated dressings are easy to detect and, by collecting serial pictures, can be shown to the patient who questions what you are trying to discuss. In many ways this opens the door for communication and can help the surgeon to address any issues that are preventing or limiting the ability of the patient to comply with instructions. The surgeon should not allow the patient to dictate their treatment, because this will lead to surgical complications, prolonged treatment, and poor outcomes. Conversely, the surgeon needs to understand the psychosocial adjustment of the patient when dictating the postoperative orders and instructions.

Despite valiant efforts to satisfy the patient in the postoperative period, unpleasant situations may arise that must be appropriately addressed. Readjusting to life after surgery is likely to be challenging and can be difficult for some patients and their families. Difficulties in adjustment are typically associated with reports of depression, loss of income, marital problems, hopelessness, low self-esteem, fatigue, anxiety, and sometimes suicidal ideation; therefore, specific structured therapeutic interventions for problems such as, but not limited, to depression, anxiety, sexual difficulties, and substance addiction or drug overuse may be required. The surgeon should try to detect these problems early and arrange for intervention as soon as they are recognized. These patients should also be followed more closely during the postoperative period to reduce surgical complications. Such intervention may operate through individual, couple, family, or group therapies.

Summary

The burgeoning popularity of limb salvage surgery to prevent amputation in the diabetic patient will provide ample opportunity to study the psychosocial benefit. Despite the surgical outcomes for diabetic limb salvage surgery, there is no agreement on what constitutes success in terms of improvement in comorbidities or the overall quality of life. Often, surgeons have focused on defining postoperative success as limb salvage with little emphasis on the overall quality of life. The authors believe that the quality of life is greatly enhanced when functional limb salvage is achieved. A continued lack of consensus on postoperative success will render comparisons of studies difficult, if not impossible. This difficulty may be particularly true for comparisons of patients who have undergone amputation versus limb salvage procedures.

In addition, little is known about the psychosocial component of the patient as it pertains to predicting postoperative outcomes. Intuitively, patients with uncontrolled psychosocial issues, substance abuse, or severe depression are thought to be unlikely to have a successful outcome. At the authors' institutions, we have seen patients with a history of each of these disorders have a successful result. These patients underwent a thorough psychosocial evaluation preoperatively, were psychosocially stable at the time of surgery, and received concurrent psychosocial treatment using a multidisciplinary approach during the postoperative course. We recommend this approach for patients who present for surgery with severe psychosocial pathology.

It is hoped that additional study of psychosocial issues in the diabetic patient population will facilitate the development of standards of care that will ultimately improve patient outcomes. Many of the patients who present for surgery do so with a good understanding of the changes they will face postoperatively. Others seem to have little appreciation of these issues. These patients may benefit from more intensive preoperative counseling.

References

[1] Luscombe FA. Health-related quality of life measurement in type 2 diabetes. Value Health 2000;3(Suppl 1):15–28.

[2] Mo F, Morrison H, Choi BC, et al. Evaluation and measurement of health-related quality of life for individuals with diabetes mellitus by Health Utilities Index Mark 3 (HUI3) system. Scientific World Journal 2006;6:1412–23.

[3] Nabuurs-Franssen MH, Huijberts MS, Nieuwenhuijzen Kruseman AC, et al. Health-related quality of life of diabetic foot ulcer patients and their caregivers. Diabetologia 2005;48(9): 1906–10.

[4] Ribu L, Hanestad BR, Moum T, et al. A comparison of the health-related quality of life in patients with diabetic foot ulcers, with a diabetes group and a nondiabetes group from the general population. Qual Life Res 2007;16(2):179–89.

[5] Watkins K, Connell CM. Measurement of health-related QOL in diabetes mellitus. Pharmacoeconomics 2004;22(17):1109–26.

[6] Rafique G, Shaikh F. Identifying needs and barriers to diabetes education in patients with diabetes. J Pak Med Assoc 2006;56(8):347–52.

[7] Eakin EG, Bull SS, Glasgow RE, et al. Reaching those most in need: a review of diabetes self-management interventions in disadvantaged populations. Diabetes Metab Res Rev 2002; 18(1):26–35.

[8] Batts ML, Gary TL, Huss K, et al. Patient priorities and needs for diabetes care among urban African American adults. Diabetes Educ 2001;27(3):405–12.

[9] Boyko EJ, Ahroni JH, Stensel V, et al. A prospective study of risk factors for diabetic foot ulcer: the Seattle Diabetic Foot Study. Diabetes Care 1999;22(7):1036–42.
[10] Tom RK, Pupp GR. Talectomy for diabetic Charcot foot: an alternative to amputation. J Am Podiatr Med Assoc 1992;82(9):447–53.
[11] Roukis TS, Zgonis T. The management of acute Charcot fracture-dislocations with the Taylor's spatial external fixation system. Clin Podiatr Med Surg 2006;23(2):467–83.
[12] Zgonis T, Roukis TS, Polyzois VD. The use of Ilizarov technique and other types of external fixation for the treatment of intra-articular calcaneal fractures. Clin Podiatr Med Surg 2006; 23(2):343–53.
[13] Zgonis T, Roukis TS, Frykberg RG, et al. Unstable acute and chronic Charcot's deformity: staged skeletal and soft-tissue reconstruction. J Wound Care 2006;15(6):276–80.
[14] Zgonis T, Roukis TS. A systematic approach to diabetic foot infections. Adv Ther 2005; 22(3):244–62.
[15] Roukis TS, Zgonis T. Skin grafting techniques for soft-tissue coverage of diabetic foot and ankle wounds. J Wound Care 2005;14(4):173–6.
[16] Jolly GP, Zgonis T, Polyzois V. External fixation in the management of Charcot neuroarthropathy. Clin Podiatr Med Surg 2003;20(4):741–56.
[17] Althof JE, Beasley BD. Psychosocial management of the foot and ankle surgery patient. Clin Podiatr Med Surg 2003;20(2):199–211.
[18] Cape J. Consultation length, patient-estimated consultation length, and satisfaction with the consultation. Br J Gen Pract 2002;52(485):1004–6.
[19] Miyajima S, Shirai A, Yamamoto S, et al. Risk factors for major limb amputations in diabetic foot gangrene patients. Diabetes Res Clin Pract 2006;71(3):272–9.
[20] Cruz CP, Eidt JF, Capps C, et al. Major lower extremity amputations at a Veterans Affairs hospital. Am J Surg 2003;186(5):449–54.
[21] Pecoraro RE, Reiber GE, Burgess EM. Pathways to diabetic limb amputation: basis for prevention. Diabetes Care 1990;13(5):513–21.
[22] Taylor LM Jr, Porter JM. The clinical course of diabetics who require emergent foot surgery because of infection or ischemia. J Vasc Surg 1987;6(5):454–9.
[23] Aulivola B, Hile CN, Hamdan AD, et al. Major lower extremity amputation: outcome of a modern series. Arch Surg 2004;139(4):395–9 [discussion: 399].
[24] Cook KD, Gutowsky RB. Teaching during rounds. Clin Podiatr Med Surg 2007;24(1): 27–36.
[25] Smith RC, Hoppe RB. The patient's story: integrating the patient- and surgeon-centered approaches to interviewing. Ann Intern Med 1991;115(6):470–7.

ELSEVIER SAUNDERS

Clin Podiatr Med Surg 24 (2007) 611–616

CLINICS IN PODIATRIC MEDICINE AND SURGERY

Index

Note: Page numbers of article titles are in **boldface** type.

doi:10.1016/S0891-8422(07)00041-9 *podiatric.theclinics.com*

C

D

E

F

G

H

I

J

K

L

R

S

T